Self-Assessment & Review of

FMGE/MCI Screening Examination

Supplement

Self-Assessment & Review of

FMGE/MCI Screening Examination

Supplement

Fourth Edition

Updated Till December 2021 Exam

Kamal KV MBBS MS (Orthopedics)
Ex-Senior Resident: Safdarjung, ESI-Okhla, Fortis-Noida
Ponseti and Ilizarov Techniques Fellow (Akola)
Madhya Pradesh—Indian Orthopaedic Association
Hand Surgery Fellow—Pune, Maharashtra, India

JAYPEE
JAYPEE BROTHERS MEDICAL PUBLISHERS
The Health Sciences Publisher
New Delhi | London

Jaypee Brothers Medical Publishers (P) Ltd

Headquarters
Jaypee Brothers Medical Publishers (P) Ltd
EMCA House, 23/23-B
Ansari Road, Daryaganj
New Delhi 110 002, India
Landline: +91-11-23272143, +91-11-23272703
+91-11-23282021, +91-11-23245672
Email: jaypee@jaypeebrothers.com

Corporate Office
Jaypee Brothers Medical Publishers (P) Ltd
4838/24, Ansari Road, Daryaganj
New Delhi 110 002, India
Phone: +91-11-43574357
Fax: +91-11-43574314
Email: jaypee@jaypeebrothers.com

Overseas Office
JP Medical Ltd.
83 Victoria Street, London
SW1H 0HW (UK)
Phone: +44 20 3170 8910
Fax: +44 (0)20 3008 6180
Email: info@jpmedpub.com

Website: www.jaypeebrothers.com
Website: www.jaypeedigital.com

Self-Assessment & Review of FMGE/MCI Screening Examination—Supplement

Fourth Edition: **2022**

ISBN: 978-93-5465-738-2

Printed at

Dedicated to

I would like to dedicate this title to all those who arranged or served me during my foreign (academic) trips. I have tried my best to compile all the names (Sorry, if I forgot someone to mention).

S. N.	Countries	College	Credit to
1	Georgia	*i. Tbilisi*	Dr Amit Verma, Dr Swapna Chauhan, Dr Anish Acharya, Amaresh Panda, Anij
		ii. Batumi	-"-
2	Russia	*iii. Nalchik*	Dr Sudhakar Tiwari, Dr Sumant Pandey, Dr Nishant Atri, Dr Gaurav Soni
		iv. Cheboksary	Dr Jitendra Gurjar
		v. Stavropol	Dr Najeerul Ameen, Dr Anupam Mishra, Dr Divyesh
		vi. Kazan	Dr Atul shrivastav
3	Kyrgyzstan	*vii. Jalalabad*	Dr Shoaib Shahid, Dr Deepak, Dr Kishan Bhandari, Dr Deewakar Jha, Dr SP Saha, Dr Firoz, Dr Shubhayu
		viii. Osh	Dr Bhupendra Magarde, Dr Aftab, Dr Jitendra Chaurasiya
4	Nepal	*ix. Bhairahawa*	Dr Pranjal Kashiv, Dr Rahul Yadav, Dr Satyam Ojha
		x. Bharatpur	Dr Sanket Dewan, Dr Gautam Solanki, Dr Akshay
		xi. Dharan	Dr Sandeep Chauhan
5	Ukraine	*xii. Vinnytsia*	Dr Jashan Preet Singh, Dr Ashray Khanna
		xiii. Kiev	-"-
6	China	*xiv. Ningbo*	Dr Nimshad, Dr Jamshid, Dr Srikant
		xv. Nanchang	Dr Azlan, Dr Khalid, Dr Armaan Ansari, Dr Prashant Raghuwanshi, Dr Ravi Singh, Dr Vishal Borana
		xvi. Nanning	Dr Jazeer, Dr Pranay
		xvii. Dali	Dr Kashif Agaz, Dr Dr Mubasheer, Dr Mujahid Tyagi
		xviii. Fuzhou	Dr Chinthu MR, Dr Pooja
		xix. Guangzhou	Dr Abhimanyu, Dr Russi Singh
7	Belarus	*xx. Minsk*	Dr Rama Sah, Dr Varun Upadhyay

PREFACE

I feel much honored to present this supplement of one the most trusted book for FMGE/ MCI Screening examination. This supplement is based on MCQs of FMGE June 2019 till FMGE December 2021.

There are 4 segments in this book, which are as follows:

1. **Image Based MCQs** segment is composed of image-based questions asked in the examination.
2. **Problem Based MCQs with Explanation** contains subject wise MCQs with explanation. Only those MCQs are kept in this section, which relates to a clinical case-based problem.
   a. Explanations are short and concise and tries to highlight the fact that why a particular option is the answer to that MCQ.
   b. For the ease of studying, explanations are placed after the MCQs.
3. **All Subject MCQs** contains MCQs randomly picked from the subjects. There is no explanation with the MCQs.
4. **Quick Review Points** contains important and commonly asked one-liner type of questions, meant for quick revision. Most of these points are from the previous 3 segments.

As I always say, students are the best judge of an author's work. And I personally feel, there is always some room left for further improvement. So I expect my dear students to share their valuable feedbacks regarding betterment of this text in subsequent editions.

Considering the volume of the work, despite my best efforts, some errors must have crept in. I request dear readers to please forward the same to me.

Errata of this title (if any) would be updated on titles exclusive Facebook page *(https://www.facebook.com/drkamalkvselfassessment/)*. Please follow the Facebook page for all relevant updates.

Hope this title will serve its purpose.

drkamalkv
E-mail: *drkamalkvgroup@gmail.com*
Website: *www.drkamalkvgroup.co.in*
Facebook: *drkamalkvgroup*
WhatsApp: 84 7000 4333

ACKNOWLEDGEMENTS

All thanks to almighty (for imparting me with this passion of writing books and teaching), to my parents (for imparting qualities of a good human being), my brothers and sister (for giving me some wonderful memories of childhood), my wife (for supporting me in all my endeavors), my daughters (for allowing me to use their share of time with my students) and my dear students (for accepting my all titles with equal enthusiasm and also, who made me academically strong, to an extent).

Thanks are due for everyone behind this project, from the publication house.

Special thanks to Shri Jitendar P Vij (Group Chairman), Mr. Ankit Vij (Group President) and Ms Chetna Malhotra Vohra (Senior Director—Professional Publishing, Marketing and Business Development), for accepting all my work, without any hesitancy or objection.

CONTENTS

Image Based MCQs

Image-based Questions

1. **A dead body was recovered from a pond with the following appearance. This is known as:**

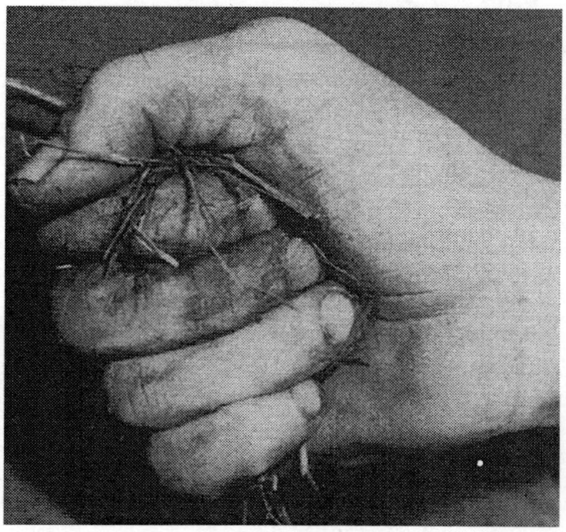

   a. Algor mortis
   b. Cadaveric spasm
   c. Mummification
   d. Saponification

Ans. b. Cadaveric spasm

2. **Odour of such a body, which is brought for autopsy:**

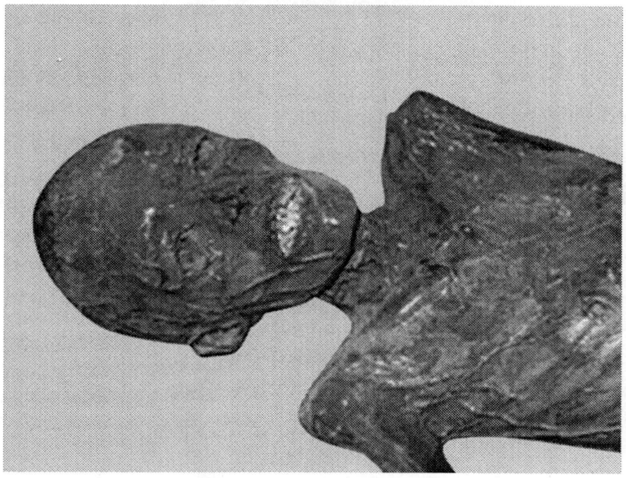

   a. Garlic
   b. No odour
   c. Bitter almond
   d. Ammoniacal

Image shows mummification.

Ans. b. No odour

3. **Such a microscopic appearance is seen in:**

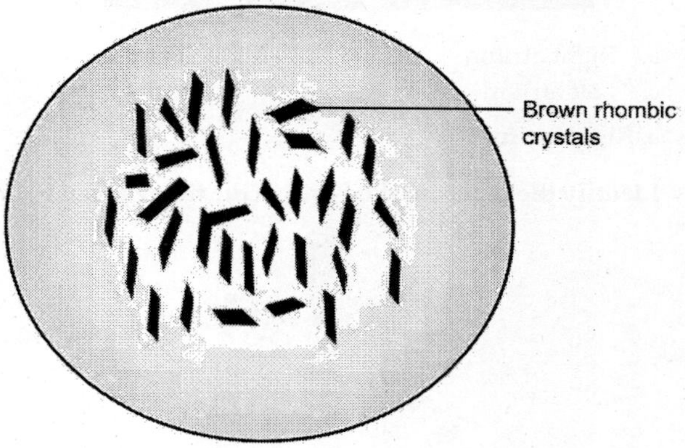

   a. Berberio test
   b. Takayama reagent
   c. Teichman test
   d. Spectroscopy

Ans. c. Teichman test

4. **Identify the image:**

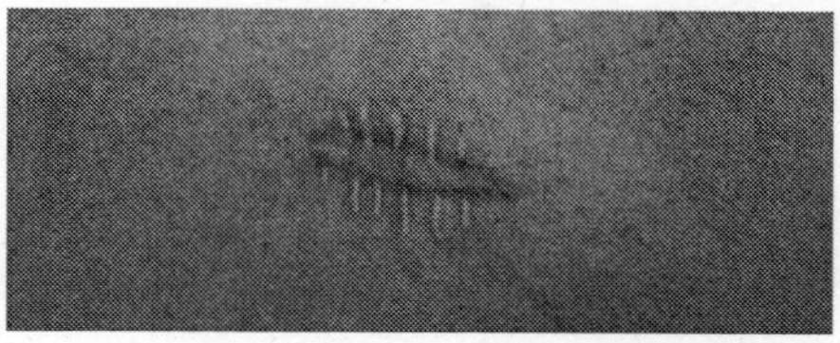

   a. Tattoo
   b. Ligature mark
   c. Tentative cuts
   d. Surgical scar

Ans. d. Surgical scar

5. **Identify the dermatome for the area marked by black arrow:**

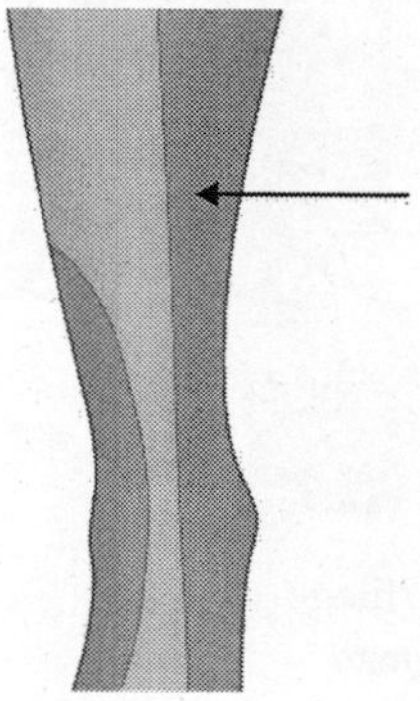

   a. L3
   b. L4
   c. L5
   d. S1

Ans. b. L4

6. **Identify the structure marked with number 1 in the image given below:**

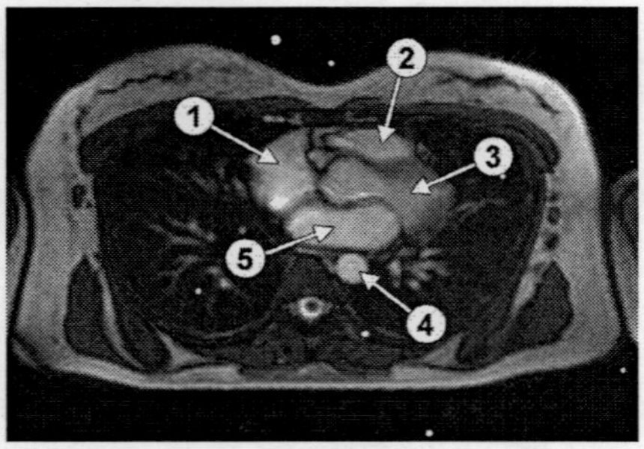

a. Right atrium
b. Right ventricle
c. Left atrium
d. Left ventricle

Ans. a. Right atrium

7. **Identify the plane marked as A in the figure given below:**

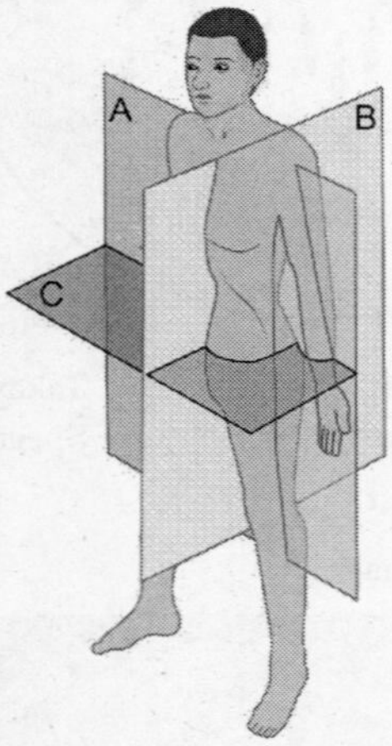

a. Coronal section
b. Sagittal section
c. Transverse section
d. Paramedian section

Ans. a. Coronal section

8. **Identify the structure marked with black arrow:**

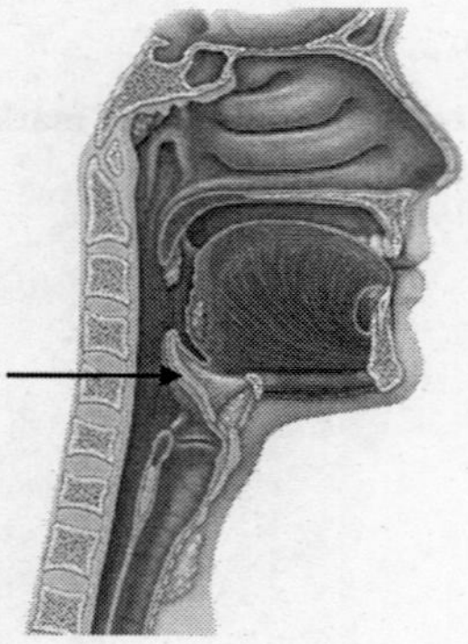

a. Arytenoid cartilage
b. Thyroid cartilage
c. Epiglottis
d. Base of tongue

Ans. c. Epiglottis

9. **Study the image given below and identify the embryological basis of the condition shown:**

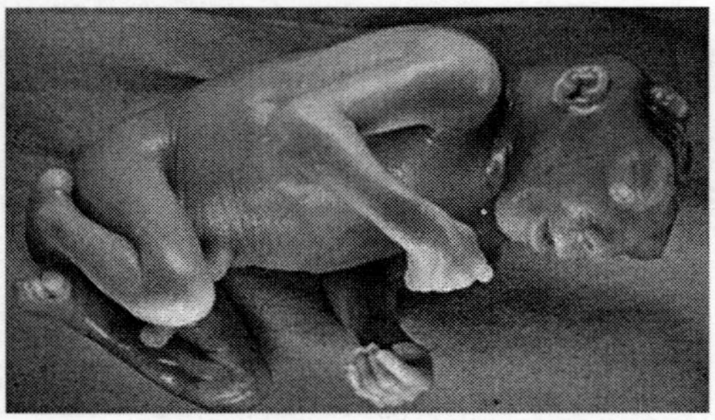

a. Failure of closure of anterior neuropore
b. Failure of closure of posterior neuropore
c. Failure of closure of both anterior and posterior neuropore
d. Failure of fusion of caudal neuropore

Image shows anencephaly.

Ans. a. Failure of closure of anterior neuropore

10. **Identify the type of joint discussed in the given X-ray of pelvis:**

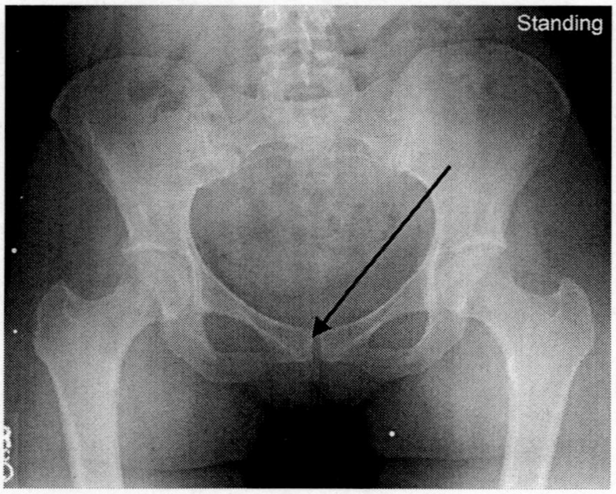

a. Fibrous
b. Pivot synovial
c. Primary cartilaginous
d. Secondary cartilaginous

Red arrow shows pubis symphysis.

Ans. d. Secondary cartilaginous

11. **Study the transverse section of trachea and identify the structure marked as 4:**

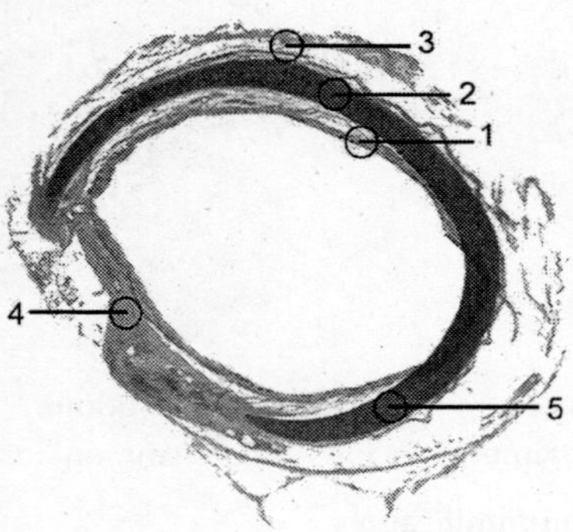

a. Tracheal cartilage b. Trachealis
c. Esophagus d. Mucosal glands

Ans. b. Trachealis

12. In the given image, physician is trying to palpate which artery?

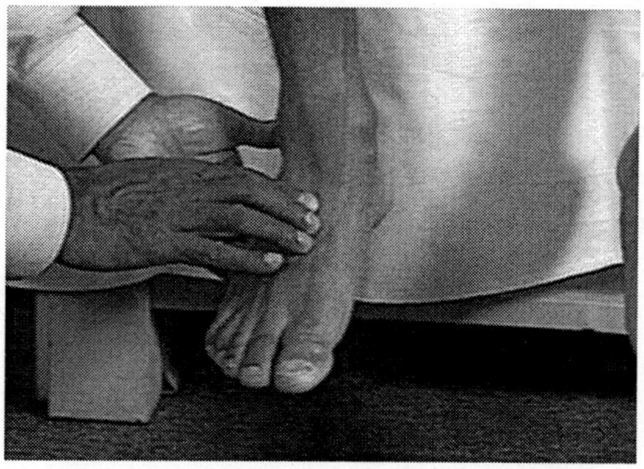

a. Anterior tibial artery b. Posterior tibial artery
c. Dorsalis pedis artery d. Lateral plantar artery

Ans. c. Dorsalis pedis artery

13. Identify the tarsal bone marked with white arrow on X-ray of foot:

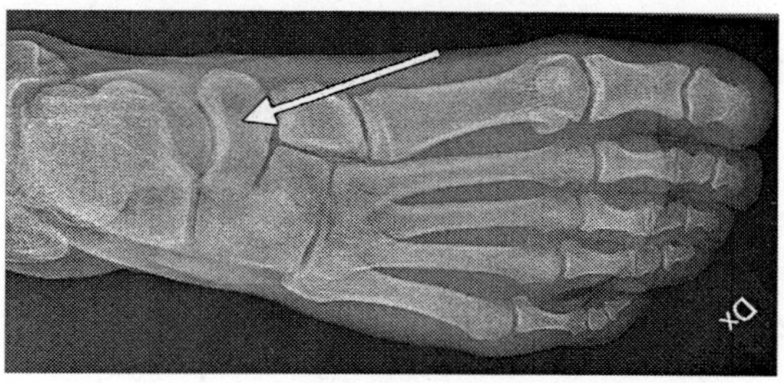

a. Calcaneum b. Cuboid
c. Navicular d. Talus

Ans. c. Navicular

14. Identify the location of the foreign body in the given X-ray:

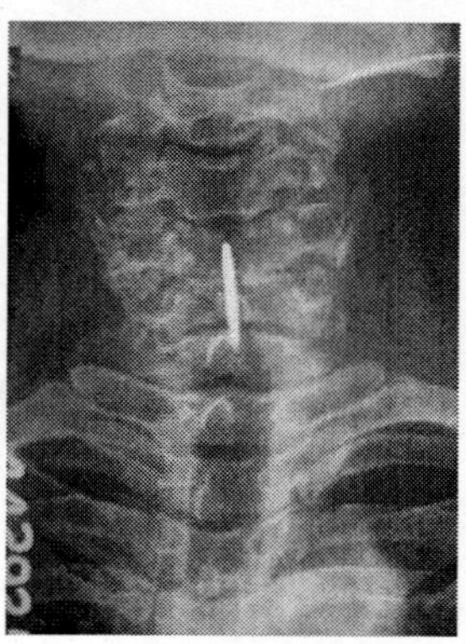

a. Oral cavity b. Trachea
c. Esophagus d. Aorta

Ans. b. Trachea

15. Study the image given below and choose the correct statement regarding the location of auscultatory areas:

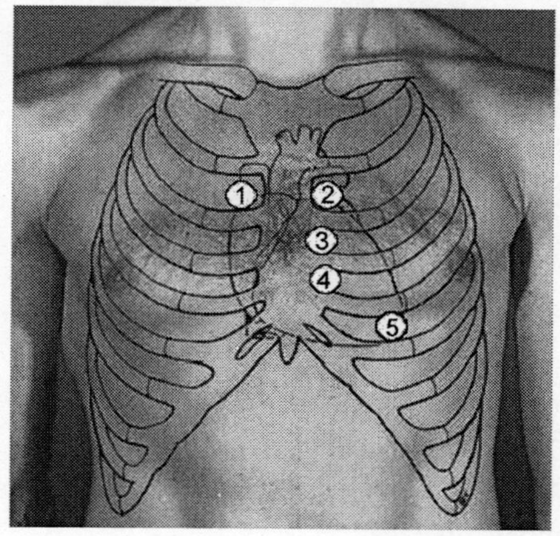

a. 2 is pulmonic area b. 3 is aortic area
c. 4 is mitral area d. 5 is tricuspid area

Ans. a. 2 is pulmonic area

16. A known case of leprosy presented to the Dermatology OPD with the complaints of deformity in his left hand as shown in the figure. Such a deformity is because of palsy of:

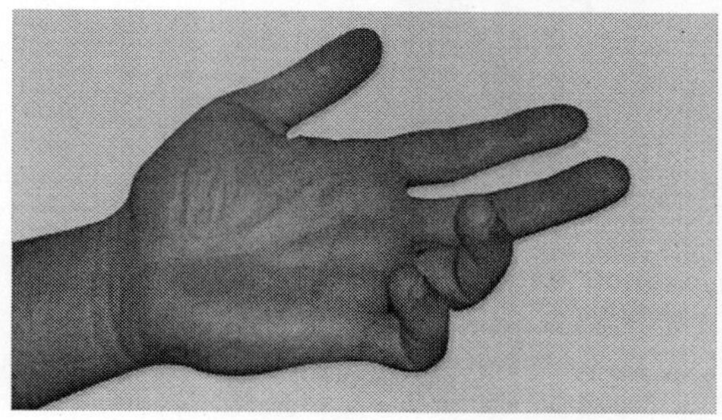

a. Ulnar nerve b. Radial nerve
c. Musculocutaneous nerve d. Median nerve

Image shows ulnar clawing.

Ans. a. Ulnar nerve

17. Identify the marked muscle:

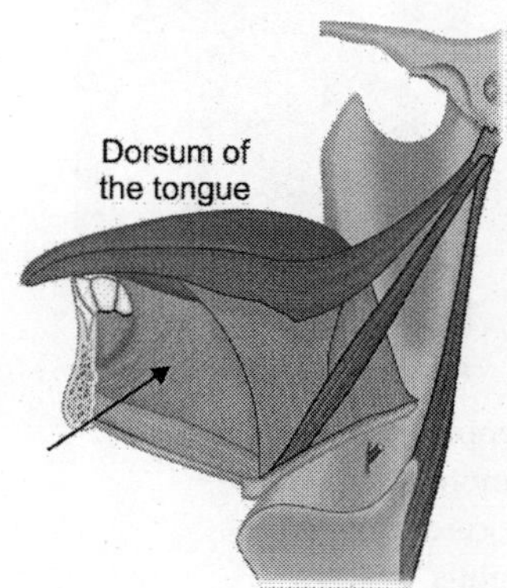

a. Palatoglossus b. Genioglossus
c. Styloglossus d. Hyoglossus

Ans. b. Genioglossus

18. **Identify the marked area:**

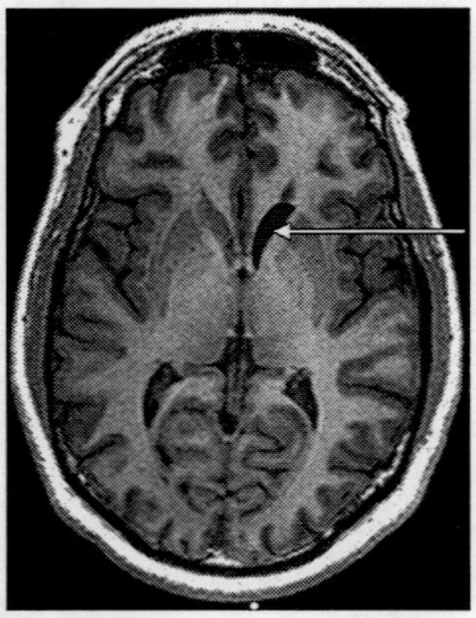

a. Caudate nucleus
b. Putamen
c. Internal capsule
d. Globus pallidus

Ans. a. Caudate nucleus

19. **All of the following branches of axillary artery are correctly labelled, *except*:**

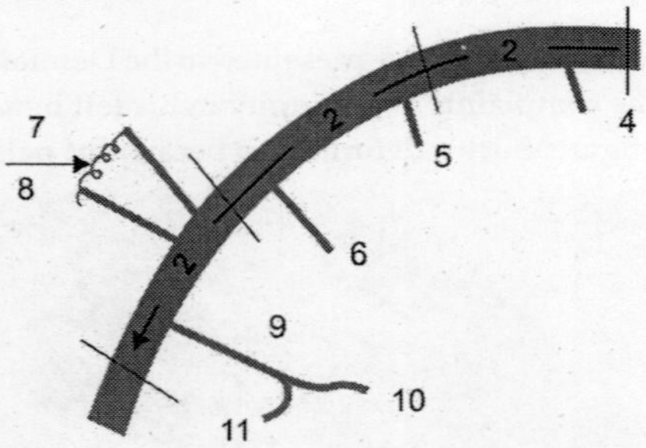

a. 4: Superior thoracic artery
b. 5: Thoraco-acromial artery
c. 6: Lateral thoracic artery
d. 9: Posterior circumflex humeral artery

Number 9 is Subscapular artery (from 3rd part)

Ans. d. 9: Posterior circumflex humeral artery

20. **What is the source of bleeding in such kind of presentation?**

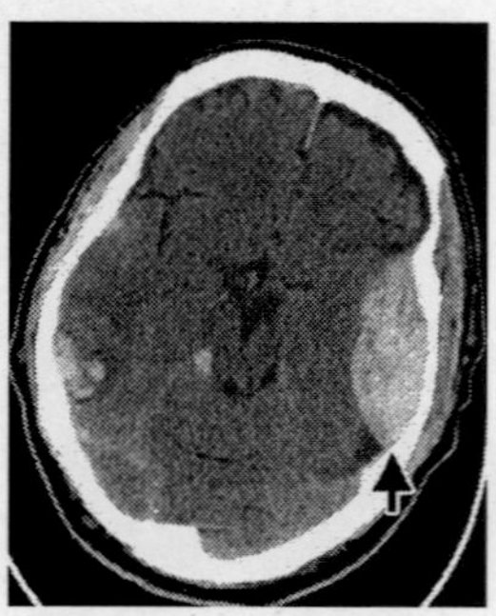

a. Dural venous sinuses
b. Middle meningeal artery
c. Anterior cerebral artery
d. Lateral sinus

CT scan shows extradural hemorrhage.

Ans. b. Middle meningeal artery

21. **Identify the nerve marked as 2:**

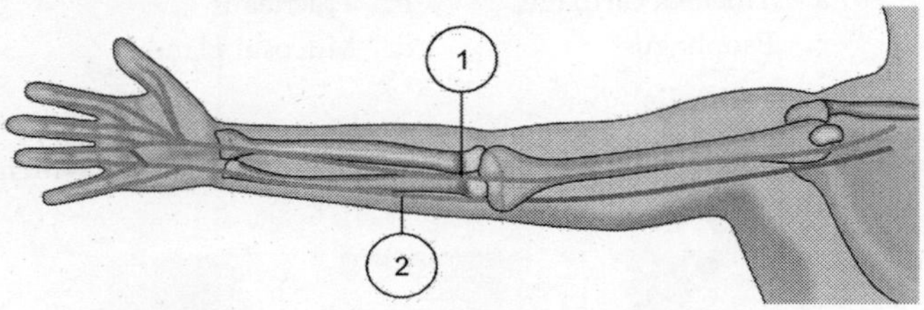

a. Ulnar nerve
b. Median nerve
c. Radial nerve
d. Musculocutaneous nerve

Ans. a. Ulnar nerve

22. **Which muscle is attached at the encircled landmark?**

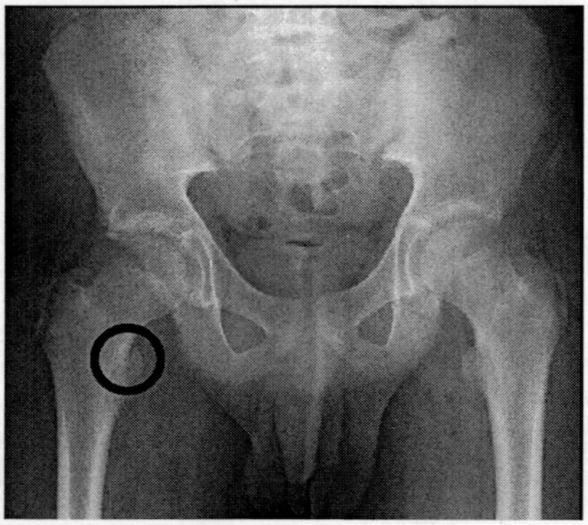

a. Gluteus maximus
b. Gluteus medius
c. Iliopsoas
d. Gluteus minimus

Encircled landmark is lesser trochanter (avulsed).

Ans. c. Iliopsoas

23. **After breast surgery, a female presented with deformity as shown below. Which nerve is most likely to be paralyzed?**

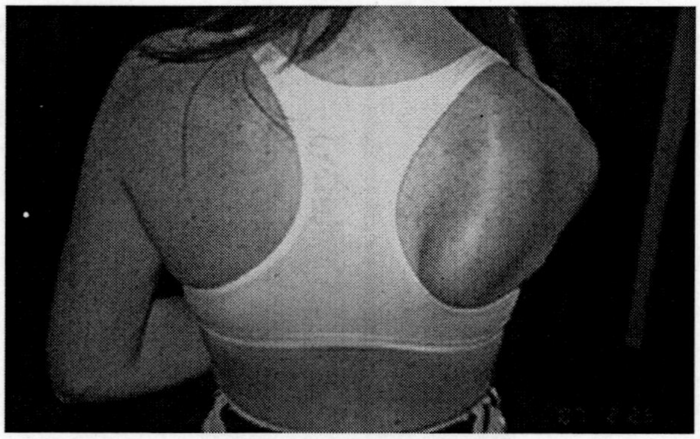

a. Axillary nerve
b. Median nerve
c. Long thoracic nerve
d. Suprascapular nerve

Image shows winging of scapula.

Ans. c. Long thoracic nerve

24. Identify the tendon marked with red arrow:

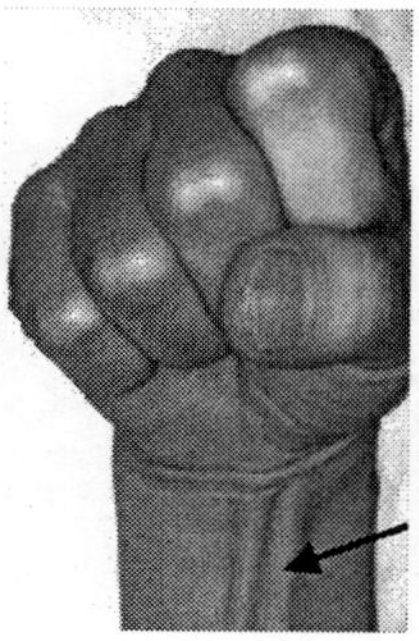

a. Palmaris longus b. Flexor carpi ulnaris
c. Flexor carpi radialis d. Flexor pollicis longus

Ans. c. Flexor carpi radialis

25. A patient presented with paraesthesia of inner aspect arm of arm. X-ray shows the following picture. Most likely diagnosis:

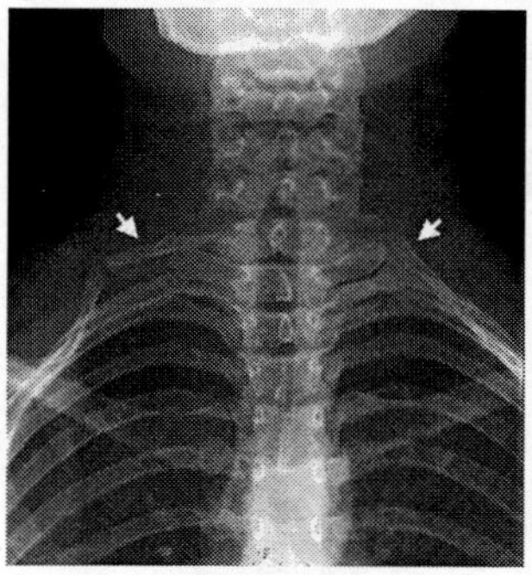

a. Superior vena cava syndrome
b. Intervertebral disc prolapse
c. Cervical rib
d. Fracture clavicle

Ans. c. Cervical rib

26. Marked area terminates at:

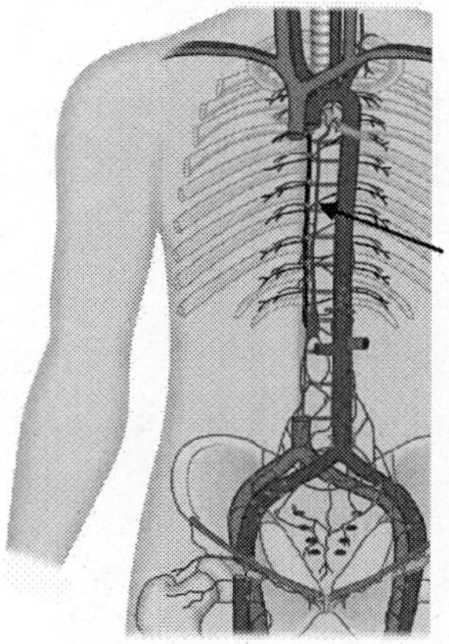

a. Right atrium b. Superior vena cava
c. Junction of left jugular vein and left subclavian vein
d. Junction of right jugular vein and right subclavian vein

Yellow coloured structure is thoracic duct

Ans. c. Junction of left jugular vein and left subclavian vein

27. Active principle of the substance shown in the figure is:

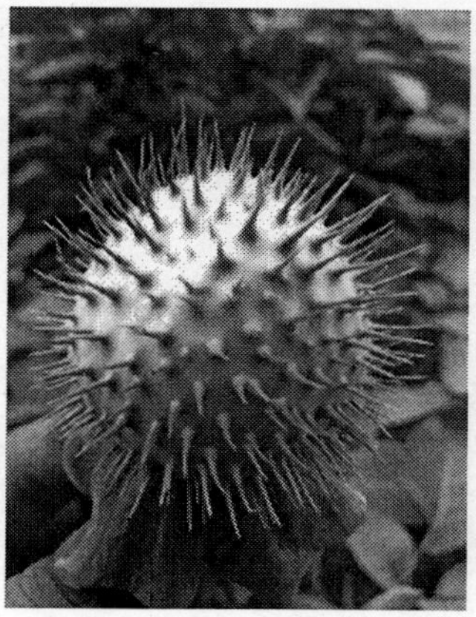

a. Tetra-hydro-cannabinol b. Abrin
c. Hyoscine d. Semicarpol

Image shows dhatura.

Ans. c. Hyoscine

28. A patient presented to the skin OPD with drying of skin and appearance as shown in the image below. Such a presentation is because of deficiency of:

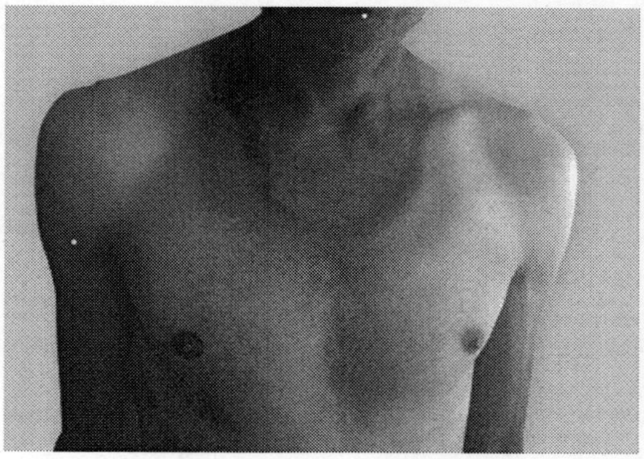

a. Thiamine b. Riboflavin
c. Niacin d. Biotin

Image shows Casal's necklace.

Ans. c. Niacin

29. Identify the condition:

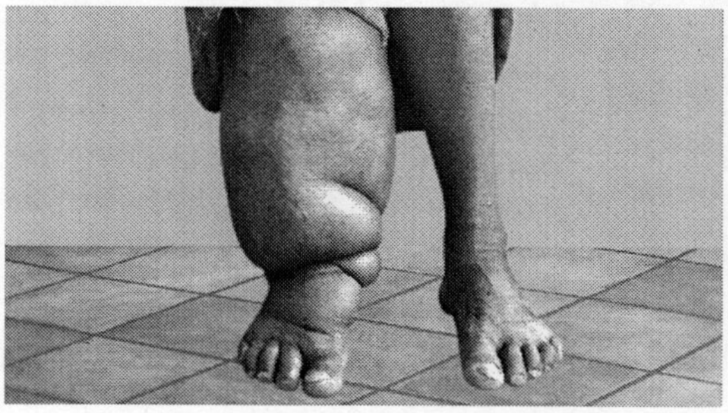

a. Lupus vulgaris b. Psoriasis
c. Leprosy d. Elephantiasis

Ans. d. Elephantiasis

30. What are the characteristic nail findings shown in this patient of psoriasis?

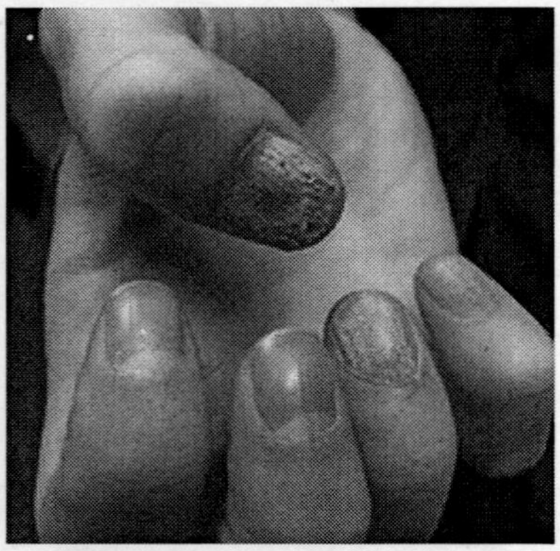

a. Onycholysis
b. Koilonychia
c. Subungual hyperkeratosis
d. Mees line

Ans. c. Subungual hyperkeratosis

31. After few months of injury by a thorn, a patient presented with a swelling in palm as shown in the figure. This is:

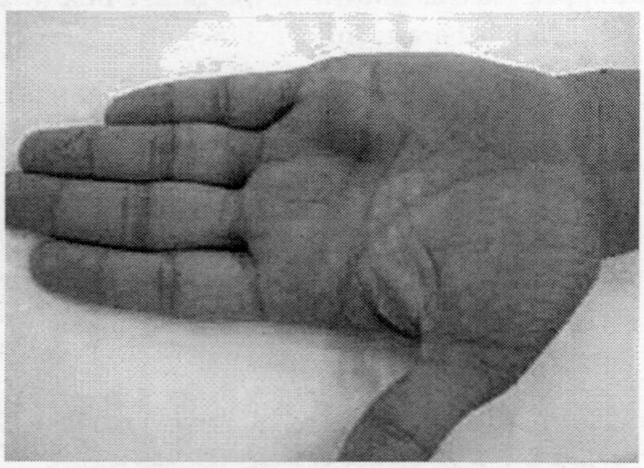

a. Implantation dermoid
b. Ganglion
c. Enchondroma
d. Dupuytren's contracture

Ans. a. Implantation dermoid

32. Identify the condition:

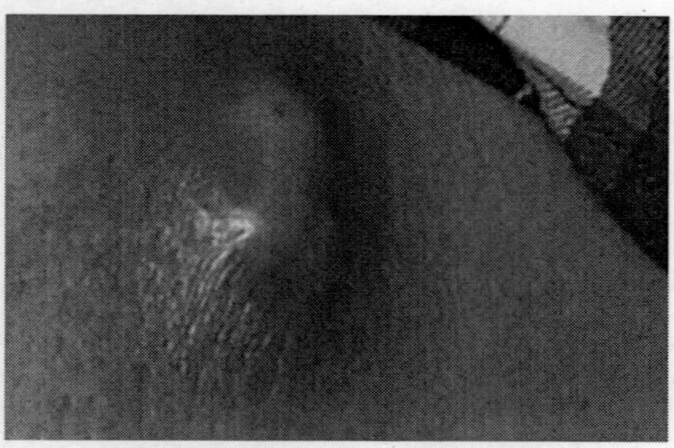

a. Carbuncle
b. Sebaceous cyst
c. Lipoma
d. Dermoid cyst

Ans. a. Carbuncle

33. A truck driver developed painless ulcer over genitals for which he was undergoing treatment. Now he developed symptoms as shown in the figure. Most likely diagnosis:

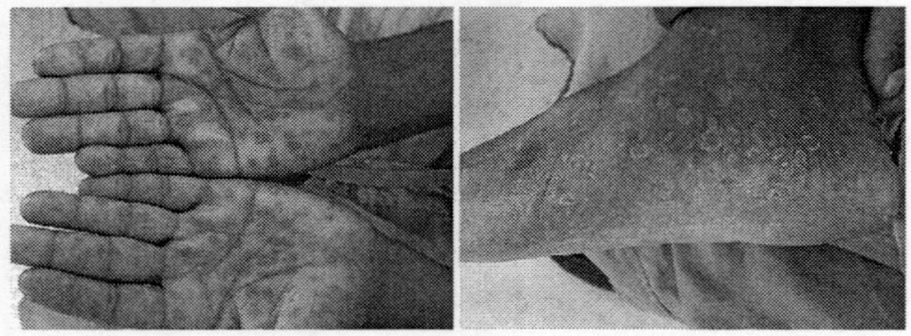

a. Fungal infection
b. HIV
c. Drug eruptions
d. Secondary syphilis

Image shows rashes.

Ans. d. Secondary syphilis

34. Identify the condition shown in the image:

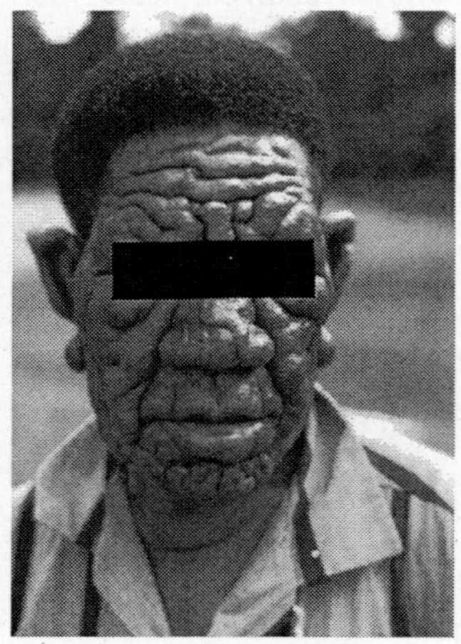

a. Anaphylaxis
b. Kala-azar
c. Lepromatous leprosy
d. Tuberculoid leprosy

Ans. c. Lepromatous leprosy

35. A patient presented with hypopigmented rash and satellite lesions as shown in the figure. Most likely diagnosis:

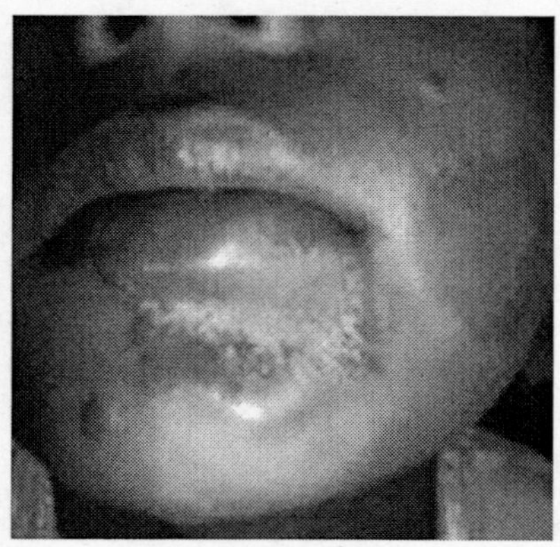

a. TT leprosy
b. LL leprosy
c. BL leprosy
d. BT leprosy

Ans. d. BT leprosy

36. A patient on anti-convulsant developed some skin problem as shown in the figure. Most likely diagnosis:

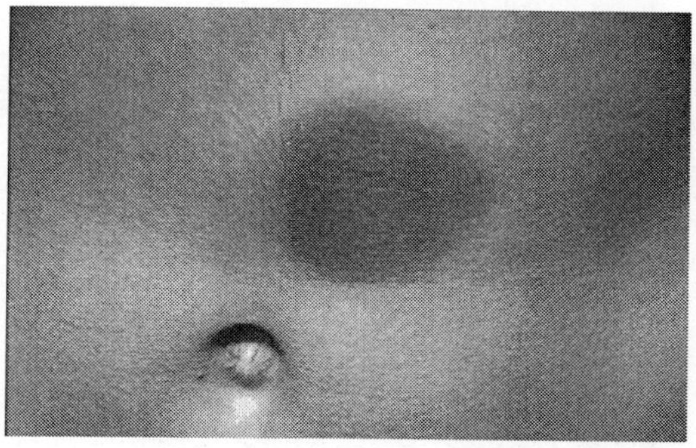

a. Pseudo-lymphoma b. Urticaria
c. Dermatitis d. Fixed drug eruptions

Ans. d. Fixed drug eruptions

37. Which sign is demonstrated in the image given below?

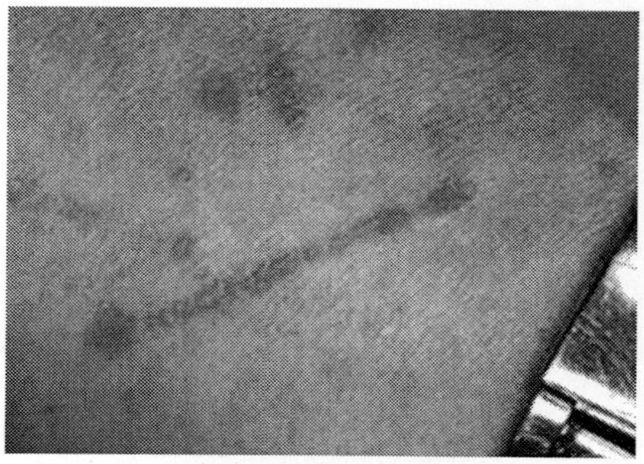

a. Koebner's phenomenon b. Auspitz sign
c. Darrier's sign d. Nikolsky's sign

Area of injury develops psoriatic lesions.

Ans. a. Koebner's phenomenon

38. An infant presented to the ENT OPD with inspiratory stridor. On examination, the epiglottis was found to be like this. Most likely condition:

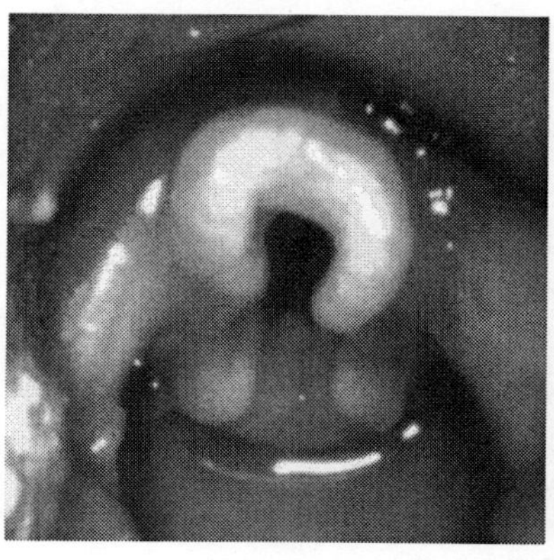

a. Croup b. Acute epiglottitis
c. Abductor palsy d. Laryngomalacia

Image shows omega shaped epiglottis.

Ans. d. Laryngomalacia

39. Identify the condition:

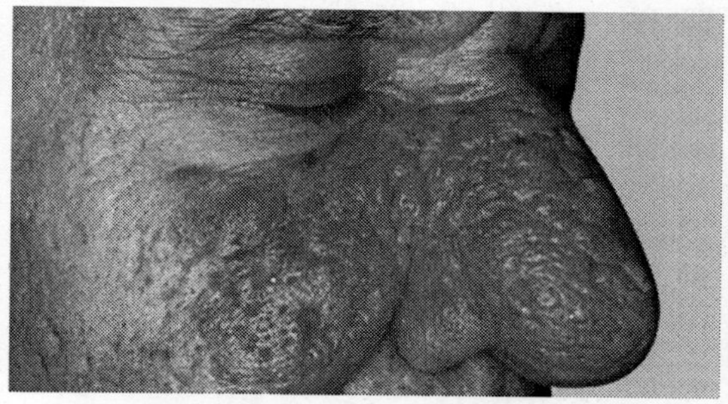

a. Rhinoscleroma b. Atrophic rhinitis
c. Rhinophyma d. Rhinosporodiosis

Ans. c. Rhinophyma

40. Identify the test performed in the image given below:

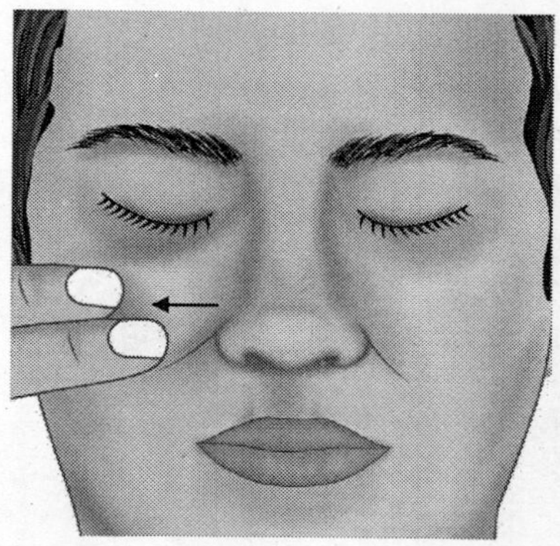

a. Epley's test
b. Heimlich manoeuvre
c. Cottle's test
d. Massaging of nasolacrimal duct

Ans. c. Cottle's test

41. A patient met with RTA and had fracture base of skull with CSF rhinorrhoea. When the fluid was taken on a white tissue paper, it showed the following appearance. Such a sign is known as:

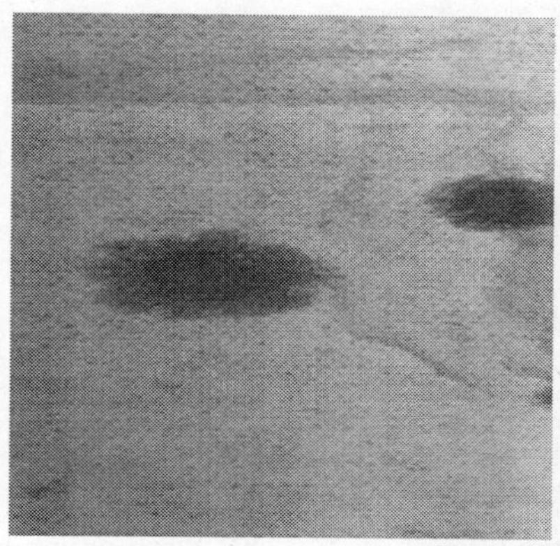

a. Halo sign b. Schwartz sign
c. Tobey Ayer's sign d. Brown sign

Ans. a. Halo sign

42. A child complains of perianal itching. Slide was prepared and examined under microscope. It demonstrates the eggs of:

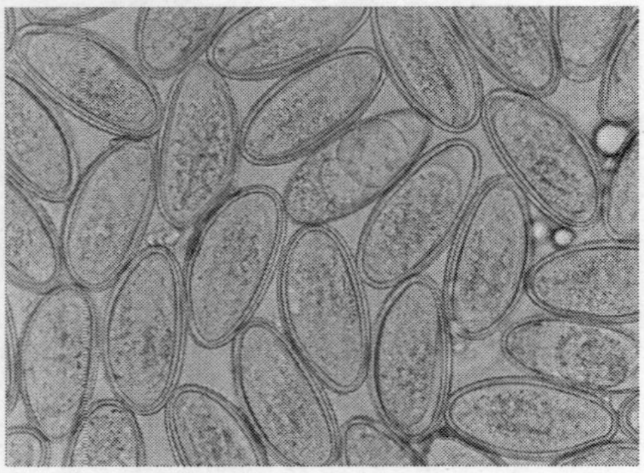

a. Enterobius vermicularis b. Ancylostoma duodenale
c. Trichuris trichura d. Ascaris lumbricoides

Ans. a. Enterobius vermicularis

43. India ink staining of the organism showed the following appearance. Which is the likely organism?

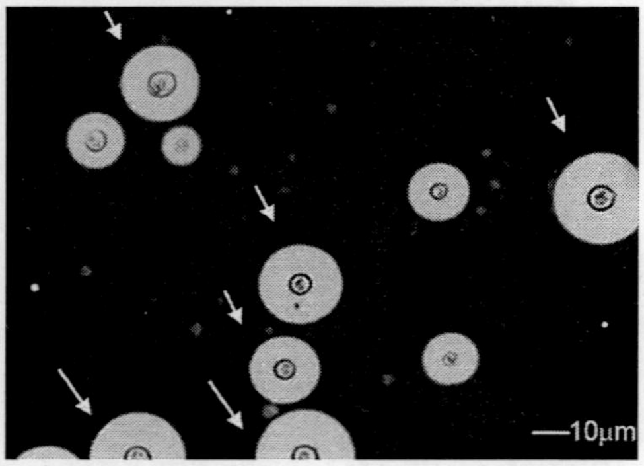

a. Cryptosporodium b. Cryptococcus
c. Chlamydia d. Campylobacter

Ans. b. Cryptococcus

44. A lady with malaria was investigated. Microscopic examination of blood showed the following picture. Such a gametocyte indicates that malaria is caused by:

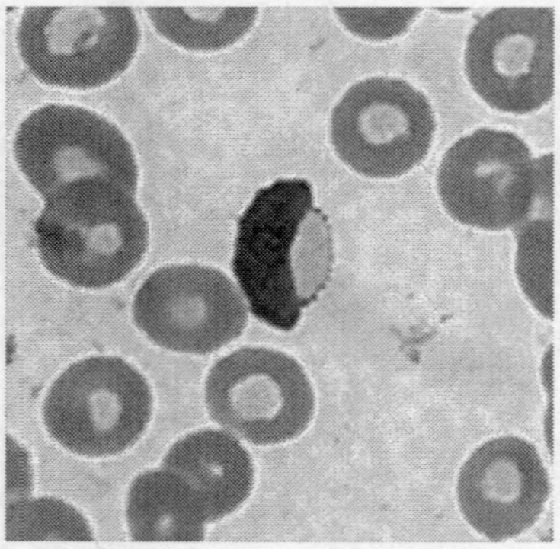

a. Plasmodium vivax b. Plasmodium falciparum
c. Plasmodium malariae d. Plasmodium ovale

Ans. b. Plasmodium falciparum

45. A 45-years-old lady presented with the complaints of post-coital bleeding. She had a history of early marriage and has 6 live children. Colposcopic examination showed an inflamed cervix which bleed on touch. Most likely diagnosis:

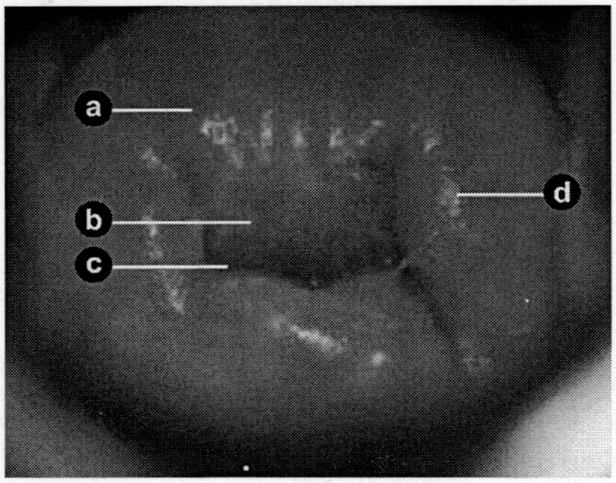

a. Chronic endometritis b. Cervical fibroid
c. Endometrial carcinoma d. Cervical carcinoma

Ans. d. Cervical carcinoma

46. Identify the type of Leopold's manoeuvre:

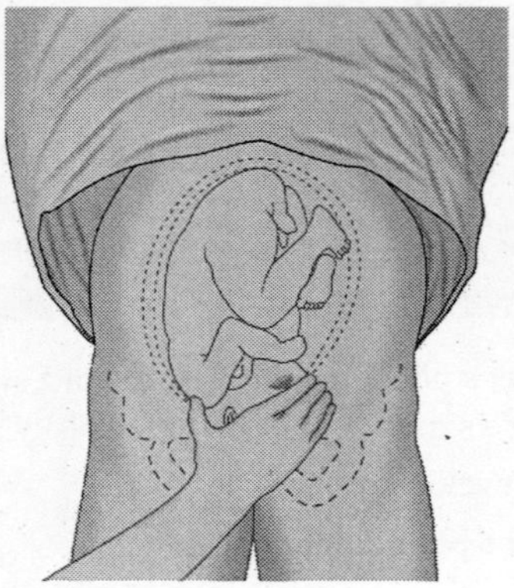

a. I b. II c. III d. IV

Ans. c. III

47. Identify the condition:

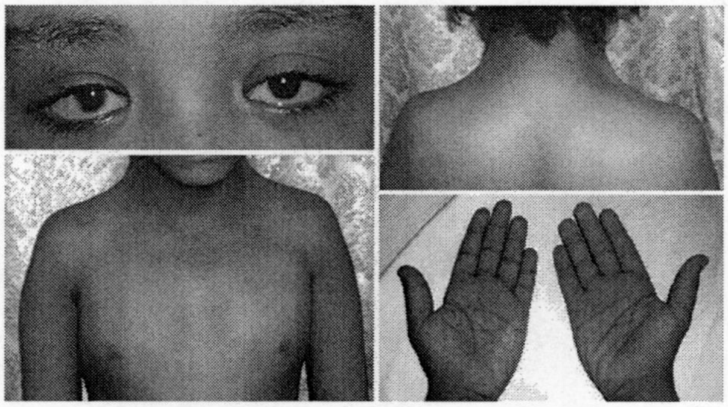

a. Down's syndrome b. Turner's syndrome
c. Klinefelter's syndrome
d. Congenital adrenal hyperplasia

Ans. b. Turner's syndrome

48. Hysterosalpingography suggest the diagnosis of:

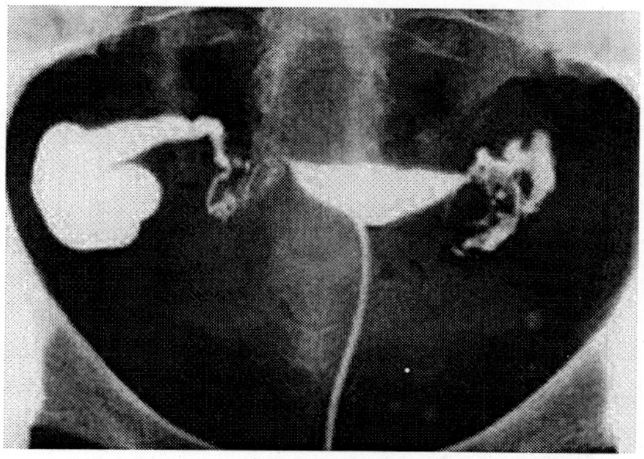

a. Right hydrosalpinx b. Left hydrosalpinx
c. Unicornuate uterus d. Bicornuate uterus

Ans. a. Right hydrosalpinx

49. A young boy develops hemarthrosis in right knee after a history of fall. Such a clinical presentation may occur because of deficiency of:

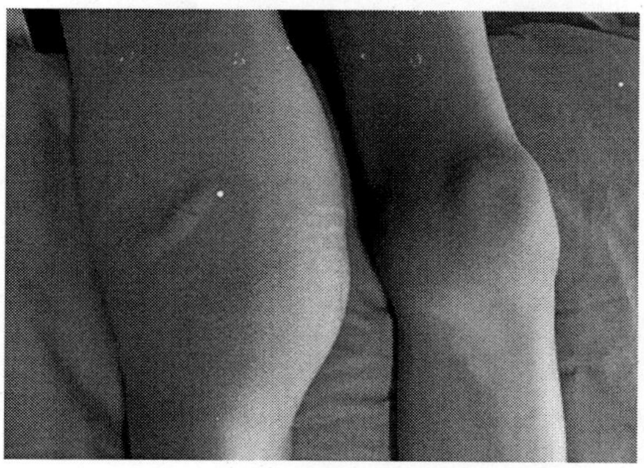

a. Vitamin K b. Vitamin C
c. Platelets d. Factor VIII

Ans. d. Factor VIII

50. Which type of intestinal movement is this:

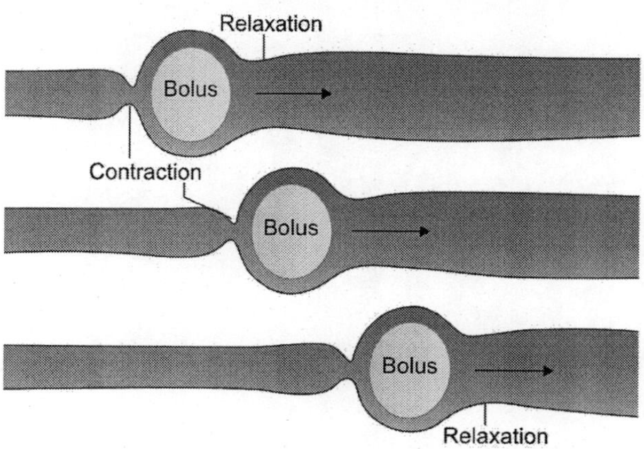

a. Peristalsis b. Anti-peristalsis
c. Mass reflex d. Segmental contraction

Ans. a. Peristalsis

51. Study the left ventricular Pressure–left ventricular Volume graph. Which phenomenon occurs at point C?

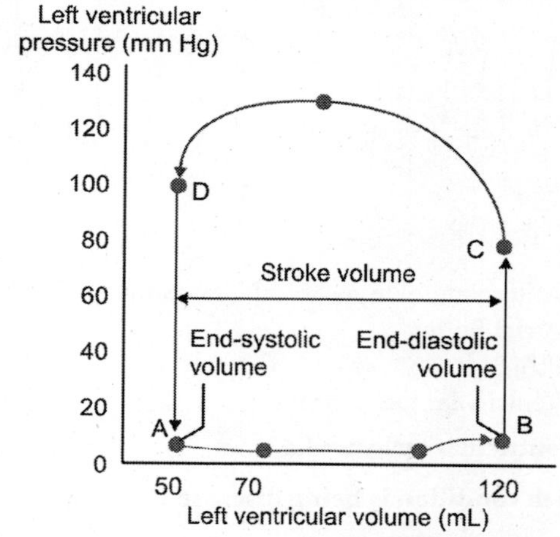

a. Mitral valve opening b. Mitral valve closure
c. Aortic valve opening d. Aortic valve closure

Ans. c. Aortic valve opening

52. Water is maximally reabsorbed at:

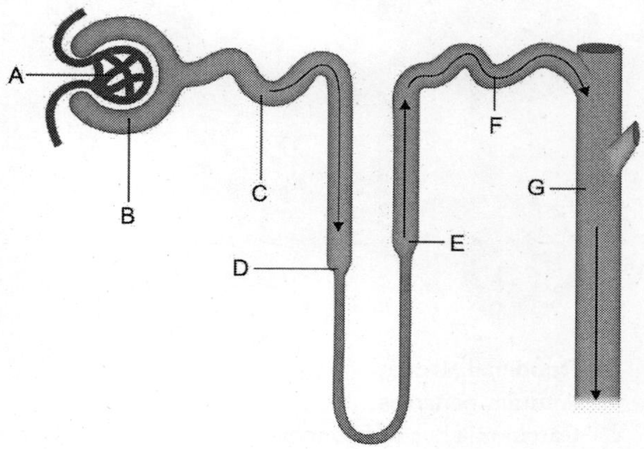

a. A b. B
c. C d. D

C denotes proximal convoluted tubules.

Ans. c. C

53. Identify the logo:

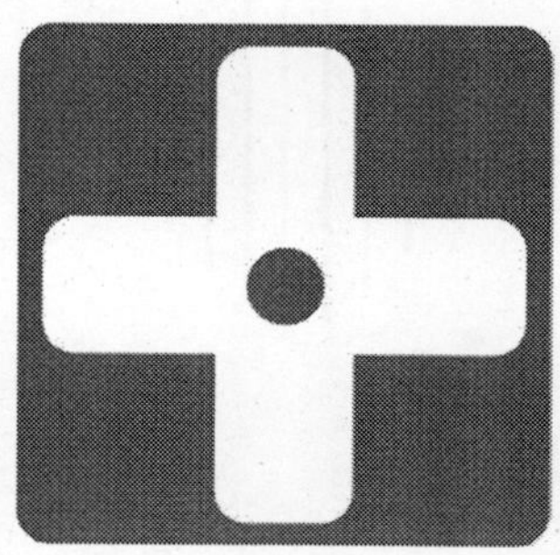

a. Red cross emblem b. Hospital
c. Suraksha clinic d. WHO

Ans. c. Suraksha clinic

54. ECG is suggestive of:

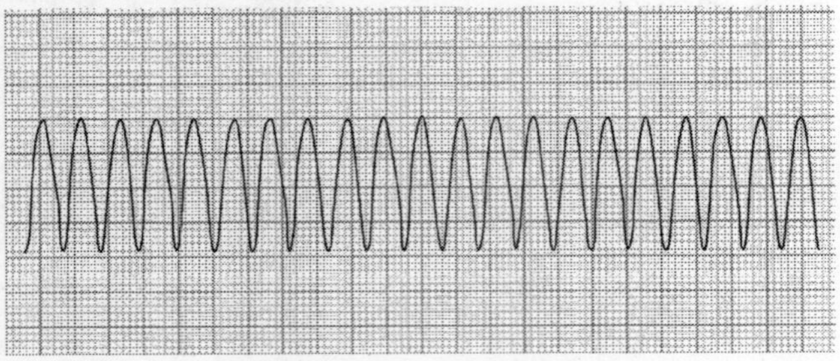

a. Anterolateral myocardial infarction
b. Atrial flutter
c. PSVT
d. Ventricular tachycardia

Ans. d. Ventricular tachycardia

55. Which condition is being discussed?

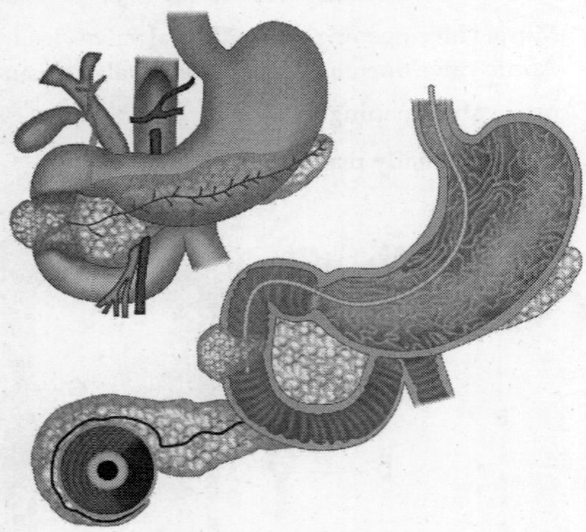

a. Duodenal atresia
b. Annular pancreas
c. Carcinoma head of pancreas
d. Pancreatic divisum

Ans. b. Annular pancreas

56. Which type of murmur is this?

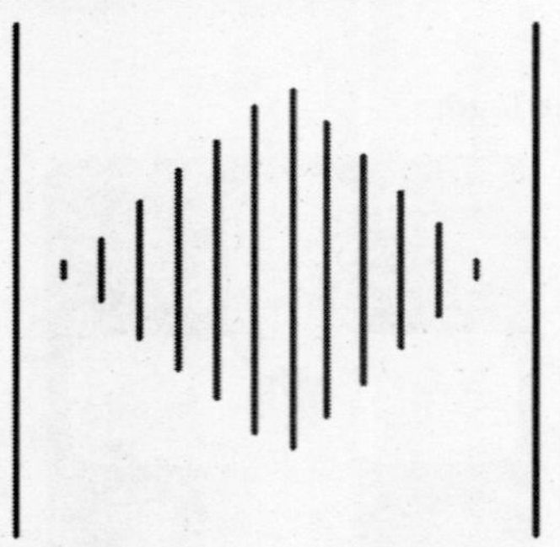

a. Diastolic murmur
b. Ejection systolic murmur
c. Pansystolic murmur
d. Continuous murmur

Ans. b. Ejection systolic murmur

57. ECG is suggestive of:

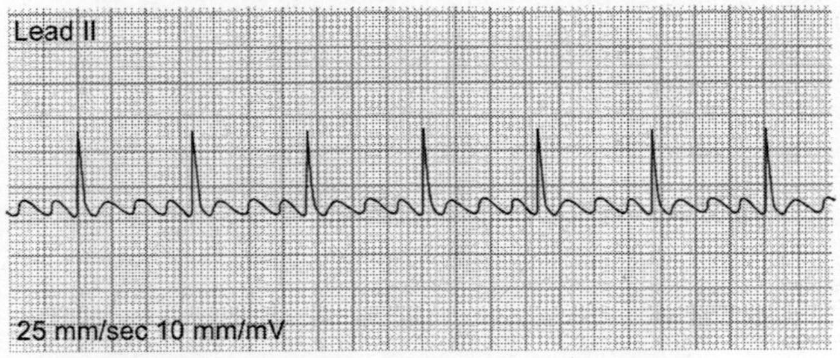

a. Atrial flutter
b. Atrial fibrillation
c. Ventricular tachycardia
d. Ventricular fibrillation

ECG shows sawtooth pattern.

Ans. a. Atrial flutter

58. Such a clinical picture is suggestive of:

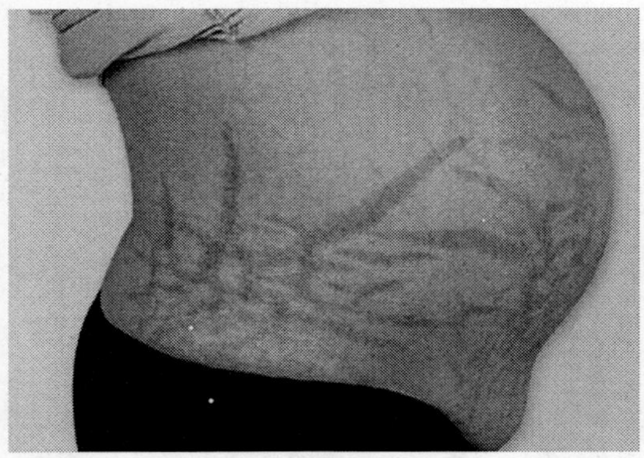

a. Addison's disease
b. Cushing's syndrome
c. Hypothyroidism
d. Morbid obesity

Image shows purple striae.

Ans. b. Cushing's syndrome

59. Identify the clinical sign shown in the image:

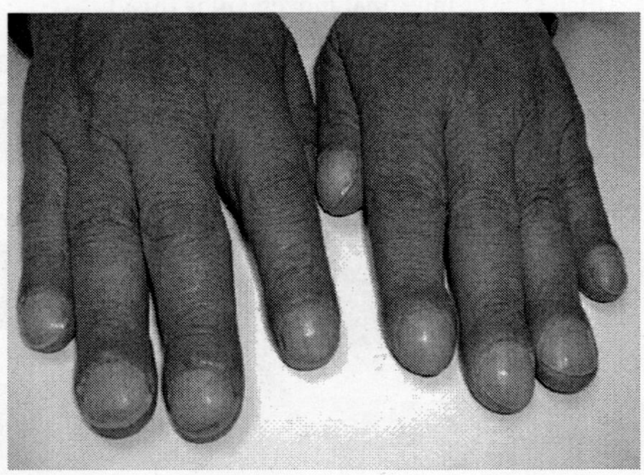

a. Cyanosis
b. Clubbing
c. Koilonychia
d. Pterygium of nail

Ans. b. Clubbing

60. **Such a presentation in AIDS patient suggest:**

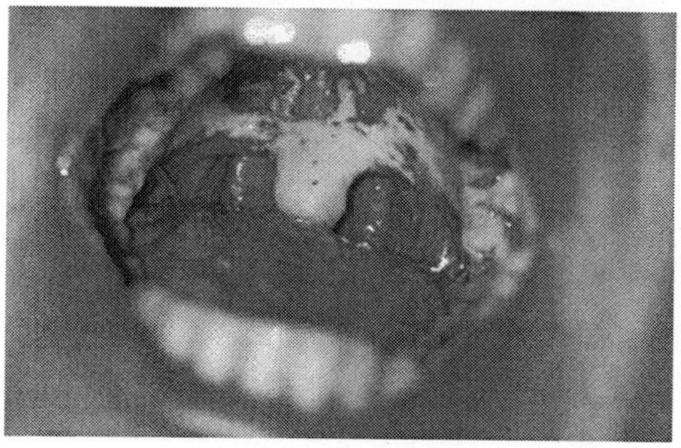

a. Stage I
b. Stage II
c. Stage III
d. Stage IV

Image shows oral candidiasis.

Ans. c. Stage III

61. **Such a jugular venous pulse suggest:**

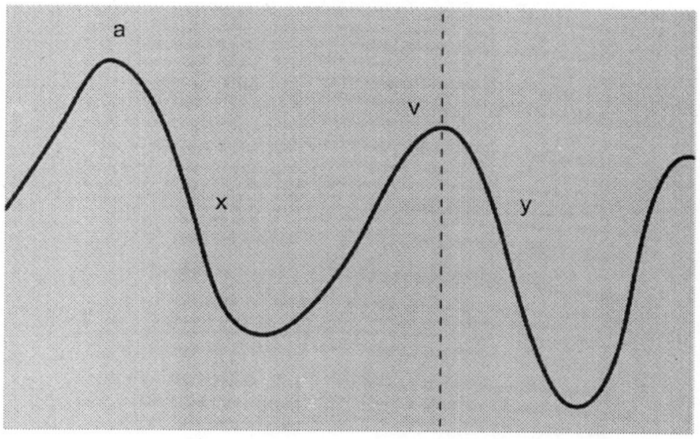

a. Cardiac tamponade
b. Constrictive pericarditis
c. Left heart failure
d. Dilated cardiomyopathy

JVP shows prominent x descent and rapid y descent.

Ans. b. Constrictive pericarditis

62. **Management of such a condition:**

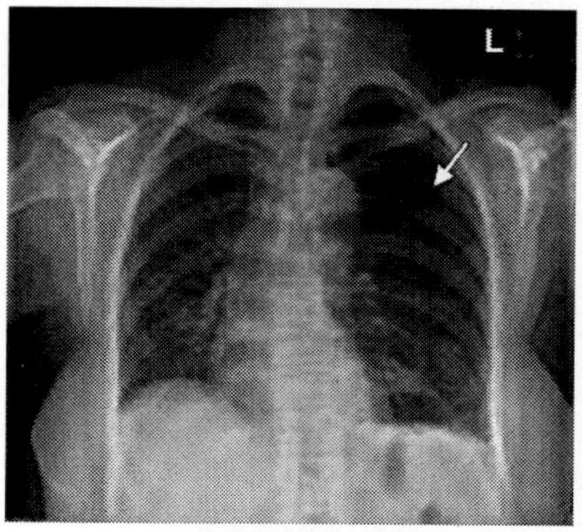

a. Right sided needle thoracostomy
b. Left sided needle thoracostomy
c. Wait and watch
d. Chest strapping

X-ray shows left sided pneumothorax and right shift of trachea.

Ans. b. Left sided needle thoracostomy

63. **A young patient developed high-grade fever. Lumbar puncture revealed CSF protein level of 220 mg/dL and CSF sugar of 35 mg/dL. The clinical image of the patient is shown below. Such a presentation is because of:**

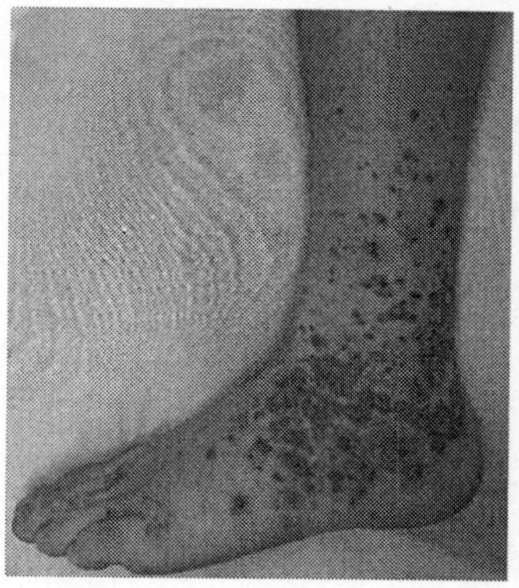

a. Staphylococcus aureus
b. Streptococcus pneumoniae
c. Neisseria meningitidis
d. Neisseria gonorrhoea

Clinical history is suggestive of Waterhouse–Friderichsen syndrome, which is associated with Neisseria meningitidis.

Ans. c. Neisseria meningitidis

64. **Such a clinical picture suggest:**

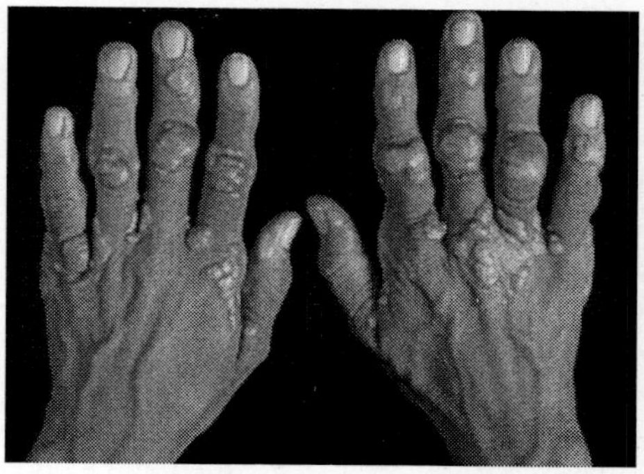

a. Hypercholesterolemia
b. Rheumatoid arthritis
c. Osteoarthritis
d. Hyperglycaemia

Image shows xanthomas.

Ans. a. Hypercholesterolemia

65. **Identify the condition:**

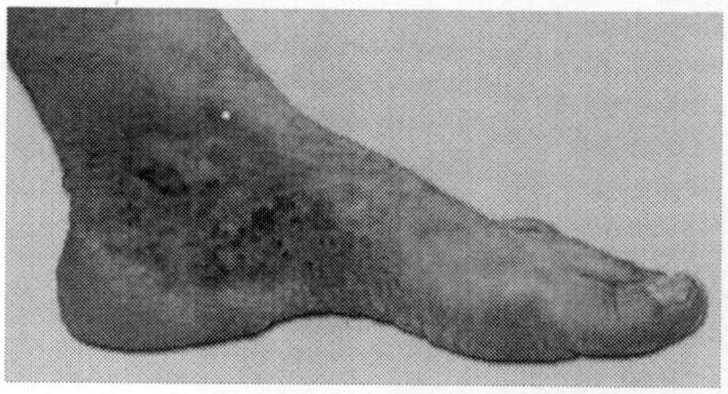

a. Arterial ulcer
b. Trophic ulcer
c. Venous ulcer
d. Pressure sore

Ans. c. Venous ulcer

66. While assessing a patient admitted in neurology ward, doctor had drawn figures on the left side and the patient was told to copy them on the right side. Condition of the patient can be labelled as:

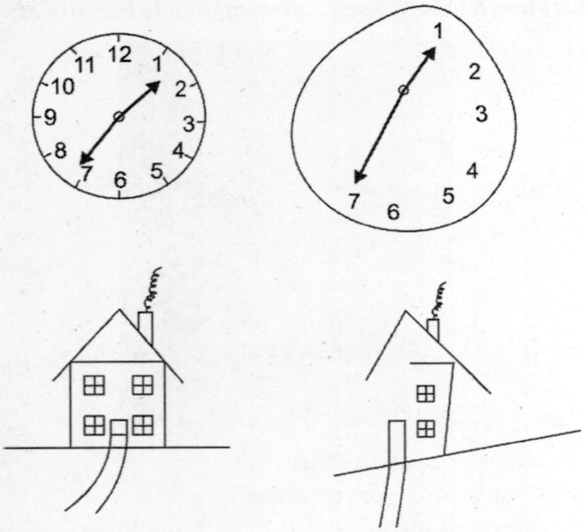

a. Apraxia b. Hemineglect
c. Agraphia d. Dyslexia

Ans. b. Hemineglect

67. Such color changes on exposure to cold are best described in:

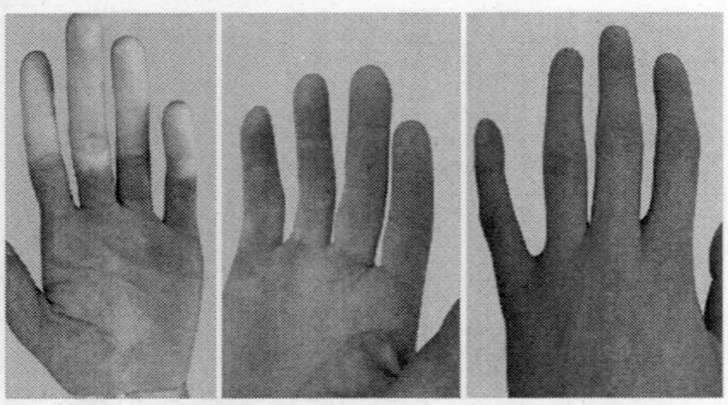

a. Virchow's triad b. Raynaud's phenomenon
c. Niacin deficiency d. Tetralogy of Fallot

Ans. b. Raynaud's phenomenon

68. During an abdominal surgery, surgeon found an incidental finding as shown in the image below, which was 2 feet proximal to ileocecal valve. This is:

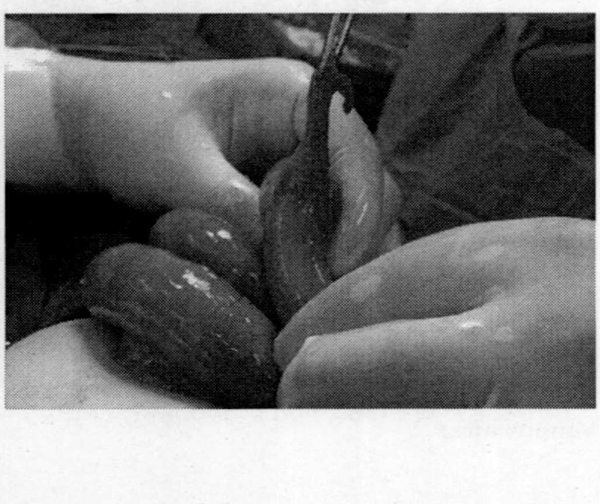

a. Intussusception b. Duodenal atresia
c. Jejunal adhesions d. Meckel's diverticulum

Ans. d. Meckel's diverticulum

69. Identify the surgical procedure:

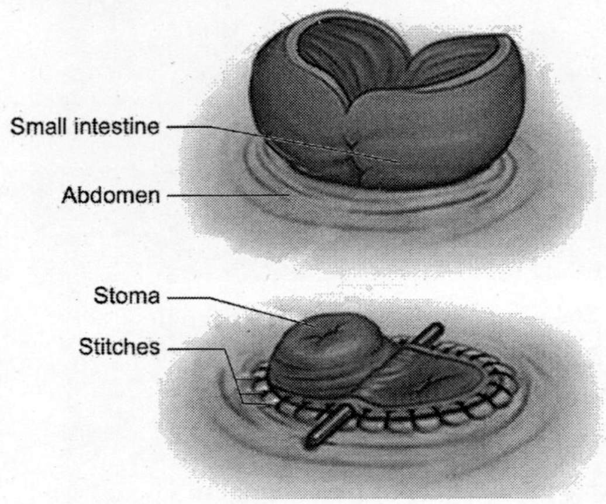

a. Loop ileostomy
b. Duodeno-jejunostomy
c. Duodeno-duodenostomy
d. Roux-en-Y procedure

Ans. a. Loop ileostomy

70. Identify the instrument:

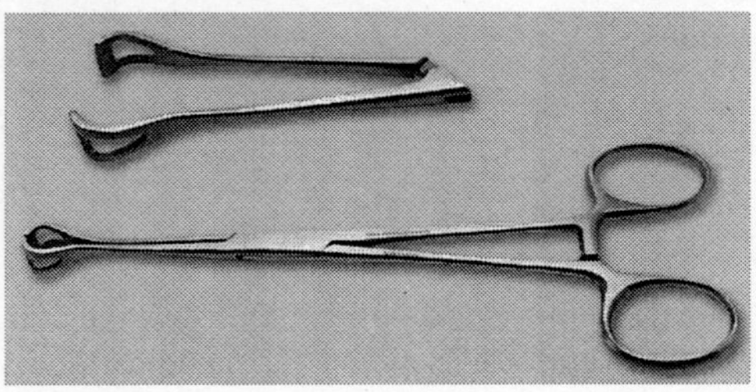

a. Artery forceps b. Babcock forceps
c. Sponge holding forceps d. Allis forceps

Ans. b. Babcock forceps

71. Such a clinical sign is seen in:

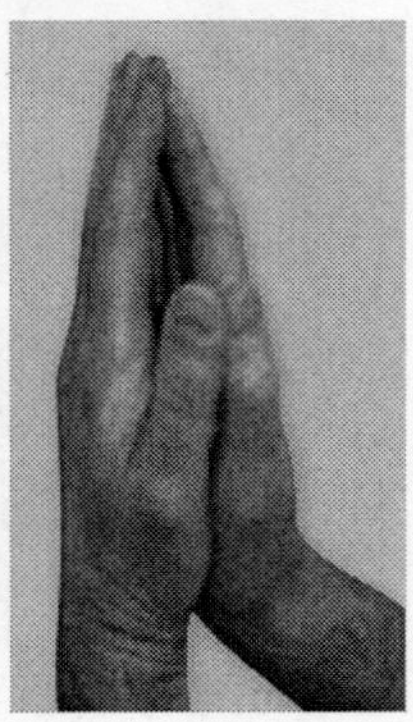

a. Diabetes mellitus b. Dupuytren's contracture
c. Carpal tunnel syndrome d. Leprosy

Image shows prayer sign.

Ans. a. Diabetes mellitus

72. A patient presented with loss of appetite, evening rise of fever and cough for 1 month. Neck examination showed the following picture. Most likely diagnosis:

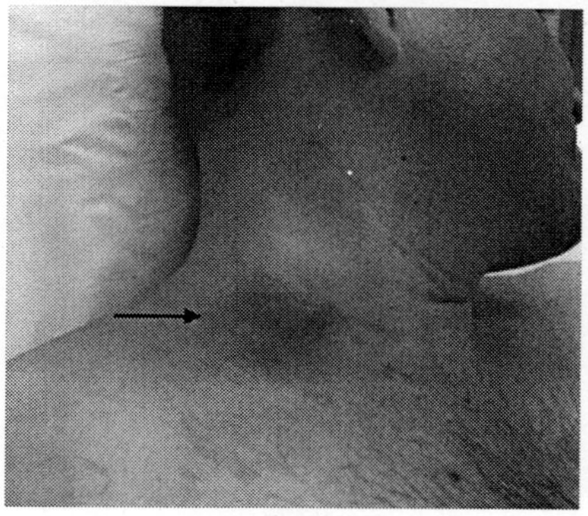

a. Hodgkin's lymphoma
b. Non-Hodgkin's lymphoma
c. Tuberculous lymphadenitis
d. Bezold's abscess

Ans. c. Tuberculous lymphadenitis

73. Identify the surgical procedure being done in a patient who underwent RTA, for maintaining airway:

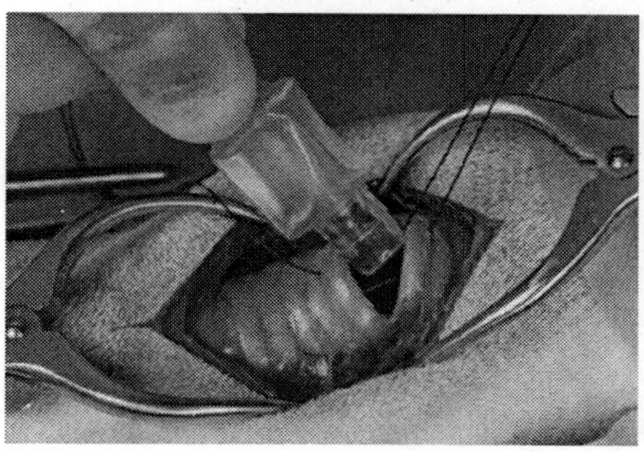

a. Tracheostomy b. Intubation
c. Radical neck dissection d. Thyroidectomy

Ans. a. Tracheostomy

74. An African patient was operated on chest for some surgical condition but later on he developed scar as shown in the figure. This is:

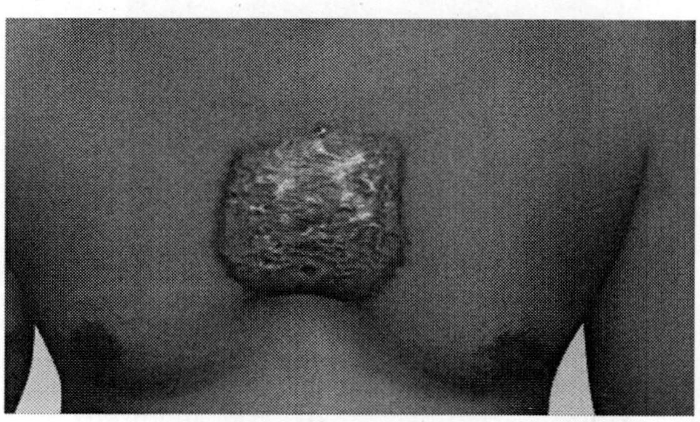

a. Hypertrophic scar b. Keloid
c. Marjolin's ulcer d. Skin TB

Ans. b. Keloid

75. Identify the condition:

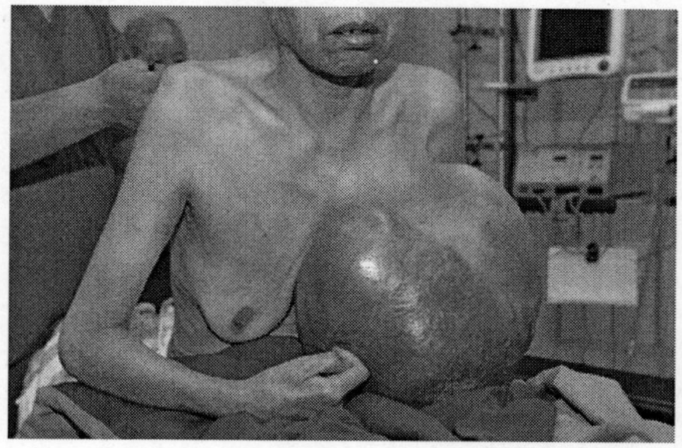

a. Paget's disease b. Phylloides tumour
c. Breast abscess d. Fibroadenoma

Ans. b. Phylloides tumour

76. A patient presented to the Surgery OPD with complains of fluid discharge per anum. Clinical image is shown below. Most likely diagnosis:

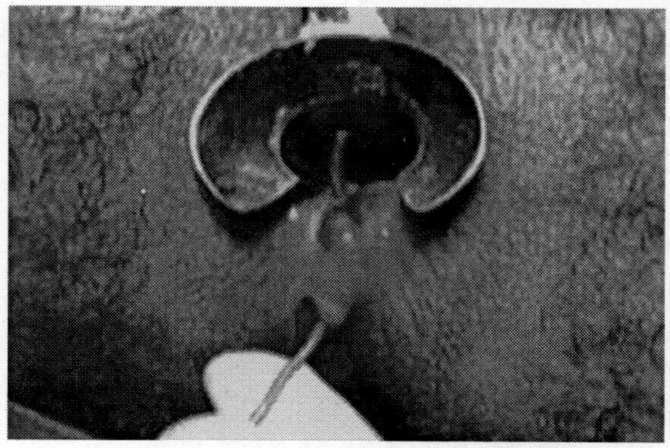

a. Anal fissure b. Fistula-in-ano
c. Hemorrhoids d. Carcinoma anus

Ans. b. Fistula-in-ano

77. Such a mispositioned IUCD is best removed by:

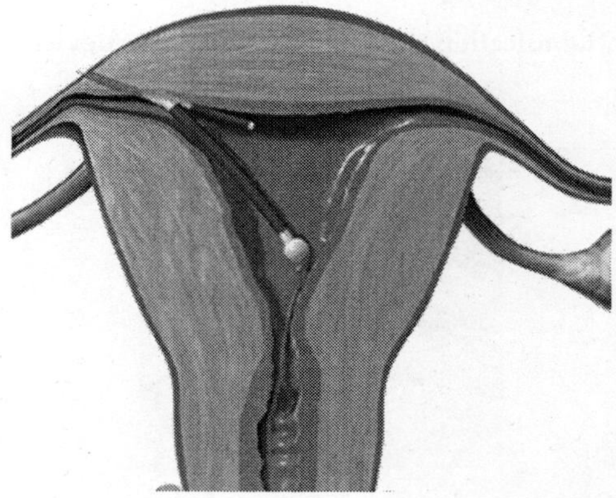

a. Laparoscopy b. Laparotomy
c. Hysterectomy d. Hysteroscopy

Ans. d. Hysteroscopy

78. What kind of twins?

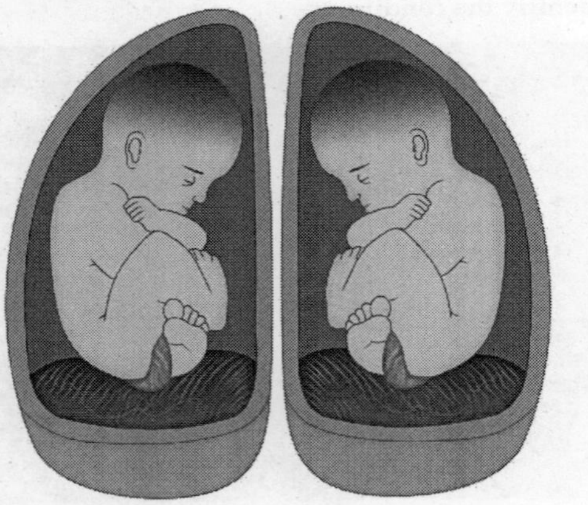

a. Monochorionic Monoamniotic
b. Monochorionic Diamniotic
c. Dichorionic Monoamniotic
d. Dichorionic Diamniotic

Ans. d. Dichorionic Diamniotic

79. A 14-years-old female presented with primary amenorrhoea and cyclical abdominal pain for last 6 months. She is having urinary retention as well. Clinical image is shown below. Most likely diagnosis:

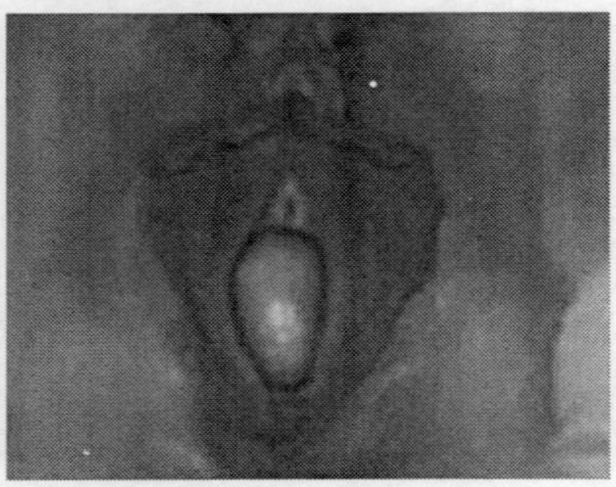

a. Congenital adrenal hyperplasia
b. Mullerian agenesis
c. Imperforate hymen
d. Uterine prolapse

Ans. c. Imperforate hymen

80. Contraindication of such a contraceptive device:

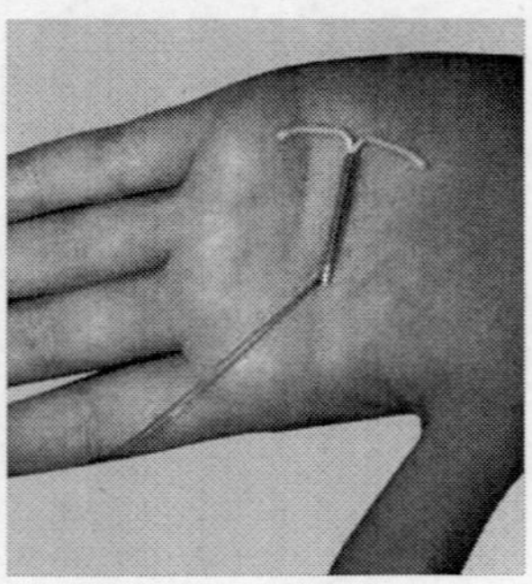

a. Obesity
b. Anemia
c. Hypertension
d. Pelvic inflammatory disease

Ans. d. Pelvic inflammatory disease

81. Lesion at site number 2 will result in:

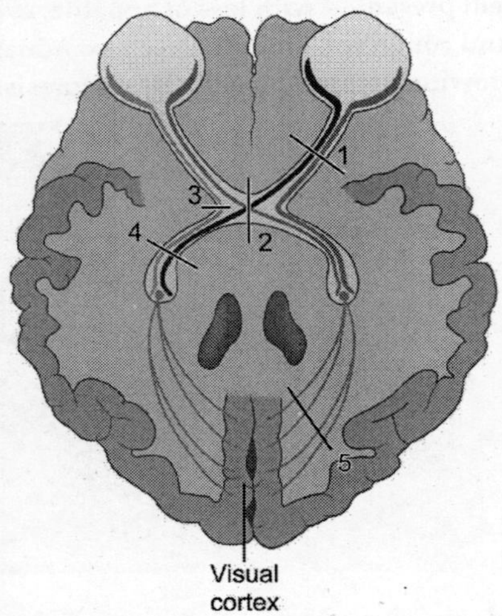

a. Bitemporal hemianopia
b. Homonymous hemianopia
c. Monocular blindness
d. Homonymous hemianopia with macular sparing

Site 2 is optic chiasm.

Ans. a. Bitemporal hemianopia

82. Use of the ophthalmological instrument shown below:

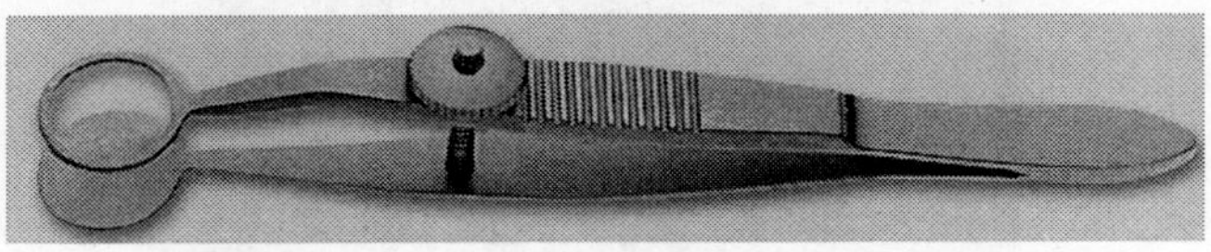

a. For strabismus surgery
b. For chalazion surgery
c. For entropion surgery
d. For cataract surgery

Image shows chalazion forceps.

Ans. b. For chalazion surgery

83. A patient presents with opacification of cornea and decreased vision. Clinical image is shown below. Next line of management:

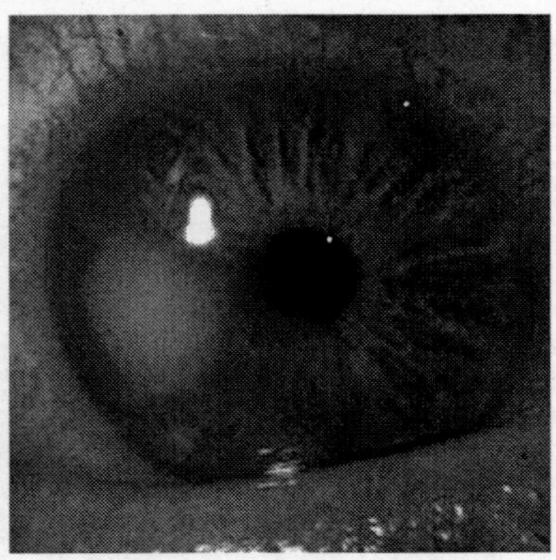

a. Keratoplasty
b. Radial keratotomy
c. LASIK
d. Wait and watch

Image shows a healed cornel ulcer.

Ans. a. Keratoplasty

84. Histological image suggest:

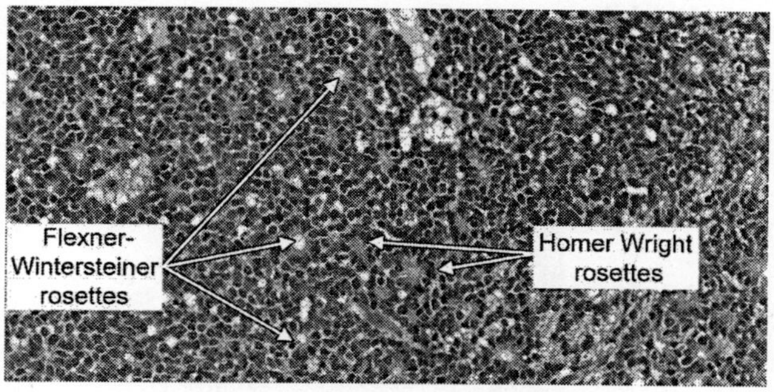

a. Craniopharyngioma
b. Optic nerve glioma
c. Malignant melanoma of choroid
d. Retinoblastoma

Ans. d. Retinoblastoma

85. Identify the condition on left side:

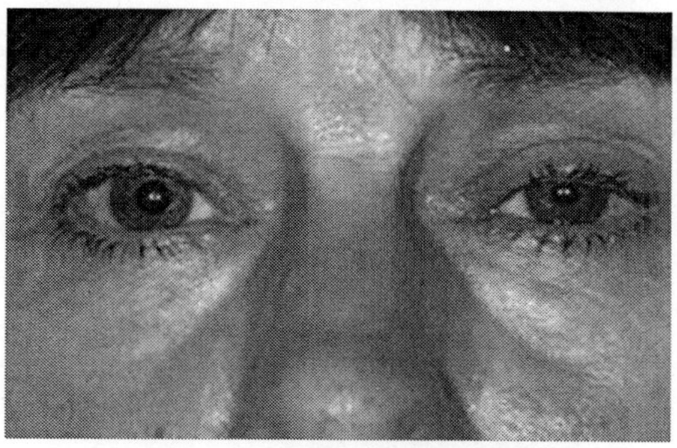

a. Entropion
b. Abducens nerve palsy
c. Horner's syndrome
d. Stye

Enophthalmos, miosis and ptosis is evident on left side.

Ans. c. Horner's syndrome

86. True statement regarding the condition shown in the image:

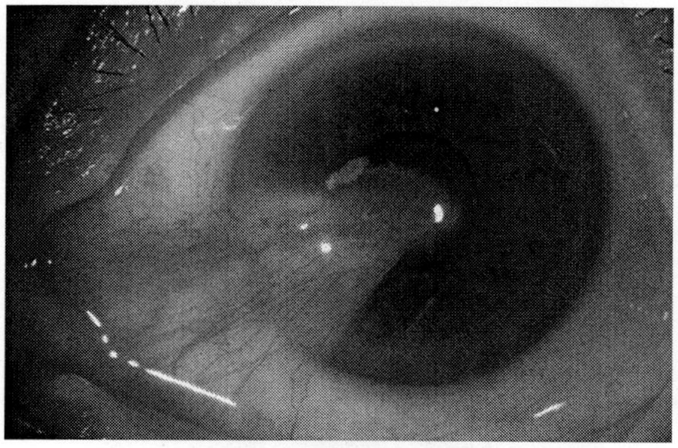

a. Degeneration of conjunctiva
b. Degeneration of cornea
c. Degeneration of lens
d. Degeneration of sclera

Image shows pterygium.

Ans. a. Degeneration of conjunctiva

87. As a result of copper deposition, a ring is formed in the cornea, as shown below. Most likely diagnosis:

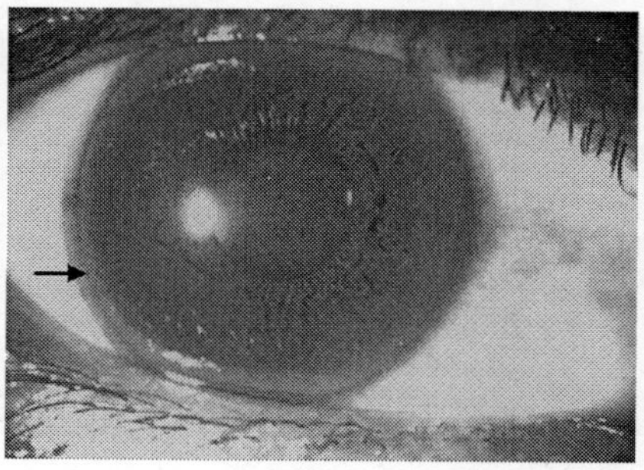

a. Trauma
b. Wilson disease
c. Retinoblastoma
d. Keratoconus

Image shows Kayser–Fleischer ring.

Ans. b. Wilson disease

88. A child presented with the complaints of fatigue and lethargy. He was found to be anemic and his liver and spleen were also enlarged. Peripheral smear shows the following presentation. Most likely diagnosis:

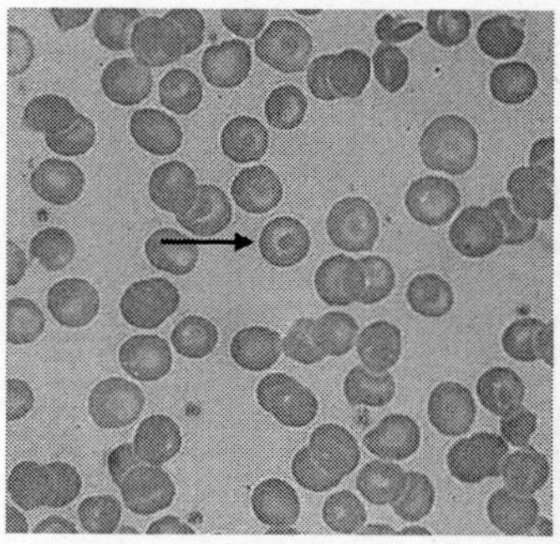

a. Sickle cell anemia
b. Iron deficiency anemia
c. Anemia of chronic diseases
d. Thalassemia

Arrow shows target cell.

Ans. d. Thalassemia

89. Such cells are derived from:

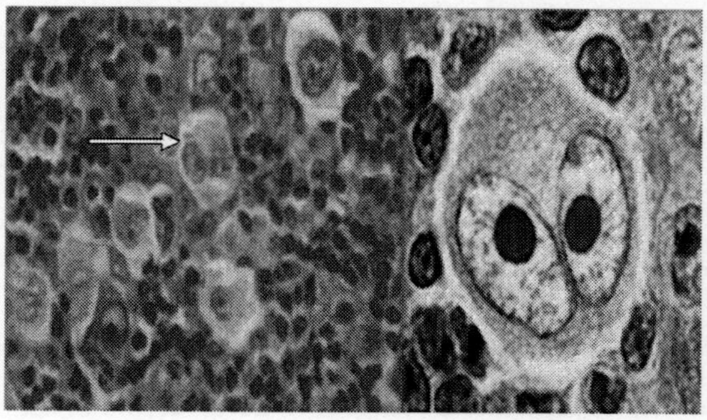

a. T cells
b. B cells
c. RBC
d. Platelets

White arrow shows Reed–Sternberg cell.

Ans. b. B cells

90. Peripheral blood smear is suggestive of:

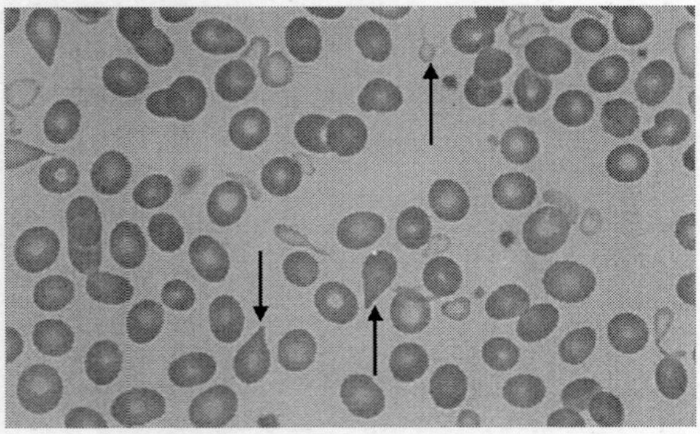

a. Thalassemia
b. Aplastic anemia
c. AML
d. Myelofibrosis

Black arrows show tear drop cell.

Ans. d. Myelofibrosis

91. A 55-years-old male presented with anemia and gum bleeding. There is marked leucocytosis. Peripheral smear is shown below. Most likely diagnosis:

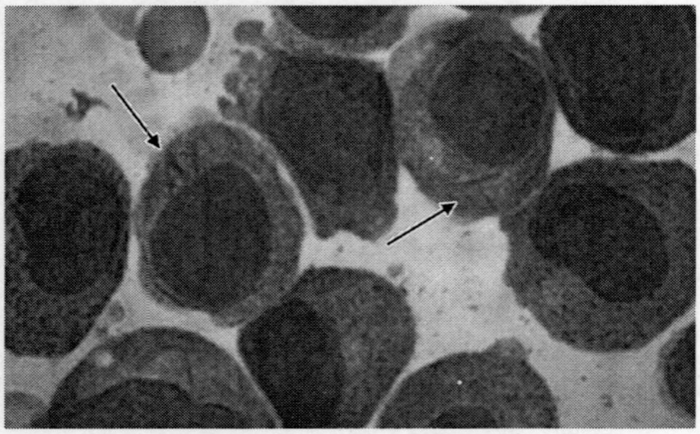

a. AML
b. CML
c. ALL
d. CLL

Black arrows show Auer rods.

Ans. a. AML

92. Such a condition is best managed by:

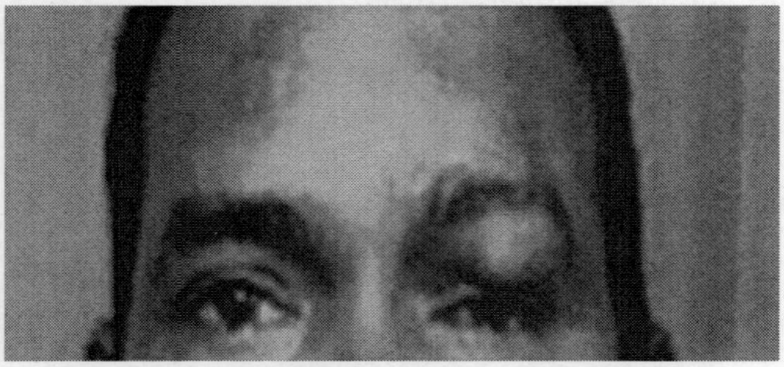

a. Wait and watch
b. Local steroid injection
c. Excision
d. Antibiotics

Image shows eyelid lipoma

Ans. c. Excision

93. Identify the condition which appears after birth. It increases in size when the child cries. A defect can be felt at umbilicus by the finger:

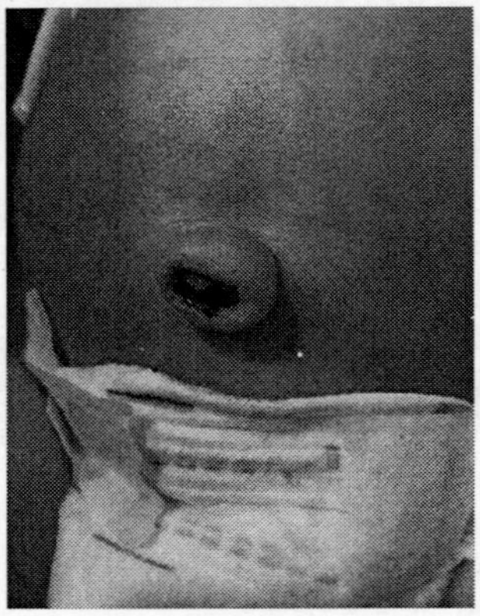

a. Gastroschisis
b. Omphalocele
c. Umbilical hernia
d. Raspberry tumour

Ans. c. Umbilical hernia

94. Management of such a condition:

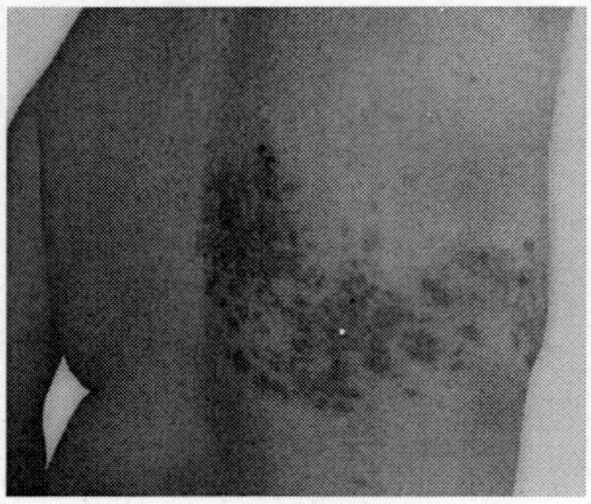

a. Penicillin
b. Atropine
c. Antihistaminics
d. Valacyclovir

Image shows herpes zoster.

Ans. d. Valacyclovir

95. Which bone is fractured?

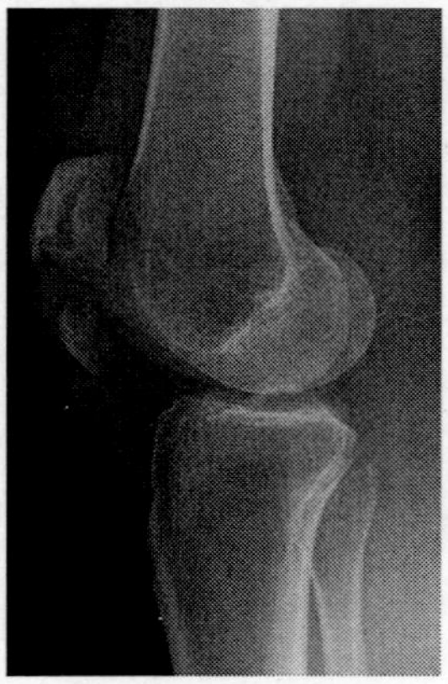

a. Femur
b. Patella
c. Tibia
d. Fibula

Ans. b. Patella

96. Identify the tumour arising from femur:

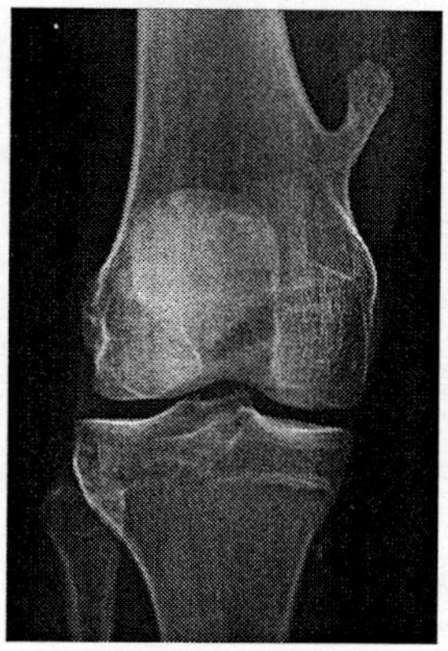

a. Ewing sarcoma
b. Osteosarcoma
c. Giant cell tumour
d. Osteochondroma

Ans. d. Osteochondroma

97. Identify the brace:

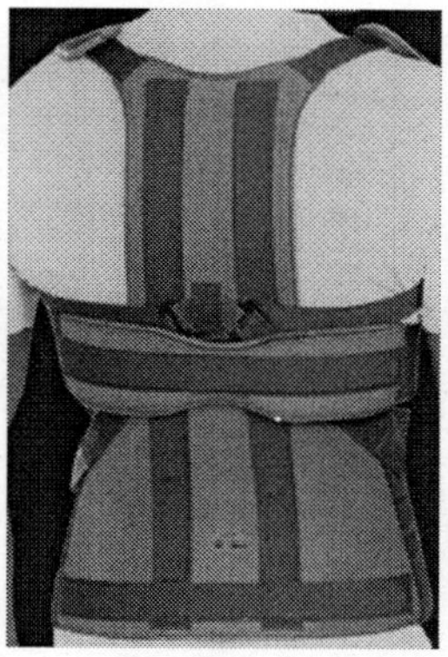

a. Boston brace
b. ASH brace
c. Taylor brace
d. Milwaukee brace

Ans. c. Taylor brace

98. Identify the injury:

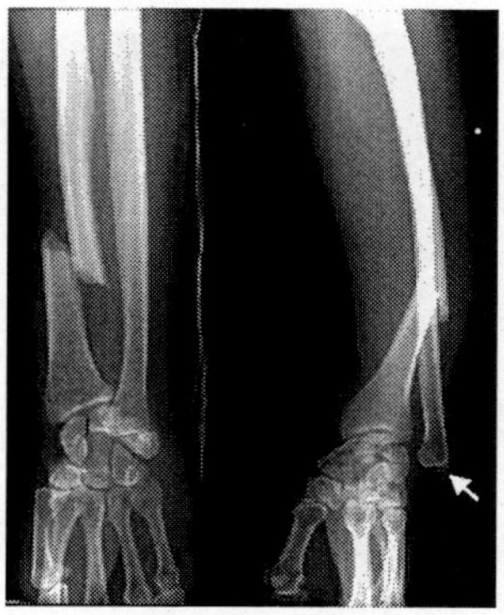

a. Monteggia fracture dislocation
b. Galeazzi fracture dislocation
c. Night stick fracture
d. Greenstick fracture

White arrow shows dislocated inferior radio-ulnar joint.

Ans. b. Galeazzi fracture dislocation

99. A patient road traffic accident presents to casualty with hypovolemia. Which of the cannula is preferred for doing rapid blood transfusion?

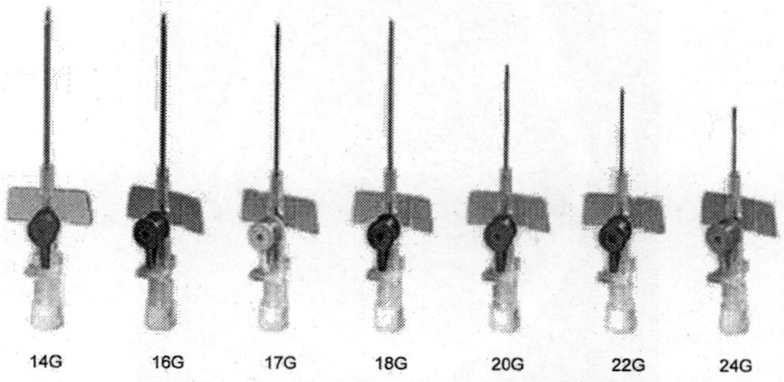

a. Yellow colored (24G)
b. Pink colored (20G)
c. Grey colored (16G)
d. Orange colored (14G)

14G is widest bore cannula. During resuscitation, we prefer a wide bore cannula so that IV fluid can be given fast.

Ans. d. Orange colored (14G)

100. Such a CT scan suggest:

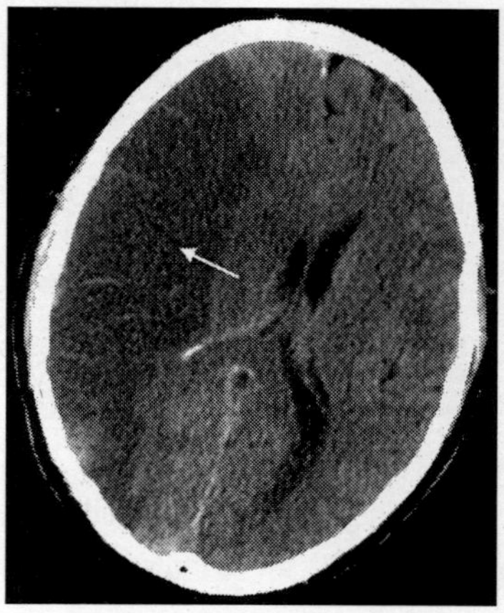

a. Infarction of anterior cerebral artery
b. Infarction of middle cerebral artery
c. Infarction of posterior cerebral artery
d. Infarction of vertebral artery

Ans. b. Infarction of middle cerebral artery

101. USG is suggestive of:

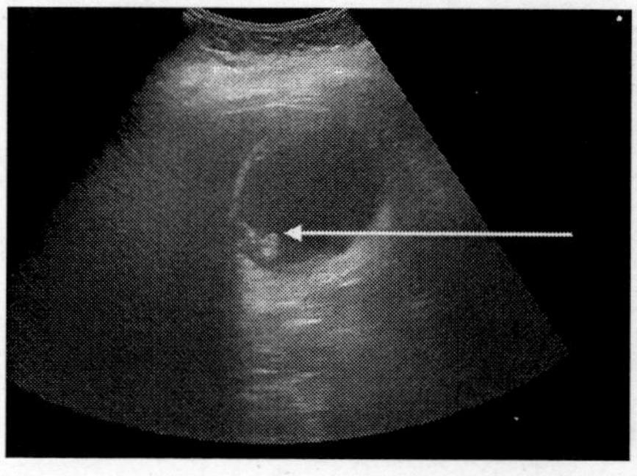

a. Gallstones
b. Renal stones
c. Hydatid cyst
d. Hepatocellular carcinoma

Ans. a. Gallstones

102. Label 50 represents:

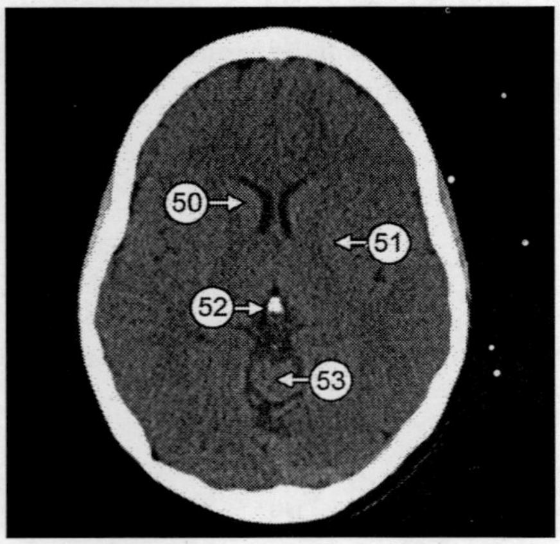

a. Caudate nucleus
b. Internal capsule
c. Globus pallidus
d. Substantia nigra

Ans. a. Caudate nucleus

103. Identify the condition:

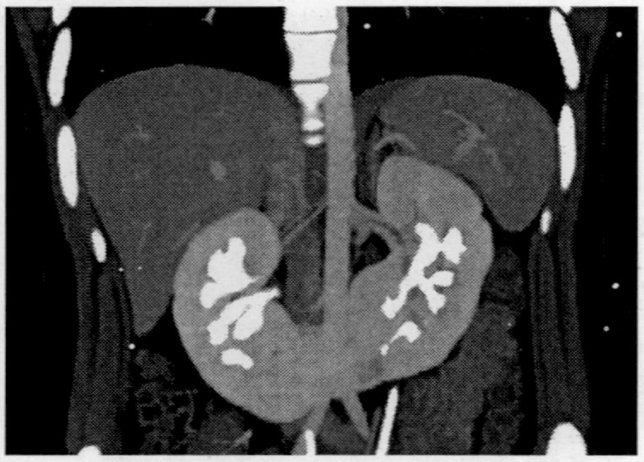

a. Renal agenesis
b. Horse shoe kidney
c. Polycystic kidney
d. Renal cell carcinoma

Ans. b. Horse shoe kidney

104. A cattle handler presented with cough. Chest X-ray was done. Most likely diagnosis:

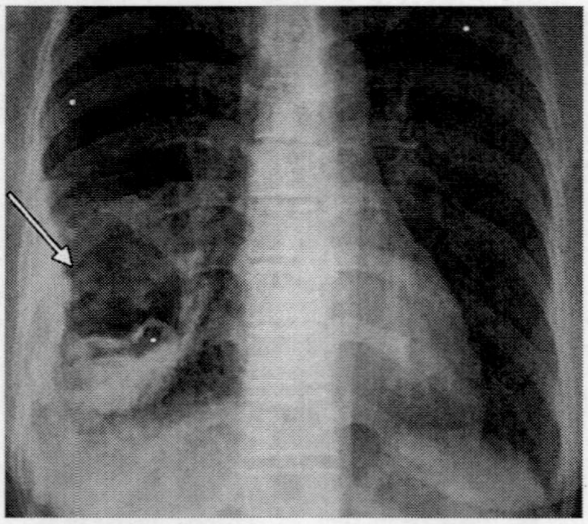

a. Tuberculosis lung
b. Hydatid cyst lung
c. Carcinoma lung
d. Silicosis

Ans. b. Hydatid cyst lung

105. X-ray pelvis of a male is shown below. Identify the condition:

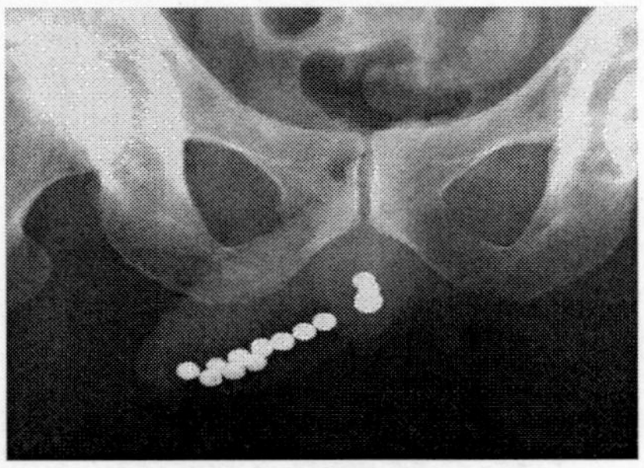

a. Implants for fracture pelvis
b. Foreign body in rectum
c. Foreign body in urethra
d. Artefacts

Ans. c. Foreign body in urethra

106. An old male presented with breathlessness and edema over both feet. Chest X-ray is shown below. Most likely condition:

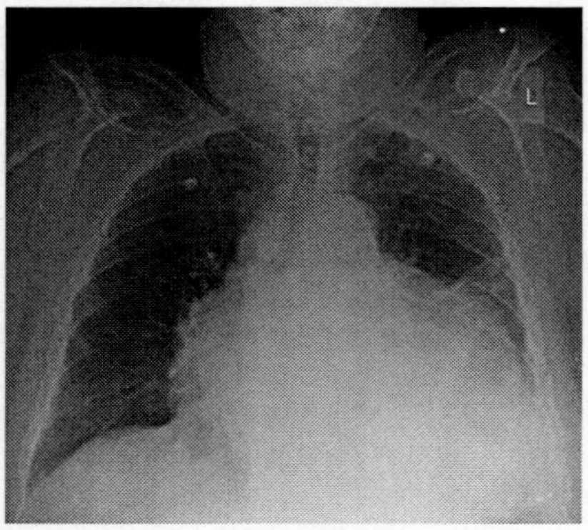

a. Pulmonary embolism
b. Pericardial effusion
c. Pneumothorax
d. Pleural effusion

Ans. b. Pericardial effusion

107. USG is suggestive of:

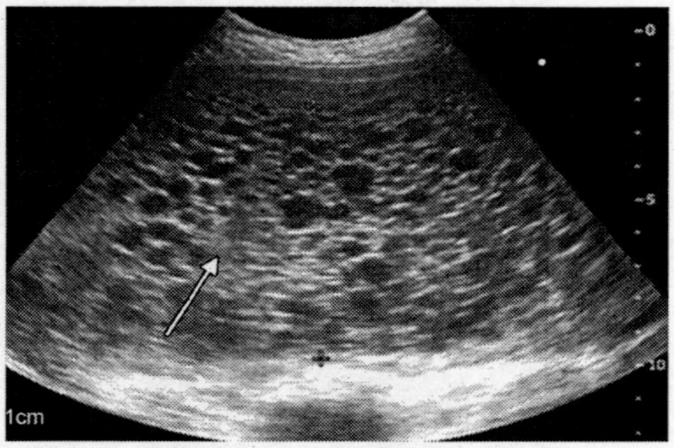

a. Hydatidiform mole
b. Retained placenta
c. Polycystic ovarian disease
d. Hydatid disease of uterus

USG shows snowstorm appearance.

Ans. a. Hydatidiform mole

108. CT scan is suggestive of:

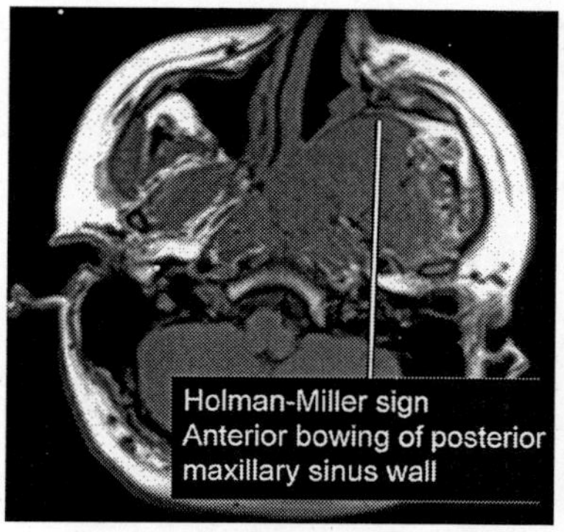

a. Nasopharyngeal angiofibroma
b. Nasopharyngeal carcinoma
c. Nasal polyp
d. Antro-choanal polyp

Ans. a. Nasopharyngeal angiofibroma

109. MRI of a known case of TB presenting with complaint of swelling in right loin region:

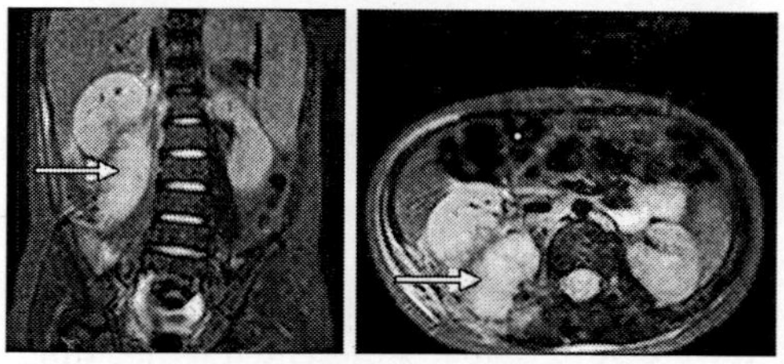

a. Renal tuberculosis
b. Psoas abscess
c. Sacro-iliac joint tuberculosis
d. TB of the right hip joint

Abscess can be seen in the region of psoas major muscle, right side.

Ans. b. Psoas abscess

110. USG abdomen in a hypertensive, obese women is suggestive of:

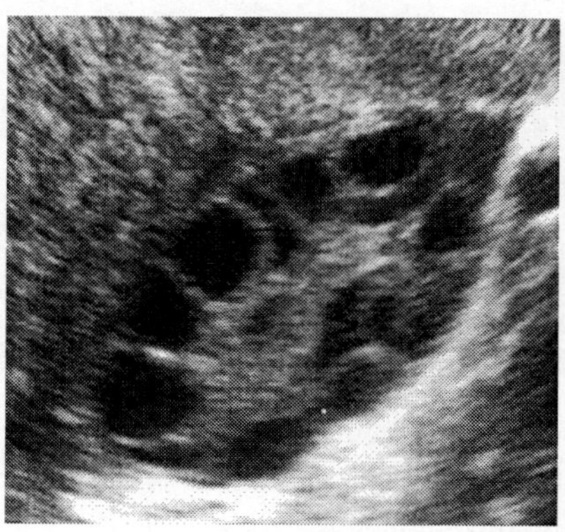

a. Hydatid cyst liver b. Polycystic ovarian syndrome
c. Adenomyosis d. Endometriosis

USG shows necklace appearance.

Ans. b. Polycystic ovarian syndrome

111. X-ray of a child suggest:

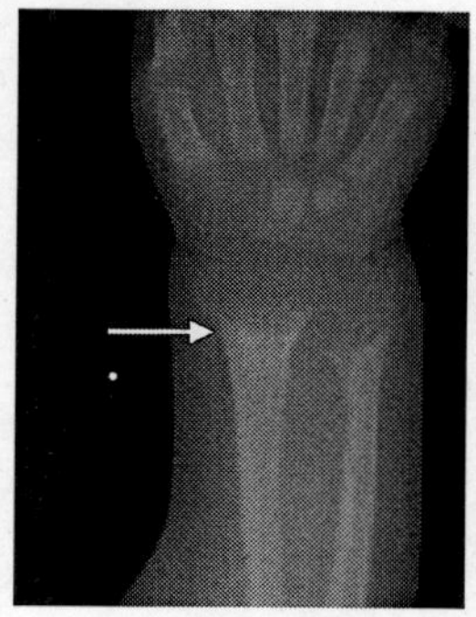

a. Scurvy b. Rickets
c. Hypothyroidism d. Osteogenesis imperfecta

White arrow shows cupping and splaying of metaphysis of radius.

Ans. b. Rickets

112. Chest X-ray of a newborn presenting with respiratory distress is suggestive of:

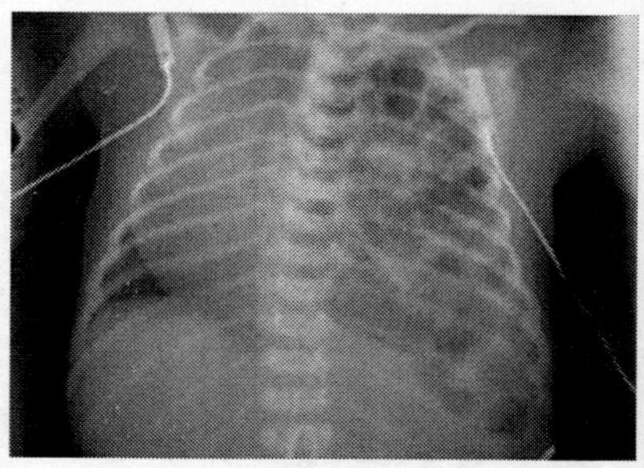

a. Hydatid cysts lung
b. Congenital diaphragmatic hernia
c. Bronchogenic cysts
d. Pleural effusion

Loops of the intestine can be seen on left side.

Ans. b. Congenital diaphragmatic hernia

113. Barium study of a 4 weeks newborn presenting with lump in the abdomen and non-bilious vomiting, is suggestive of:

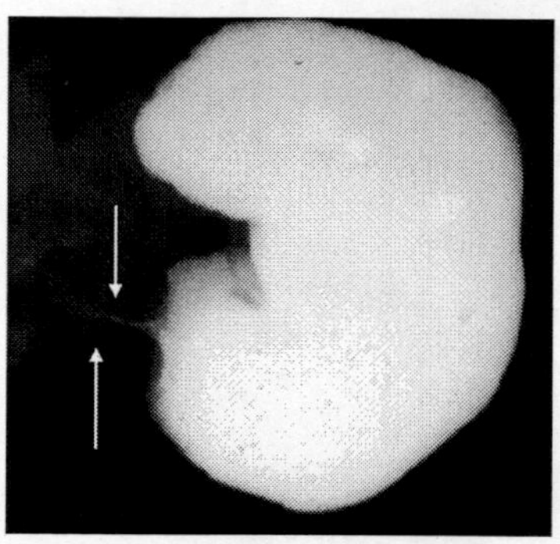

a. Achalasia cardia
b. Infantile hypertrophic pyloric stenosis
c. Perforation d. Duodenal atresia

White arrow shows narrowed pyloric canal.

Ans. b. Infantile hypertrophic pyloric stenosis

114. Such an abdominal X-ray is suggestive of:

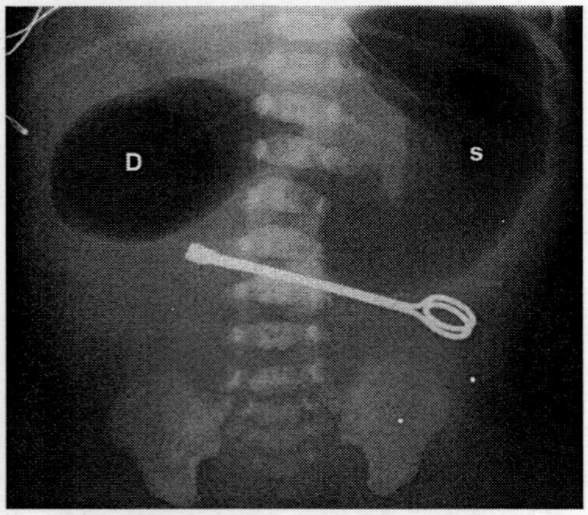

a. Infantile hypertrophic pyloric stenosis
b. Duodenal atresia
c. Jejunal atresia
d. Ileal atresia

'S' is air in stomach and 'D' is air in proximal duodenum (double bubble sign).

Ans. b. Duodenal atresia

115. Which condition is discussed?

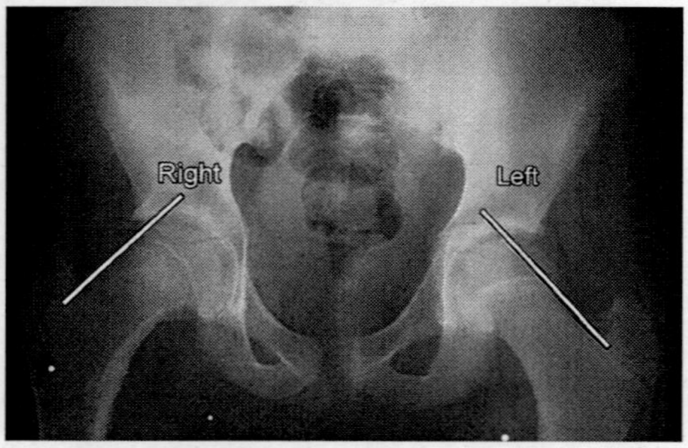

a. Perthe's disease
b. Slipped capital femoral epiphyses
c. Developmental dysplasia of the hip
d. Avascular necrosis of the femoral head

Right hip is affected (Trethowan's sign).

Ans. b. Slipped capital femoral epiphyses

116. X-ray pelvis is suggestive of:

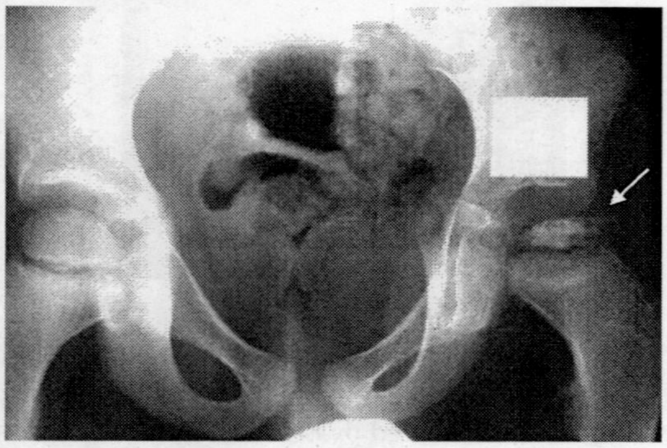

a. Perthe's disease
b. Slipped capital femoral epiphyses
c. Developmental dysplasia of the hip
d. Avascular necrosis of the femoral head

White arrow shows deformed femoral head epiphysis.

Ans. a. Perthe's disease

117. Identify the plasmodia:

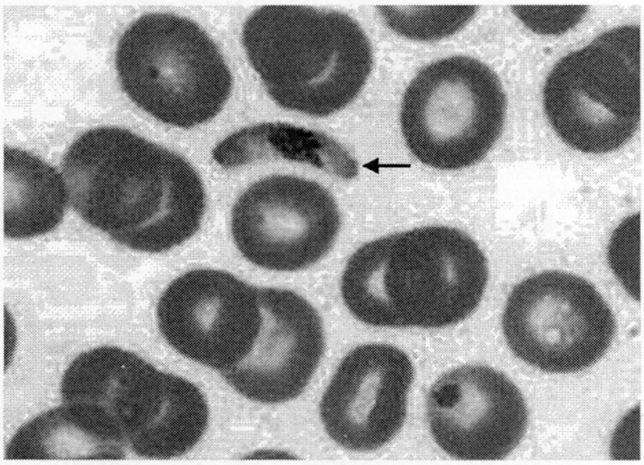

a. Plasmodium vivax
b. Plasmodium falciparum
c. Plasmodium malariae
d. Plasmodium ovale

Image shows banana shaped gametocyte.

Ans. b. Plasmodium falciparum

118. A known case of diabetes presented with painless visual loss. Fundus examination was done and the clinical image is shown below. Most likely diagnosis:

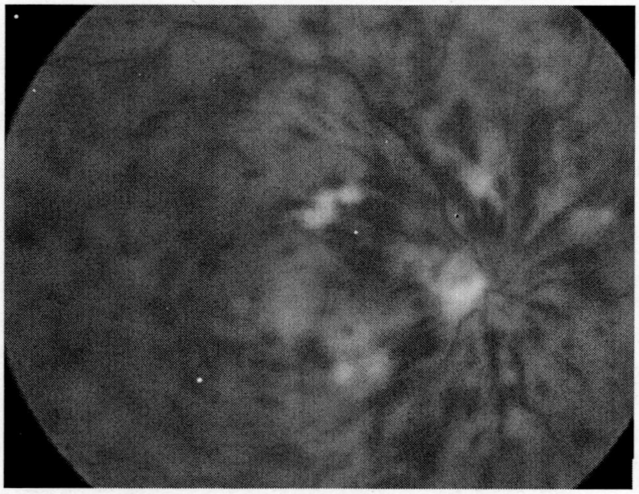

a. Central retinal vein occlusion
b. Central retinal artery occlusion
c. Proliferative diabetic retinopathy
d. Non-proliferative diabetic retinopathy

Image shows blood and thunder fundus.

Ans. a. Central retinal vein occlusion

119. Identify the bone fractured in the image given below:

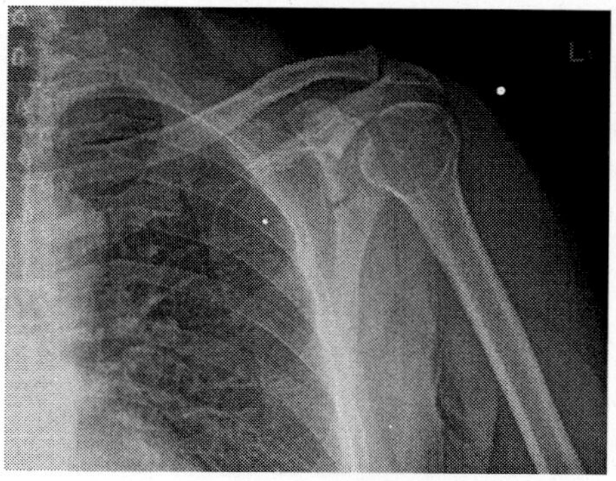

a. Clavicle
b. Humerus
c. Scapula
d. 4th rib

Ans. c. Scapula

120. A 12-years-old girl from Nigeria presented to the Pediatrics OPD with the complaints of night sweat, fever and loss of weight since last few months. There was an intra-abdominal mass and peripheral lymphadenopathy as well. Doctor advised for biopsy of the lymph node. The image is shown below. Most probable diagnosis and associated translocation:

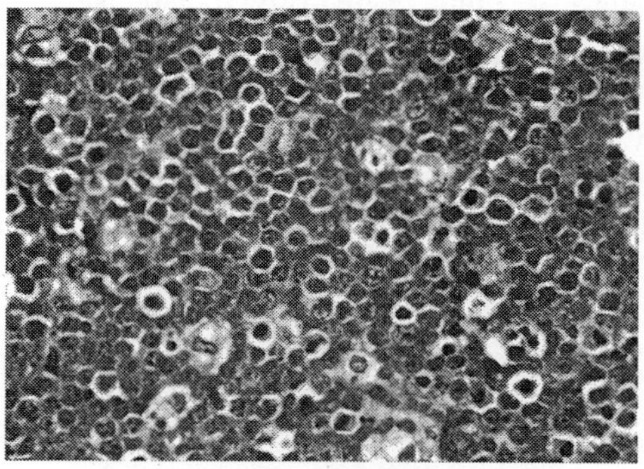

a. Burkitt's lymphoma; t(9, 22)
b. Burkitt's lymphoma; t(8, 14)
c. CML (t8, 14)
d. CML (t9, 22)

Image shows starry sky appearance.

Ans. b. Burkitt's lymphoma; t(8, 14)

121. Identify the condition shown below, which is diagnosed laparoscopically:

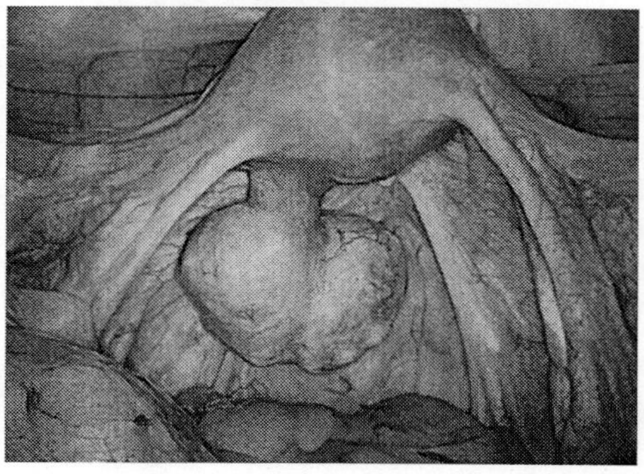

a. Uterine fibroid
b. Carcinoma fallopian tube
c. Carcinoma ovary
d. Multiple pregnancy

Ans. a. Uterine fibroid

122. A post-covid diabetic patient, with uncontrolled blood sugar, presented to the casualty with the complaint of breathlessness. The clinical finding of nasal and oral examination is shown below. Most likely diagnosis:

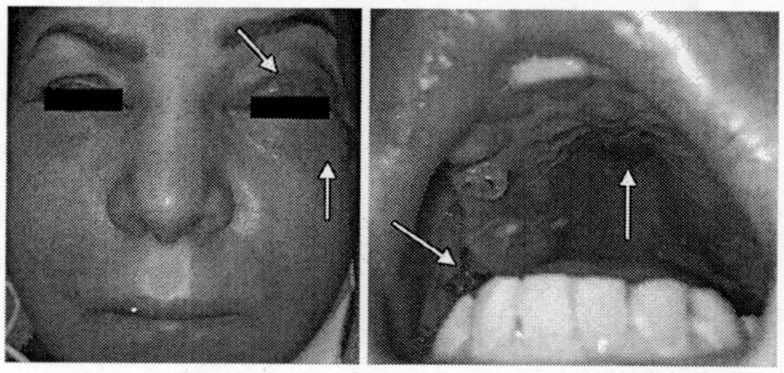

a. Mucormycosis
b. Kaposi sarcoma
c. Oral thrush
d. Diphtheria

Ans. a. Mucormycosis

123. Study the image shown below. Such a presentation occurs because of:

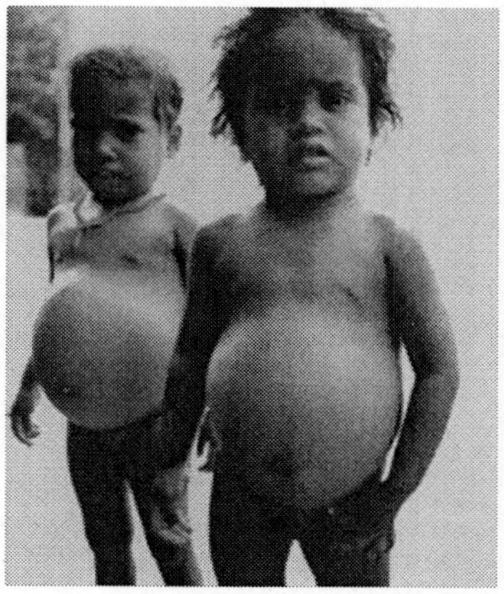

a. Less energy intake
b. Less protein intake
c. Excess energy intake
d. Excess protein intake

Image shows children with Kwashiorkor.

Ans. b. Less protein intake

124. Identify the clinical condition:

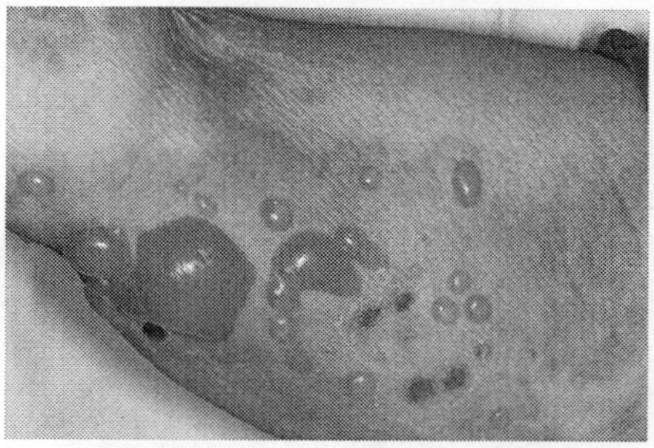

a. Bullous pemphigoid
b. Pemphigus vulgaris
c. Scalds
d. Lupus vulgaris

Ans. a. Bullous pemphigoid

125. Identify the clinical condition:

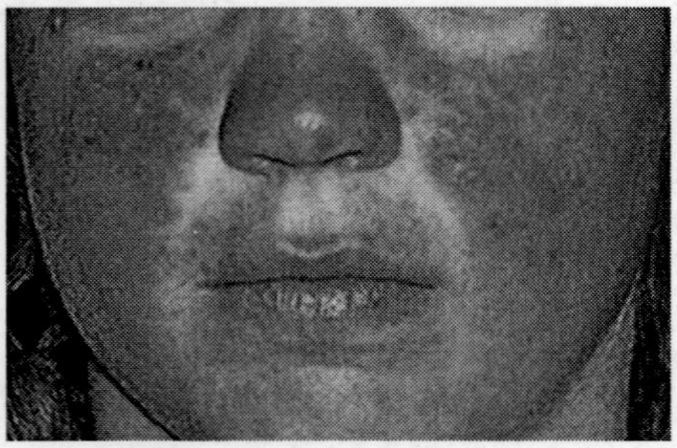

a. Erythema infectiosum
b. Photodermatitis
c. Bee sting
d. SLE

Image shows typical butterfly rash.

Ans. d. SLE

126. Study the graph and identify the correct statement:

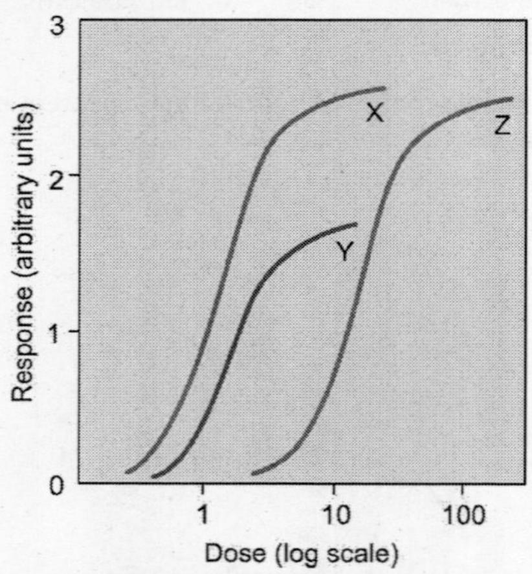

a. Drug X is more potent and efficacious than drug Y
b. Drug X is more potent but less efficacious than drug Z
c. Drug Y is more potent and more efficacious than drug Z
d. Drug Z is more potent and more efficacious than drug Y

Ans. a. Drug X is more potent and efficacious than drug Y

127. A patient is having diabetes mellitus for more than 20 years. Fundus examination was done and the clinical image is shown below. Fundus image is suggestive of:

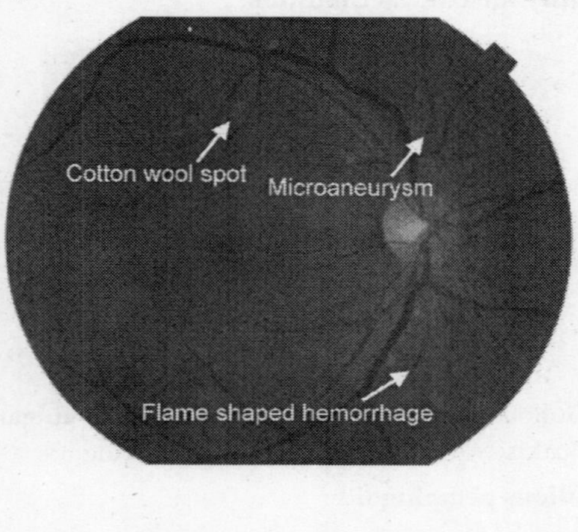

a. CRAO
b. CRVO
c. Proliferative diabetic retinopathy
d. Non-proliferative diabetic retinopathy

Ans. d. Non-proliferative diabetic retinopathy

128. Clinical image of a patient is shown below. Which enzyme deficiency would be noted in such a patient?

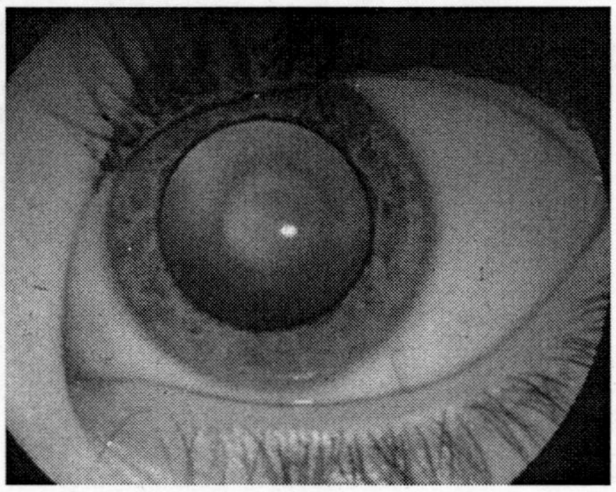

a. Phosphofructokinase
b. Hexokinase
c. Galactose-1-phosphate uridyl transferase
d. HMG CoA reductase

Image shows oil-drop cataract of Galactosemia.

Ans. c. Galactose-1-phosphate uridyl transferase

129. A 35-years-old male presented to the Medicine OPD with the complaints of itching, jaundice, mood disorder and tremors. He was referred for ophthalmological examination. Slit lamp examination of his eyes is shown below. Most likely diagnosis:

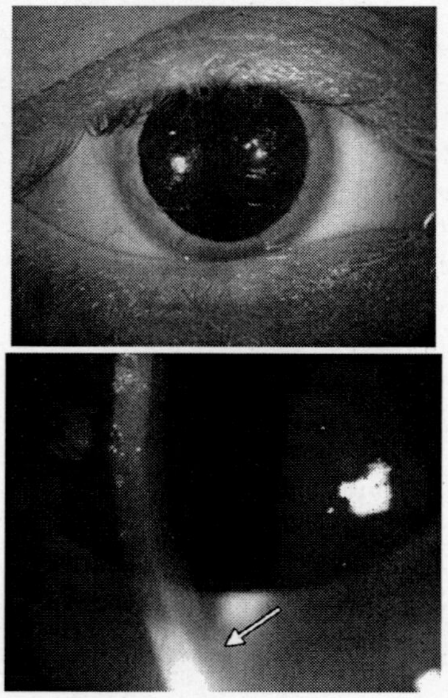

a. Primary hemochromatosis
b. Parkinson disease
c. Obstructive jaundice
d. Wilson disease

Image shows Kayser-Fleischer ring.

Ans. d. Wilson disease

130. Identify the condition:

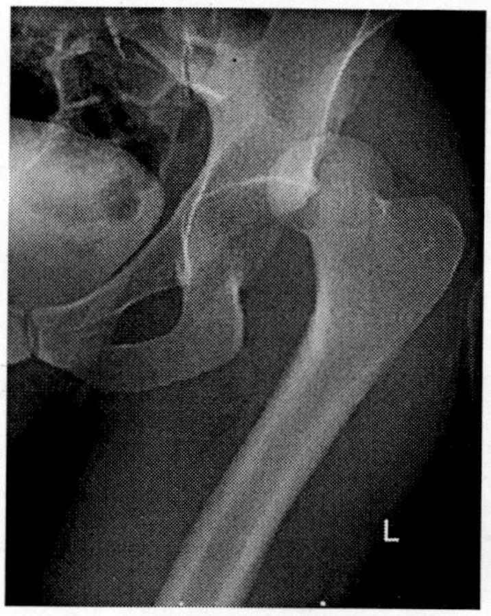

a. Anterior dislocation of the hip joint
b. Posterior dislocation of the hip joint
c. Fracture neck of femur
d. Fracture acetabulum

Ans. b. Posterior dislocation of the hip joint

131. A known case of osteoarthritis knee was on NSAIDs since last 6 months. Now she presented to the casualty with complains of severe agonising pain in right hypochondrium. There is also history of coffee ground vomiting. Per abdomen examination revealed guarding and rigidity of the abdominal wall. On percussion, liver dullness is obliterated. Chest X-ray was done, which is shown below. Most likely diagnosis:

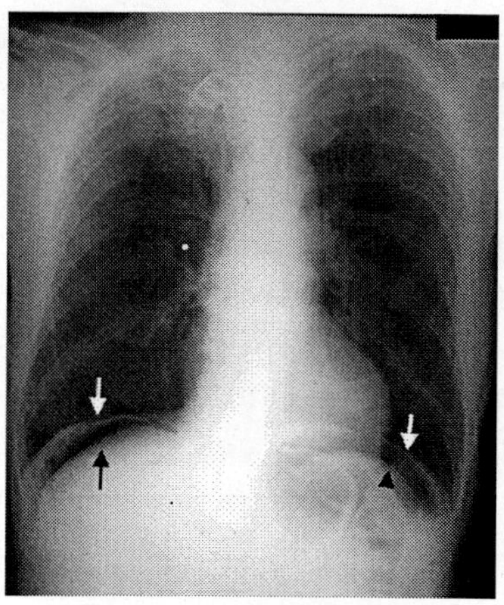

a. Liver abscess
b. Gut perforation
c. Pyloric stenosis
d. Intestinal obstruction

Ans. b. Gut perforation

132. A 65-years-old male, who is a known case of heart disease, now developed dyspnoea of exertion. Clinical photographs of the patient are shown below. Edema of such a patient is best treated with a diuretic, which acts by:

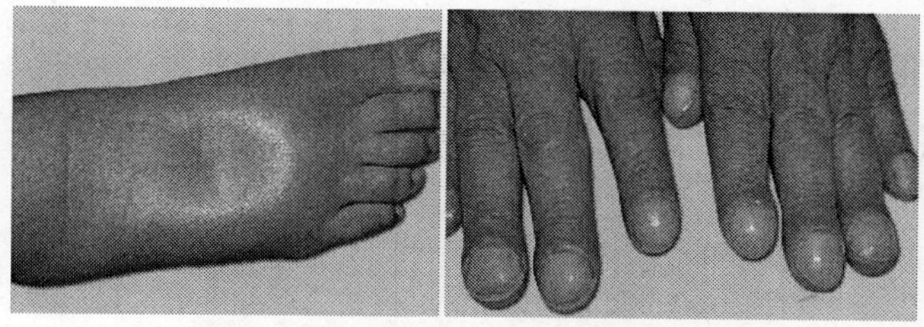

a. Inhibition of Na-K-2Cl symporter in loop of Henle
b. Inhibition of angiotensin converting enzyme
c. Antagonizing aldosterone in distal convoluted tubule
d. Inhibition of Na-Cl symporter in distal convoluted tubule

First image shows pitting edema and second image shows clubbing.

Ans. a. Inhibition of Na-K-2Cl symporter in loop of Henle

133. Identify the statistical diagram shown below:

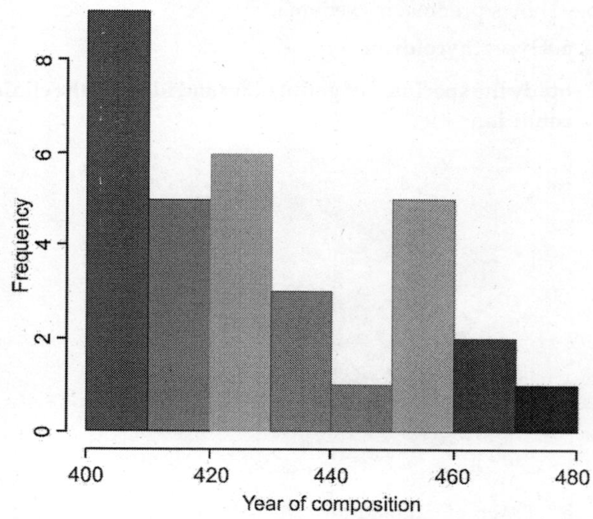

a. Histogram
b. Bar diagram
c. Scatter diagram
d. Pie chart

Ans. a. Histogram

134. Identify the logo:

मानकः पथप्रदर्शकः

a. Bureau of Indian Standards (BIS)
b. ISI standards
c. AgMark
d. FPO mark

Ans. a. Bureau of Indian Standards (BIS)

135. A young lean female presented with complains of palpitations and weight loss. On examination, sinus tachycardia was present and following finding was noticed on her legs. Clinical picture is suggestive of:

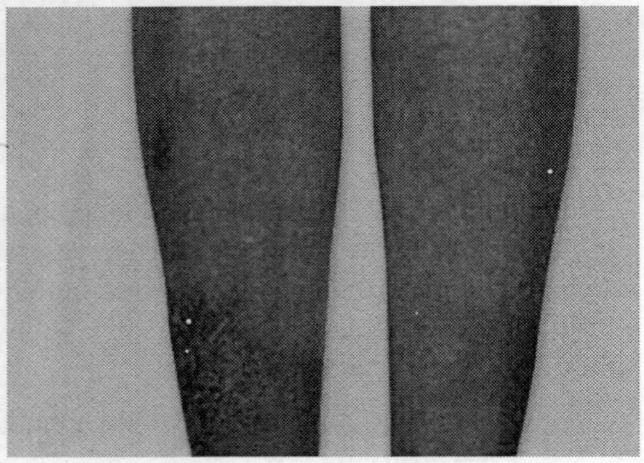

a. Hyperthyroidism
b. Hypothyroidism
c. Filariasis
d. Cushing's syndrome

Image shows pretibial myxedema.

Ans. a. Hyperthyroidism

136. Study the specimen of gallbladder and identify the clinical condition:

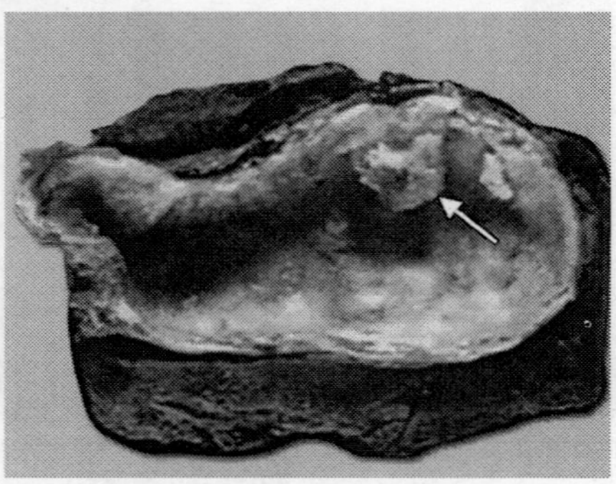

a. Polyp of gallbladder
b. Cholesterol stone in gallbladder
c. Strawberry gallbladder
d. Gallbladder carcinoma

Ans. d. Gallbladder carcinoma

137. Given flow-volume loop suggest:

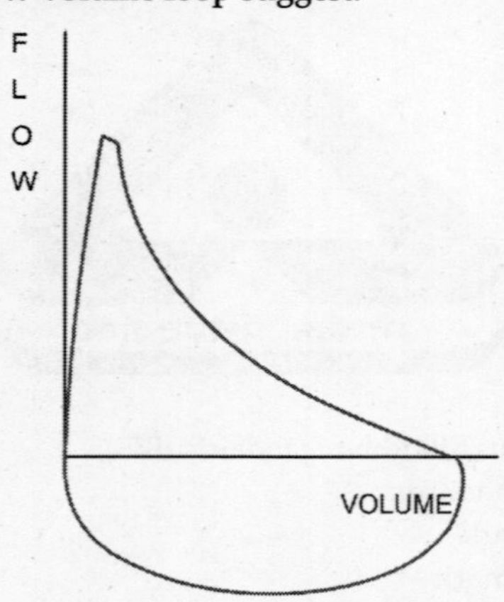

a. Normal study
b. Chronic obstructive pulmonary disease
c. Restrictive lung disease
d. Interstitial lung disease

Ans. b. Chronic obstructive pulmonary disease

138. A 50-years-old male presented to the Surgery OPD with the complaints of abdominal pain. On per abdomen examination, liver was found to be enlarged. USG abdomen was ordered which shows the findings shown in the figure. Most likely diagnosis:

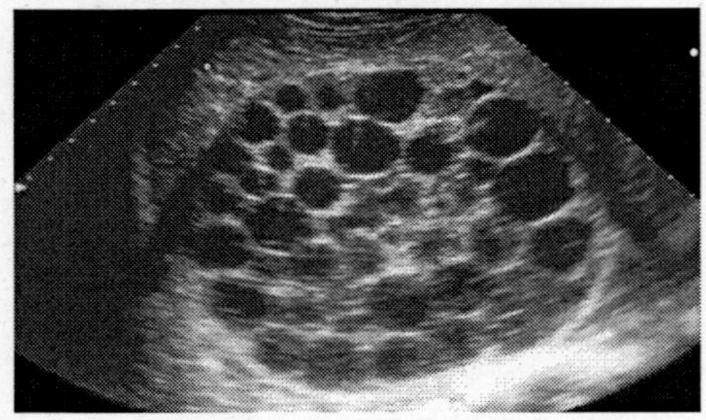

a. Simple liver cyst
b. Amoebic liver abscess
c. Pyogenic liver abscess
d. Hepatic hydatid cyst

Ans. d. Hepatic hydatid cyst

139. Histopathology of thyroid swelling was done, which is shown below. Findings are consistent with the diagnosis of:

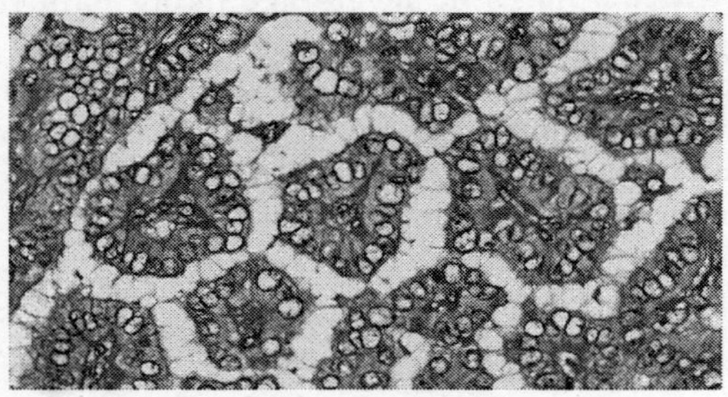

a. Medullary carcinoma of thyroid
b. Follicular carcinoma of thyroid
c. Papillary carcinoma of thyroid
d. Anaplastic carcinoma of thyroid

Image shows Orphan Annie eye nuclei.

Ans. c. Papillary carcinoma of thyroid

140. Study the chest X-ray given below and identify the finding:

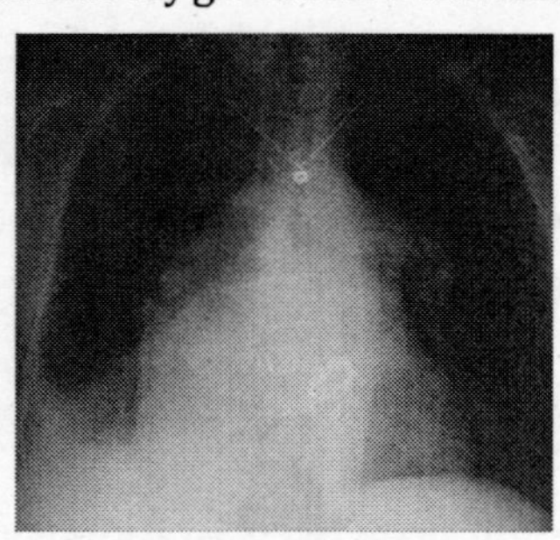

a. Prosthetic mitral valve
b. Prosthetic aortic valve
c. Native mitral valve
d. Native aortic valve

Ans. a. Prosthetic mitral valve

141. Identify the prosthesis:

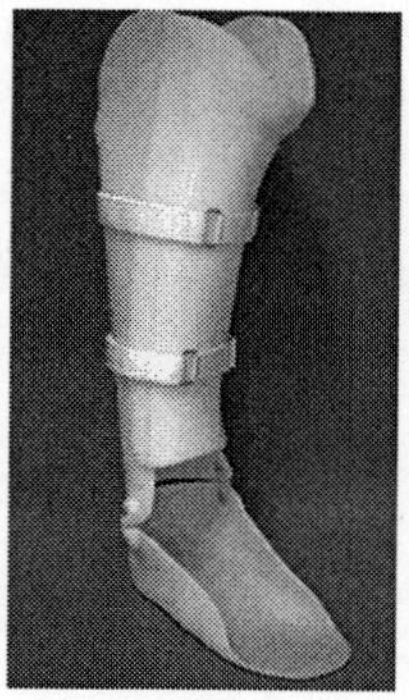

a. Patellar tendon bearing brace
b. SOMI brace
c. SACH foot
d. Jaipur foot

Ans. a. Patellar tendon bearing brace

142. A 65-years-old post-menopausal woman had a history of fall in bathroom over outstretched hand. X-ray wrist was done. Most likely diagnosis:

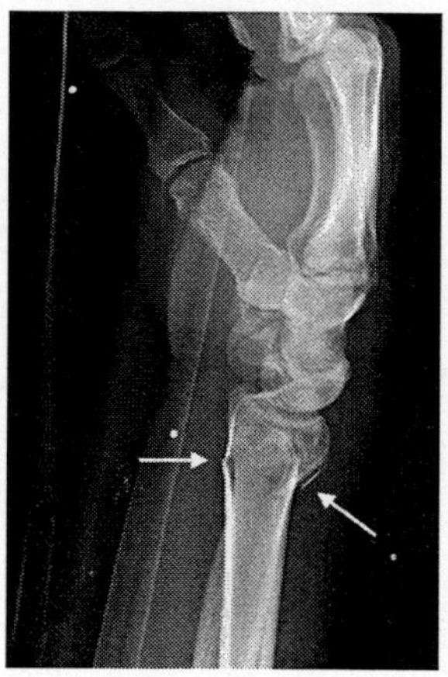

a. Colle's fracture
b. Smith's fracture
c. Dorsal Barton fracture
d. Volar Barton fracture

Arrows show fracture line and dorsal angulation of distal fragment.

Ans. a. Colle's fracture

143. Study the CT scan image given below and suggest the diagnosis:

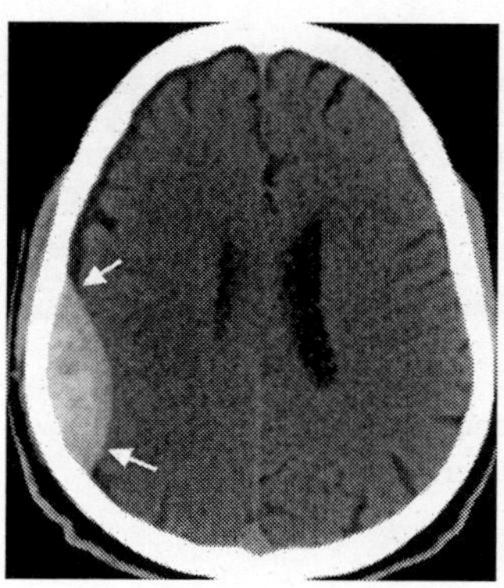

a. Subdural hemorrhage
b. Epidural hemorrhage
c. Intracerebral hemorrhage
d. Subarachnoid hemorrhage

Arrows show a biconvex lesion.

Ans. b. Epidural hemorrhage

144. Identify the condition present on the scalp in the given figure:

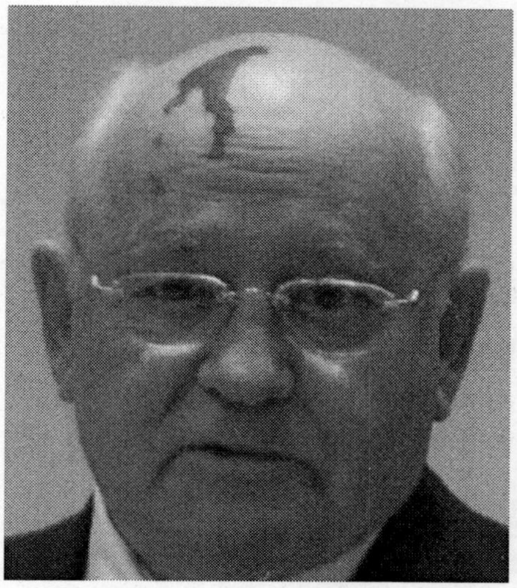

a. Strawberry nevus
b. Portwine stain
c. Allergic reaction
d. Acanthosis nigricans

Image is of Mikhail Gorbachev.

Ans. b. Portwine stain

145. Study the X-ray and identify the condition:

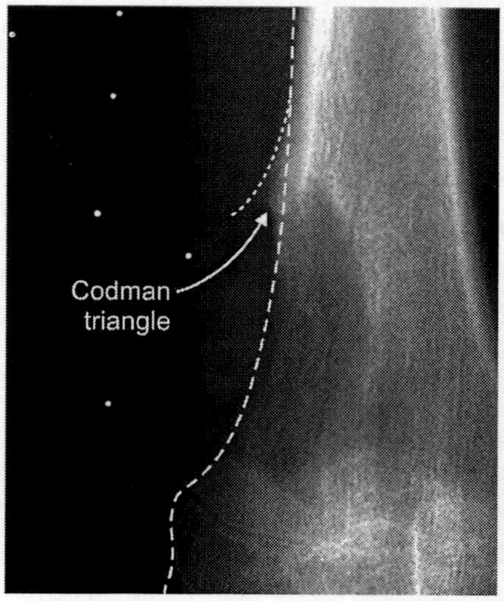

a. Ewing sarcoma
b. Giant cell tumour
c. Osteosarcoma
d. Multiple myeloma

Ans. c. Osteosarcoma

146. Identify the abnormal condition shown in the figure with arrows:

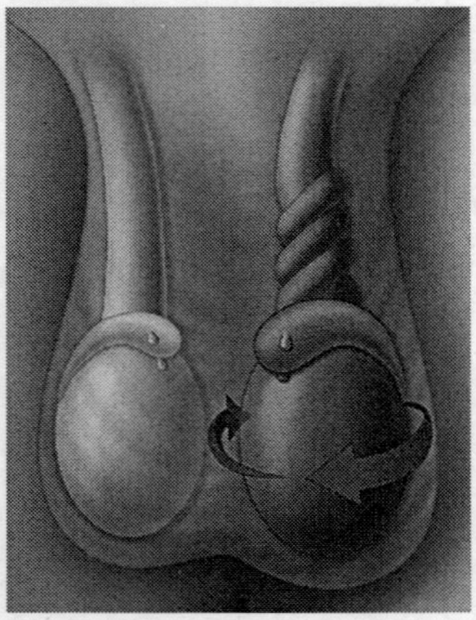

a. Hydrocele
b. Testicular cancer
c. Testicular torsion
d. Varicocele

Ans. c. Testicular torsion

147. Such a pupil is commonly seen in:

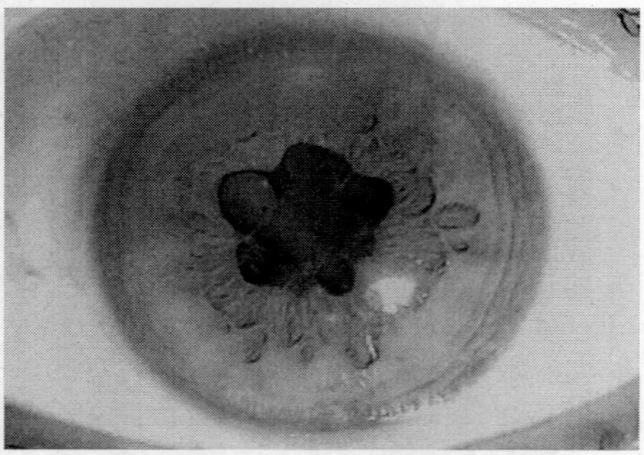

a. Glaucoma
b. Cataract
c. Anterior uveitis
d. Keratomalacia

Image shows festooned pupil.

Ans. c. Anterior uveitis

148. Identify the parasite:

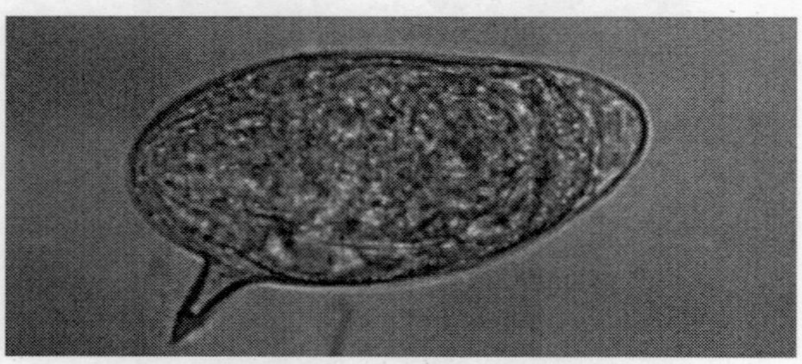

a. Clonorchis sinensis
b. Fasciola hepatica
c. Echinococcus granulosus
d. Schistosoma mansoni

Ans. d. Schistosoma mansoni

149. A child developed high-grade fever and sore throat. Oral cavity examination was done. Which of the following media is used to make a final diagnosis?

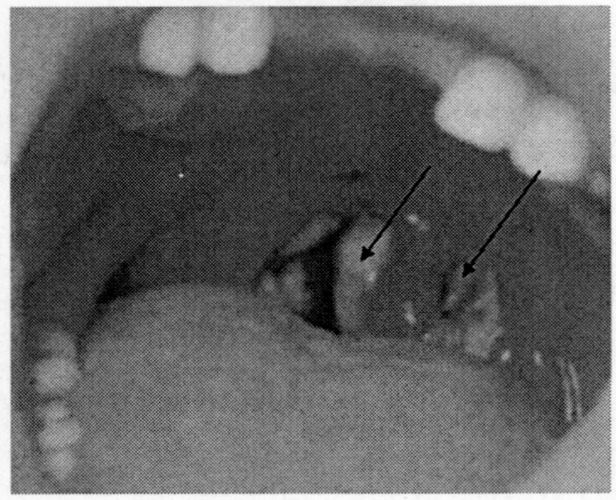

a. LJ media
b. Thayer Martin media
c. Loeffler's serum slope
d. Bordet Gengou media

Ans. c. Loeffler's serum slope

150. Identify the following parasite:

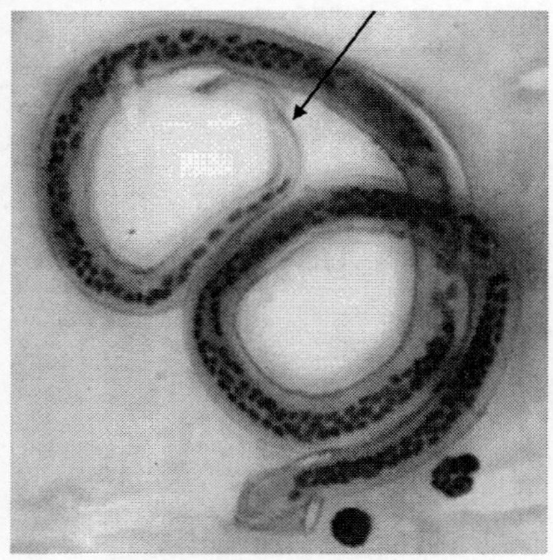

a. Tinea saginata
b. Ancylostoma duodenale
c. Ascaris lumbricoides
d. Wuchereria bancrofti

Ans. d. Wuchereria bancrofti

151. Oral examination of a patient with HIV shows the following condition, which bleeds on scrapping. Causative organism for this condition:

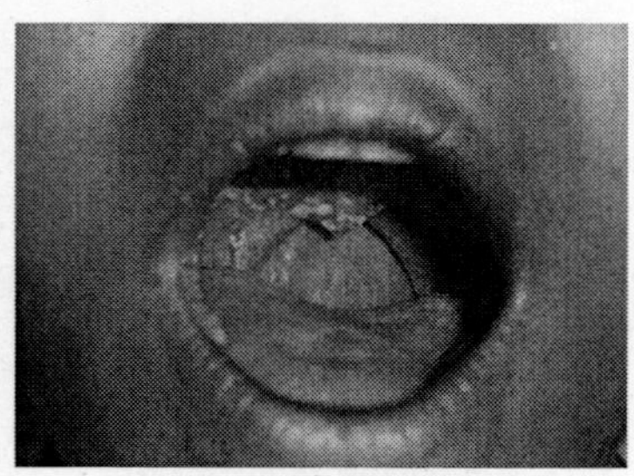

a. Candida
b. Cryptococcus
c. Corynebacterium diphtheriae
d. Mycobacterium tuberculosis

Ans. a. Candida

152. Identify the virus:

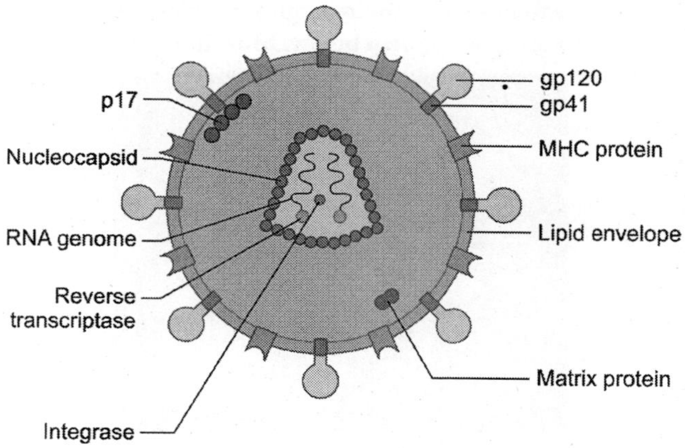

a. HIV
b. Influenza virus
c. Hepatitis B virus
d. Rabies virus

Ans. a. HIV

153. Injury of which bony landmark is shown by arrows?

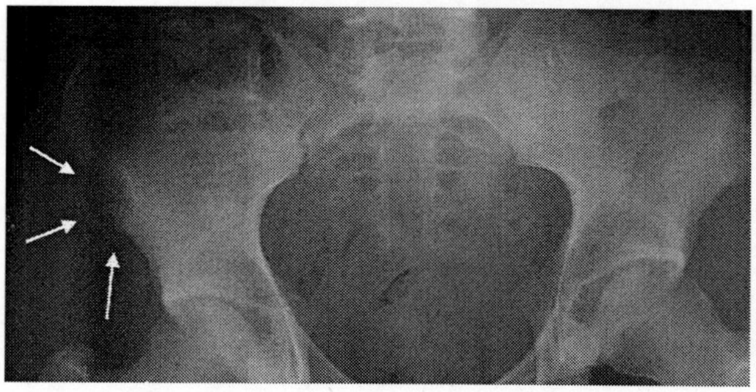

a. Iliac crest
b. Anterior superior iliac spine
c. Obturator foramen
d. Pubis symphysis

Ans. b. Anterior superior iliac spine

154. Nerve supply of the muscle shown in figure is:

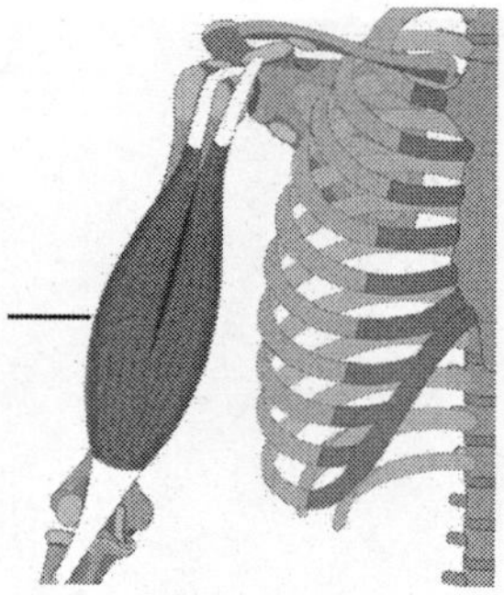

a. Musculocutaneous nerve
b. Radial nerve
c. Median nerve
d. Ulnar nerve

Muscle shown is biceps brachii.

Ans. c. Median nerve

155. Identify the area marked with a circle:

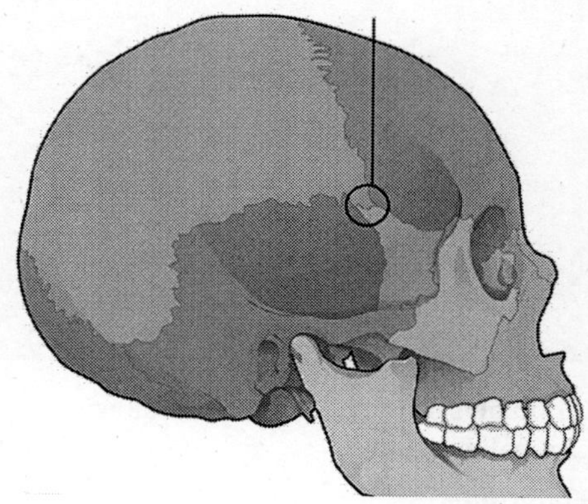

a. Nasion
b. Pterion
c. Glabella
d. Asterion

Ans. b. Pterion

156. Identify the structure marked in red:

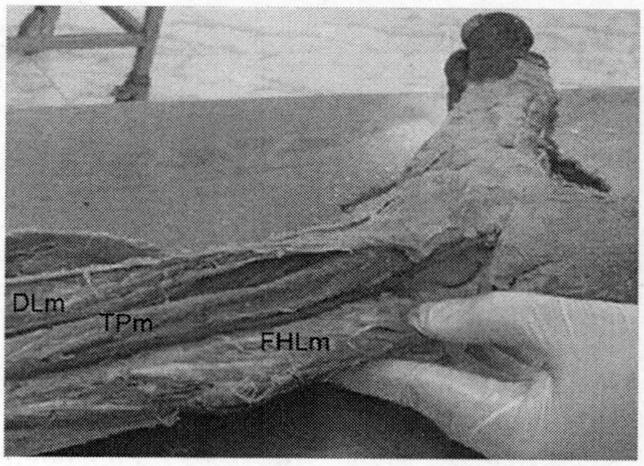

a. Flexor hallucis longus muscle
b. Posterior tibial artery
c. Extensor digitorum longus muscle
d. Tibialis posterior muscle

Ans. b. Posterior tibial artery

157. Identify the image:

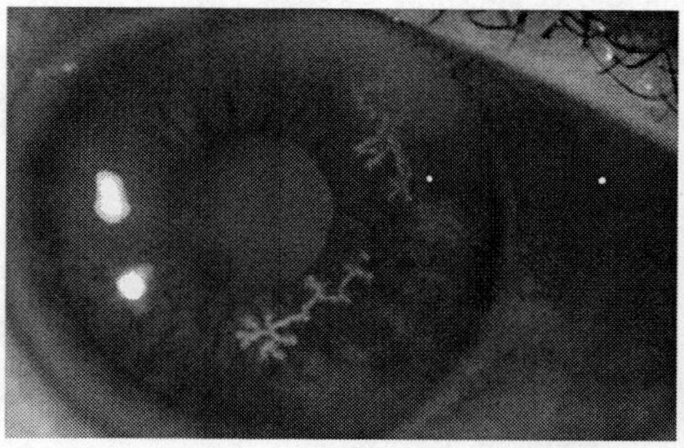

a. Vernal keratoconjunctivitis
b. Mycotic keratitis
c. Herpes simplex keratitis
d. Bacterial keratitis

Image shows dendritic ulcer.

Ans. c. Herpes simplex keratitis

158. Identify the condition shown below:

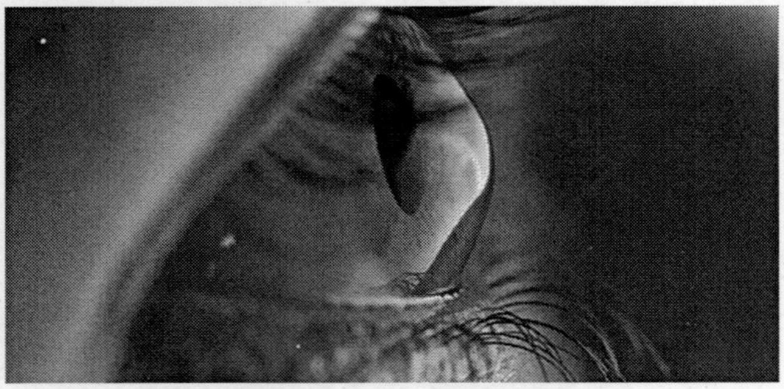

a. Iridodialysis
b. Keratoconus
c. Corneal dystrophy
d. Herpetic keratitis

Ans. b. Keratoconus

159. A known case of HIV-AIDS developed severe diarrhoea. Rectal swab showed the organism as shown in the image. Identify the organism:

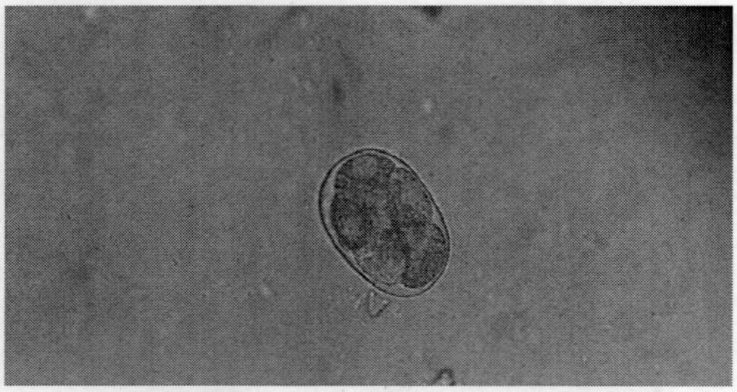

a. Cryptosporidium
b. Cryptococcus neoformans
c. Campylobacter jejuni
d. Clostridium botulinum

Ans. a. Cryptosporidium

160. A 32-years-old male presented to the Ortho OPD with the complaint swelling around left knee joint. X-ray of the right knee was done which showed a lytic lesion eroding the cortex of tibia. Doctor also ordered for histopathological examination, the image of which is shown below. Findings are suggestive of the diagnosis of:

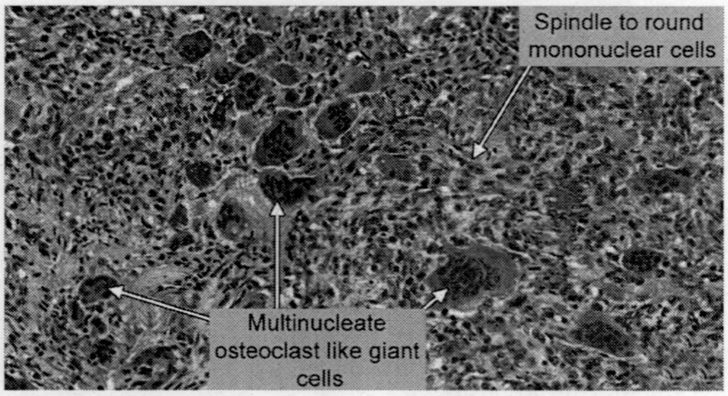

a. Osteoblastoma
b. Osteosarcoma
c. Osteoclastoma
d. Osteoid osteoma

Ans. c. Osteoclastoma

161. A young male presented to Medicine OPD with the complaints of jaundice. On examination, he was also having tremors. Ophthalmological examination was done and findings are shown below. Most likely diagnosis:

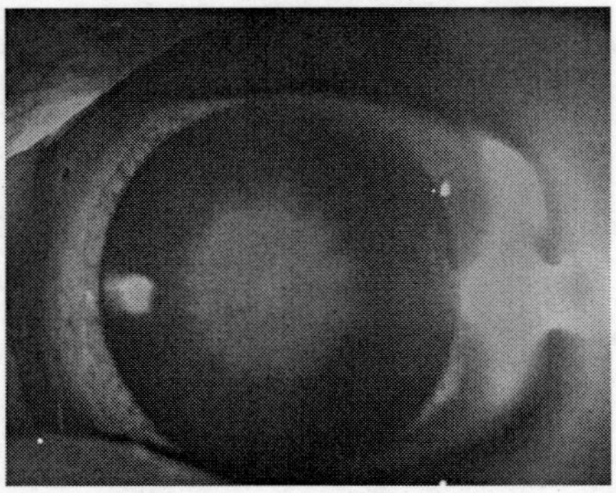

a. Hepatocellular carcinoma
b. Arsenic poisoning
c. Parkinson's disease
d. Wilson's disease

Image shows a sunflower cataract.

Ans. d. Wilson's disease

162. Identify the bacterium:

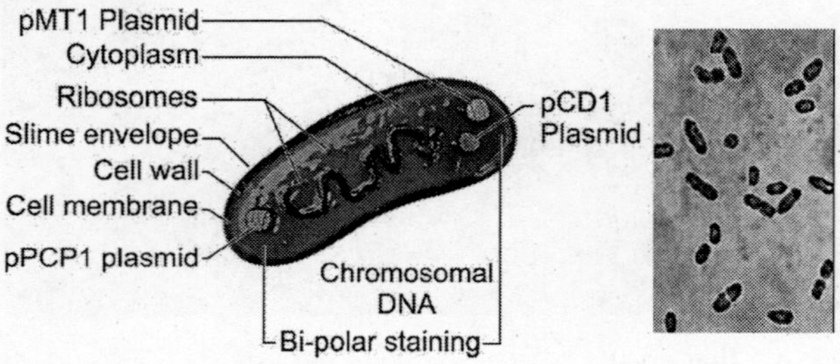

a. Yersinia pestis
b. Staphylococcus aureus
c. Shigella
d. Bacillus anthracis

Ans. a. Yersinia pestis

163. Persistence of the posterior part of the vascular sheath of the lens results in a cataract as shown below. This is:

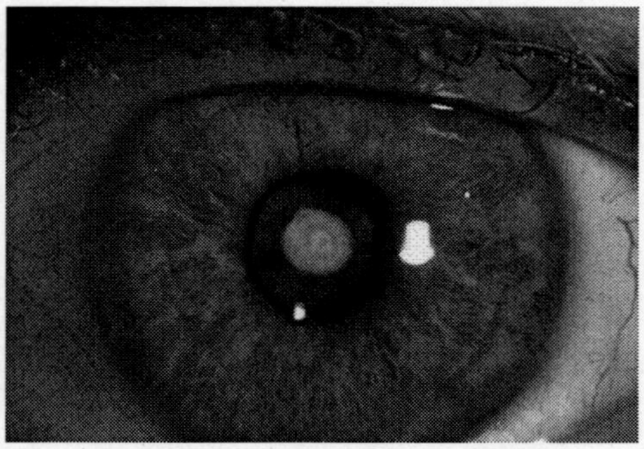

a. Posterior polar cataract
b. Posterior subcapsular cataract
c. Anterior polar cataract
d. Anterior subcapsular cataract

Ans. a. Posterior polar cataract

164. **Which condition is discussed?**

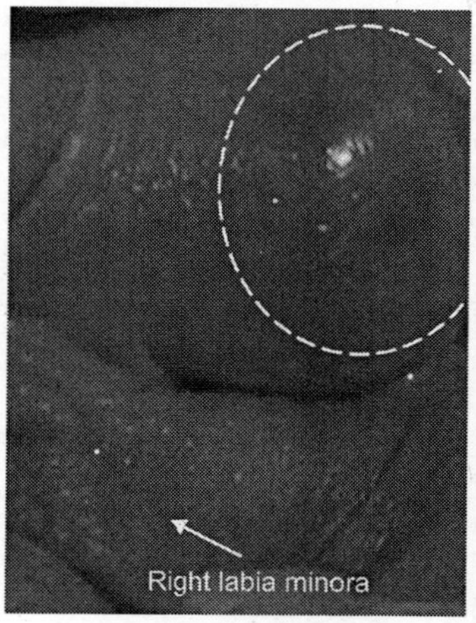

a. Bartholin gland cyst
b. Bartholin gland carcinoma
c. Bartholin gland adenoma
d. Skene's duct cyst

Ans. a. Bartholin gland cyst

165. **A specimen from kidney was stained with Congo red stain and was visualized under polarising microscope. The appearance is shown below. Identify the substance from the options given below:**

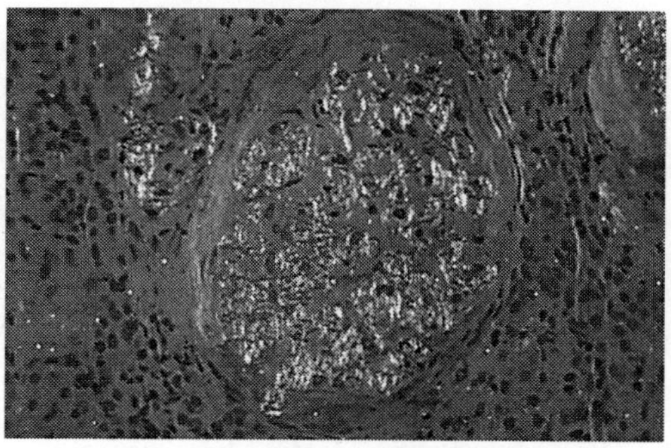

a. Collagen
b. Cellulose
c. Amyloid
d. Starch

Ans. c. Amyloid

166. **A male patient developed high-grade fever, headache, vomiting and nuchal rigidity of sudden onset. Lumbar puncture was done and CSF sample showed the growth of the micro-organism shown below in the image. Identify the organism:**

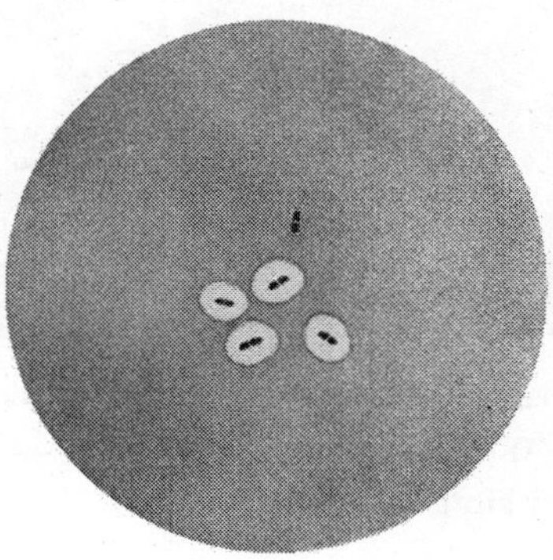

a. Pseudomonas aeruginosa
b. Neisseria meningitidis
c. Staphylococcus aureus
d. Streptococcus pneumoniae

Ans. d. Streptococcus pneumoniae

167. **A 29-years-old female, mother of 4 children, attended Medicine OPD with the complaint of tiredness. On examination, there was pallor. Nail changes are shown below in the image. Hemoglobin level came out to be 6.5 gm%. Most likely diagnosis:**

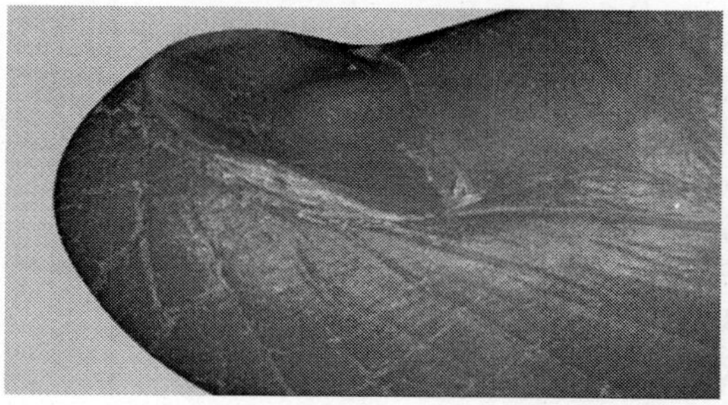

a. Arsenic poisoning
b. Iron deficiency anemia
c. Chronic liver disease
d. Chronic kidney disease

Image shows spoon shaped nail.

Ans. b. Iron deficiency anemia

168. **Study the CT scan image given below and make a diagnosis:**

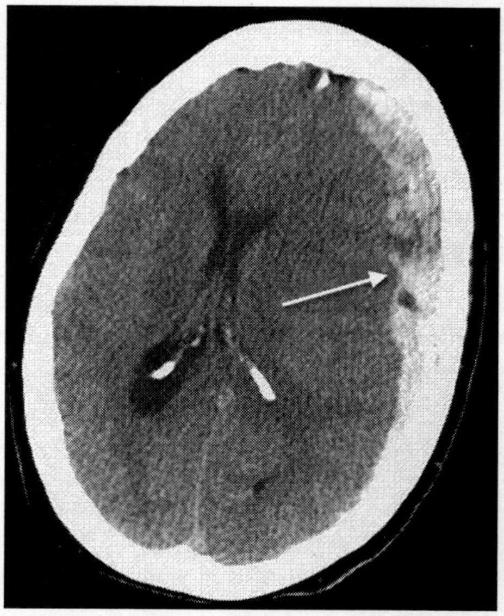

a. Subdural hemorrhage
b. Subarachnoid hemorrhage
c. Extradural hemorrhage
d. Parenchymal hemorrhage

Image shows concavo-convex deformity.

Ans. a. Subdural hemorrhage

169. Look at the congenital abnormality shown below. Such an anomaly occurs because of incomplete fusion of:

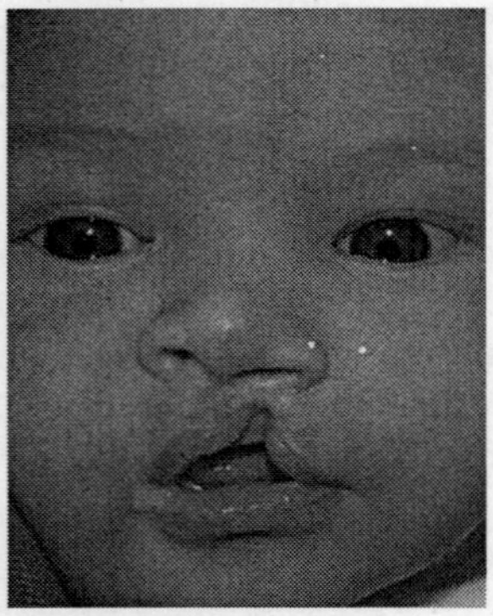

a. Palatal process with lateral nasal process
b. Palatal process with medial nasal process
c. Maxillary process with lateral nasal process
d. Maxillary process with medial nasal process

Ans. d. Maxillary process with medial nasal process

170. A patient with some ENT disease was started on some drug. Because of drug intake, later on he developed some teeth problem as shown in the clinical picture below. Identify the ENT disease:

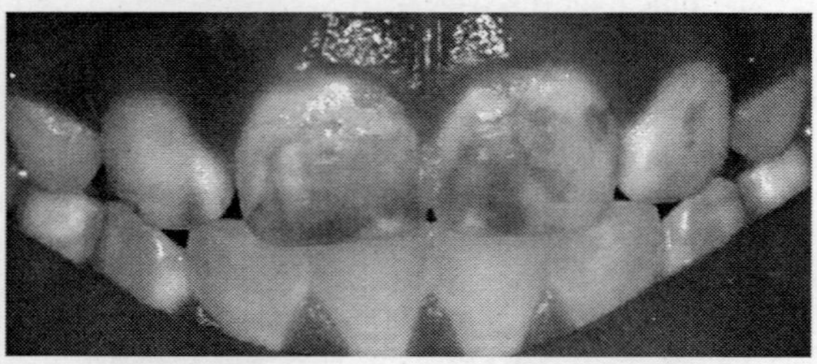

a. Otosclerosis
b. Meniere's disease
c. Acute suppurative otitis media
d. Chronic suppurative otitis media

Image shows dental fluorosis. Drug is sodium fluoride.

Ans. a. Otosclerosis

171. Clinical picture of the eye of a known case of severe malnutrition is shown below. Identify the condition:

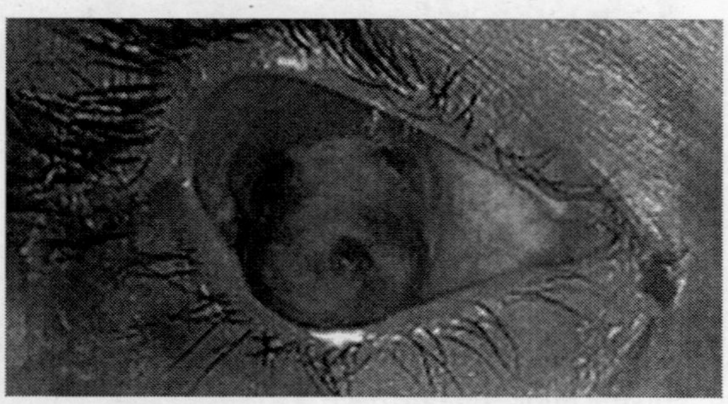

a. Bitot's spot b. Congenital cataract
c. Anterior staphyloma d. Megalocornea

Ans. c. Anterior staphyloma

172. An old trumpet player presented to the ENT OPD with the complaints of cough, change in quality of voice, difficulty in breathing and a swelling in the neck region. Neck swelling was reducible and tend to increase in size on coughing or doing Valsalva manoeuvre. X-ray of the neck region was done as shown below. Most likely diagnosis:

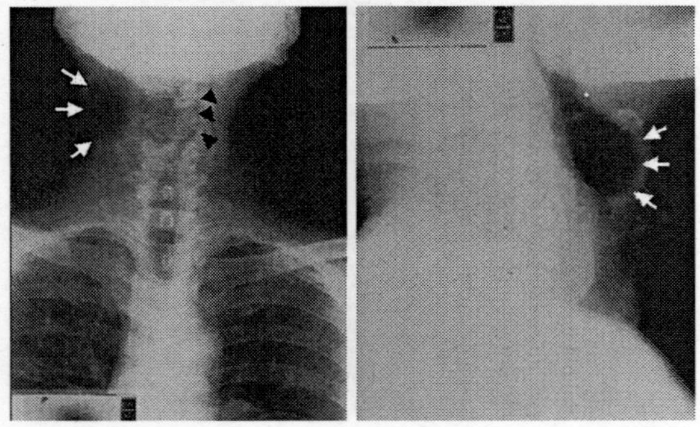

a. Laryngomalacia b. Laryngocele
c. Laryngeal TB d. Laryngeal Ca

Ans. b. Laryngocele

173. A newborn male child presented to the Ophthalmology OPD with the complaints of excessive watering from the eyes. Clinical image of the patient is shown below. Most likely diagnosis:

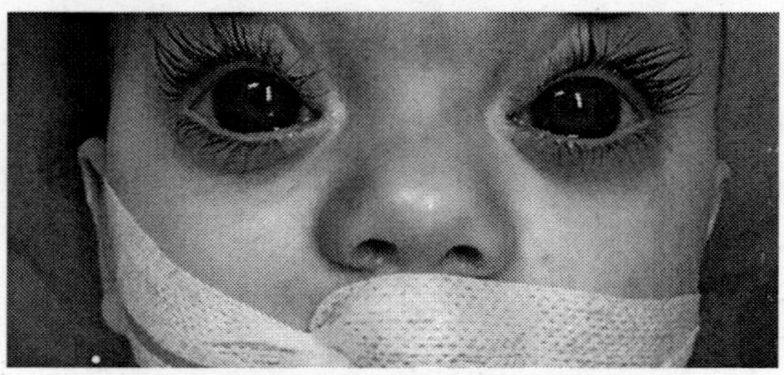

a. Buphthalmos b. Congenital cataract
c. Acute dacryocystitis d. Microcornea

Ans. a. Buphthalmos

174. Identify the structure marked as '5' in the given CT scan:

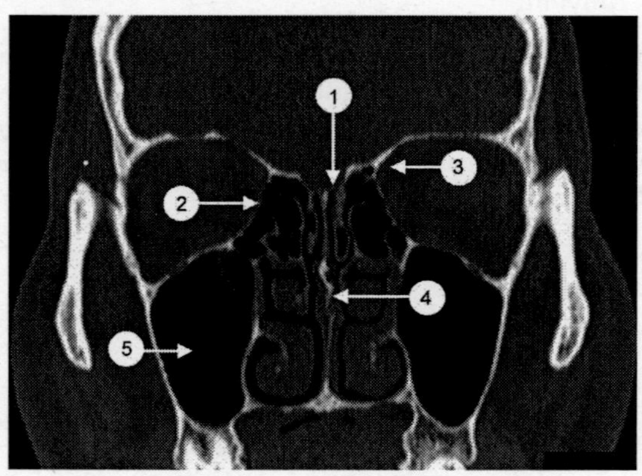

a. Frontal sinus b. Ethmoid sinus
c. Maxillary sinus d. Sphenoid sinus

Ans. c. Maxillary sinus

175. **A 12-years-old female presented with cough and low-grade fever. There was associated sore throat for 5 days. Patient was started on some antibiotic along with paracetamol for fever. After three days, sore throat resolved and fever also subsided gradually. But later on, she developed a greyish-whitish membrane in the oral cavity and neck swelling as shown in the image below. She also experienced difficulty in breathing and swallowing. Which of the following organism is associated with such a clinical disease?**

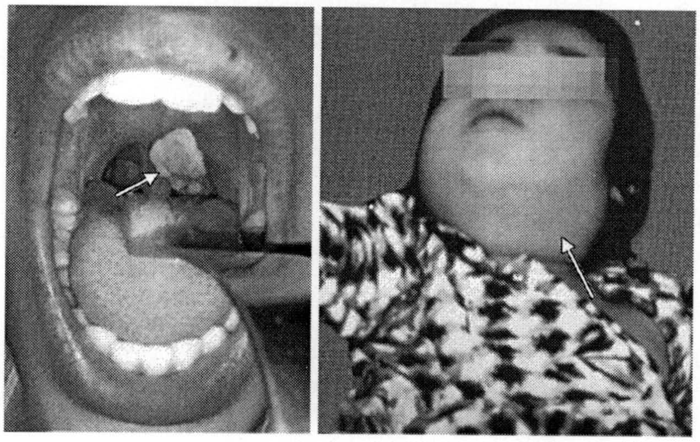

a. Corynebacterium diphtheriae
b. Mycobacterium tuberculosis
c. Streptococcus pneumoniae
d. Staphylococcus aureus

Ans. a. Corynebacterium diphtheriae

176. **A patient presented to the Ophthalmology OPD with the complaint of pain, visual loss and orbital swelling. On examination proptosis was noticed. Clinical image of the patient is given below. Findings are suggestive of:**

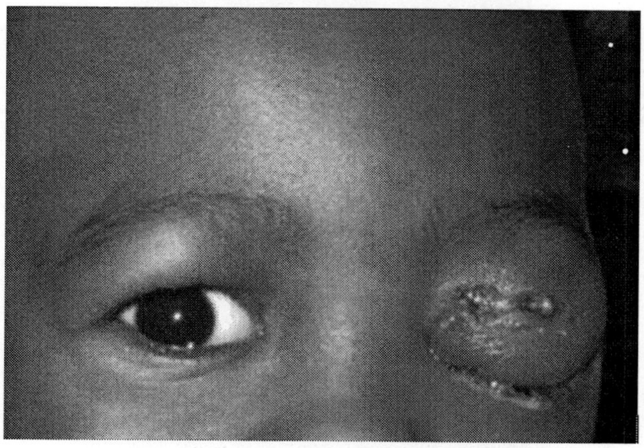

a. Internal hordeolum b. External hordeolum
c. Orbital cellulitis d. Basal cell carcinoma

Ans. c. Orbital cellulitis

177. **A young female presented with complaints of itching in eyes and watering from eyes and nose. Clinical picture of the eye is shown below. Most likely diagnosis:**

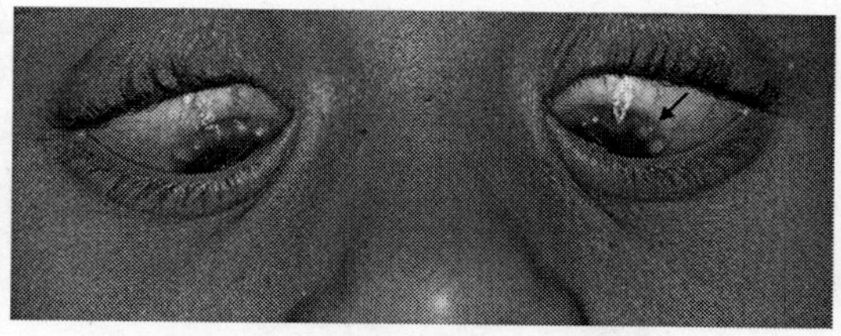

a. Vernal keratoconjunctivitis
b. Basal cell carcinoma
c. Malignant melanoma
d. Trachoma

Black arrow shows Horner-Tranta's spots.

Ans. a. Vernal keratoconjunctivitis

178. **Identify the X-ray view shown below:**

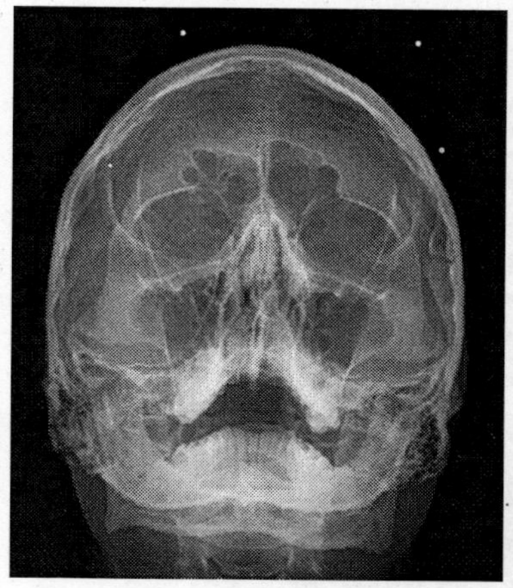

a. Pierre's view b. Caldwell's view
c. Occipito-lateral view d. Water's view

Ans. d. Water's view

179. **Identify the fracture:**

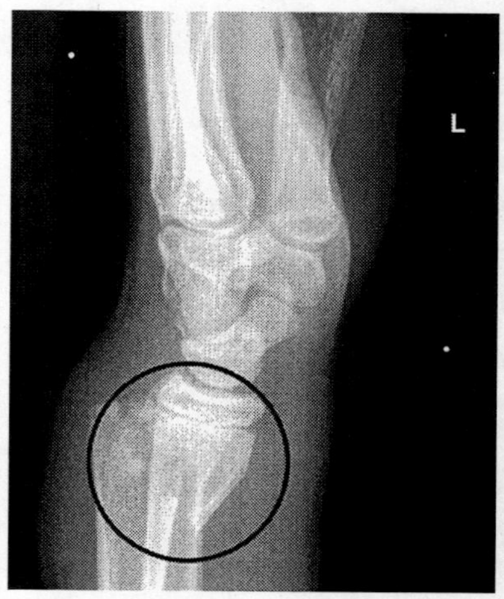

a. Colle's fracture b. Monteggia fracture
c. Galeazzi fracture d. Smith's fracture

Displacement of distal fragment is opposite to that seen in Colle's fracture.

Ans. d. Smith's fracture

180. A 29-years-old female is a known case of some valvular heart disease. She presented to the Medicine OPD with fever of 15 days duration. Physician examined the patient and the clinical findings are shown in the images below. On per-abdomen examination of the same patient, what would be the finding?

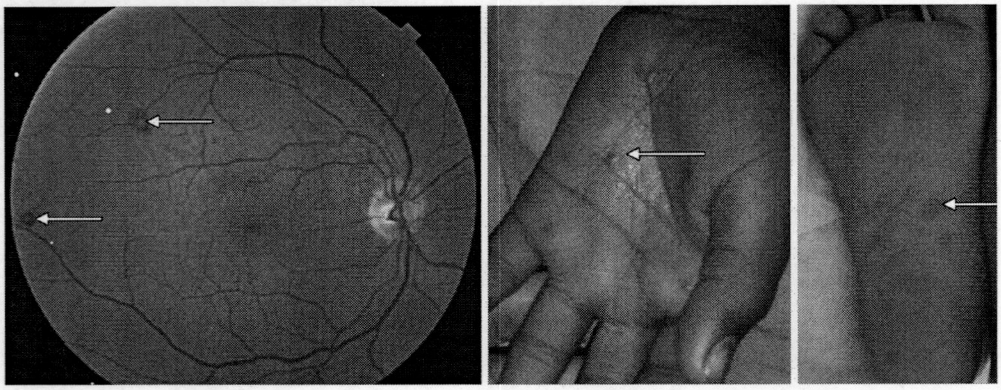

a. Intestinal obstruction
b. Ascites
c. Splenomegaly
d. Portal hypertension

Fundus examination shows Roth's spots and palm-sole shows Janeway lesions.

Ans. c. Splenomegaly

181. A 16-years-old girl with 46XX karyotype is having primary amenorrhoea. Secondary sexual characters are well developed. On per-vaginal examination, a bulging membrane is seen. Clinical image is given below. Next step in management:

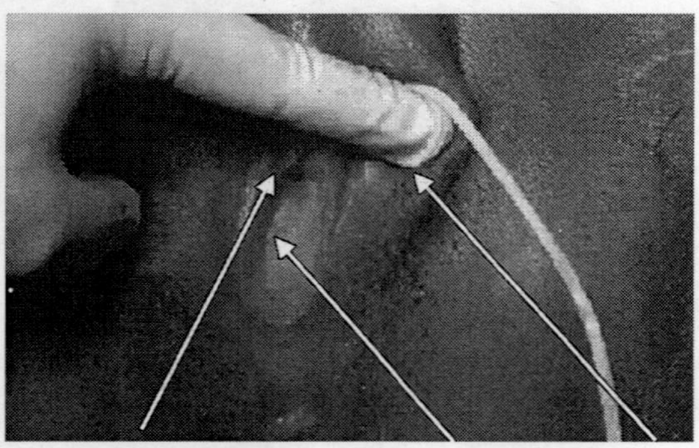

a. Wait and watch
b. Long-term estrogen therapy
c. Bilateral oophorectomy
d. Cruciate incision and drainage of blood

Image is of imperforate hymen.

Ans. d. Cruciate incision and drainage of blood

182. Identify the condition:

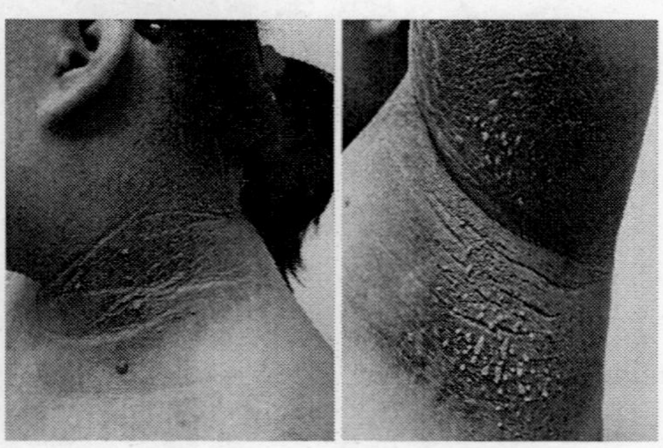

a. Dermatitis herpetiformis
b. Leprosy
c. Acanthosis nigricans
d. Lupus vulgaris

Ans. c. Acanthosis nigricans

183. A 50-years-old lady presented to the Surgery OPD with complaints of mass in breast. Examining surgeon diagnosed it as a case of carcinoma breast. Clinical picture of the breast is given below. What is the T-staging:

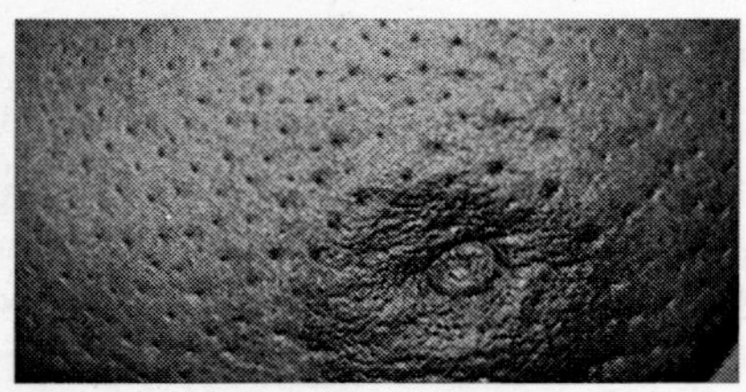

a. T4d
b. T4c
c. T4b
d. T4a

Image shows Peau'd orange.

Ans. c. T4b

184. A lady with breast lesion presented to the Surgery OPD. Examining surgeon found that the mass is NOT movable. The mass is attached to the underlying ribs. There is NO metastasis to lymph node. Clinical image is given below. Most likely diagnosis:

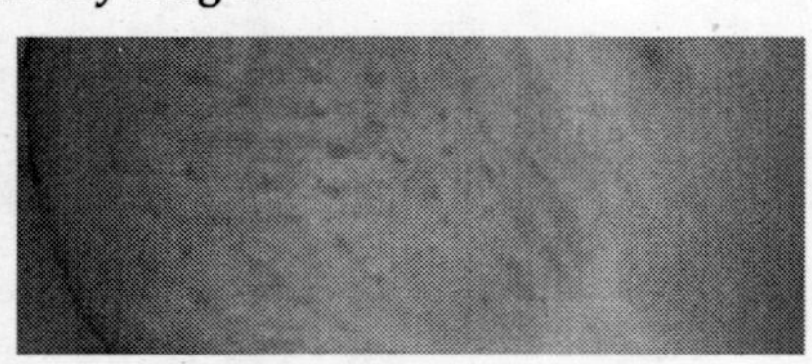

a. Inflammatory breast cancer
b. Acute mastitis
c. Phyllodes tumour
d. Scirrhous carcinoma

Ans. a. Inflammatory breast cancer

185. A 28-years-old lactating lady presented to the Surgery OPD with fever and redness over breast. Clinical image is given below. Most likely diagnosis:

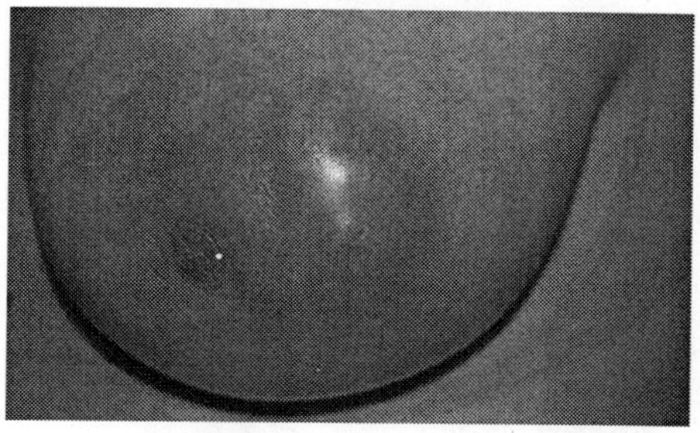

a. Carcinoma breast b. Breast abscess
c. Phyllodes tumour d. Paget's disease

Ans. b. Breast abscess

186. Identify the marked muscle:

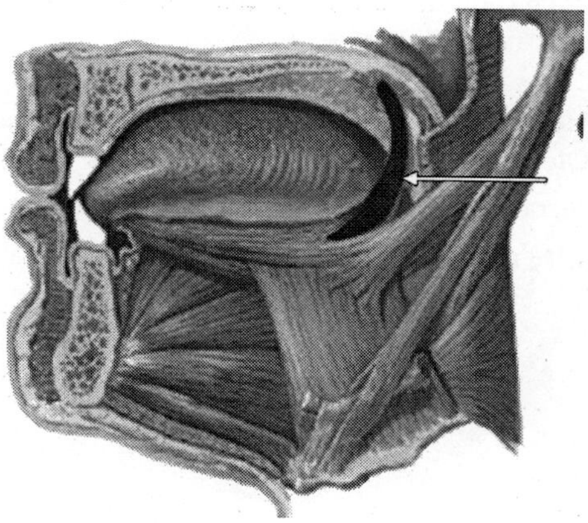

a. Genioglossus b. Hyoglossus
c. Palatoglossus d. Styloglossus

Ans. c. Palatoglossus

187. Splint shown in the figure is used for:

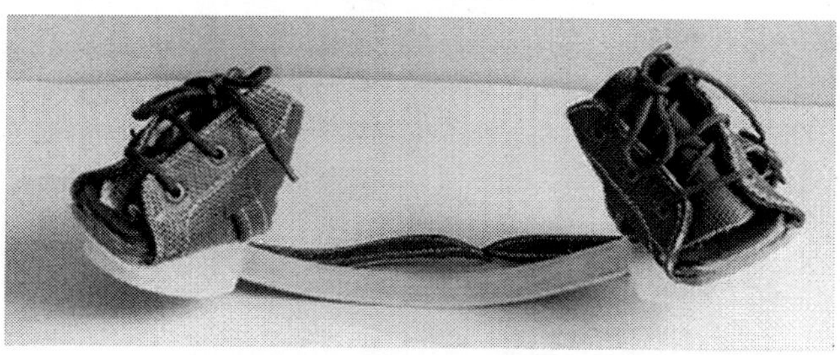

a. Slipped capital femoral epiphyses
b. Perthe's disease
c. CTEV
d. Congenital hip dislocation

Image shows DB splint.

Ans. c. CTEV

188. A young male had a road traffic accident. His right lower limb was in an attitude as shown below. Which nerve injury is most likely to occur in such a case?

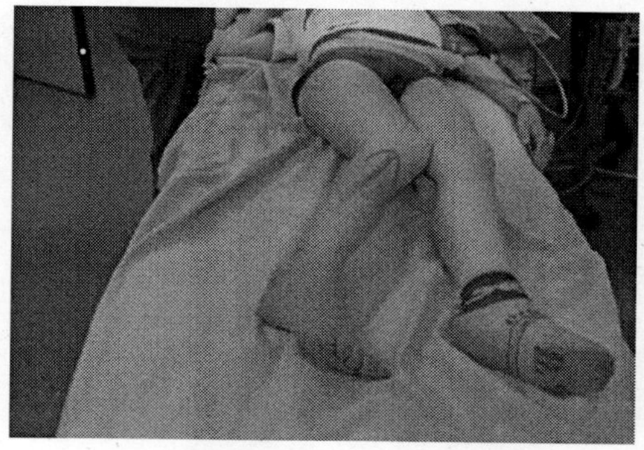

a. Common peroneal nerve b. Obturator nerve
c. Sciatic nerve d. Femoral nerve

Attitude of lower limb suggest posterior dislocation of hip joint.

Ans. c. Sciatic nerve

189. While performing the procedure, as shown in the image below, which of the following structure is NOT pierced?

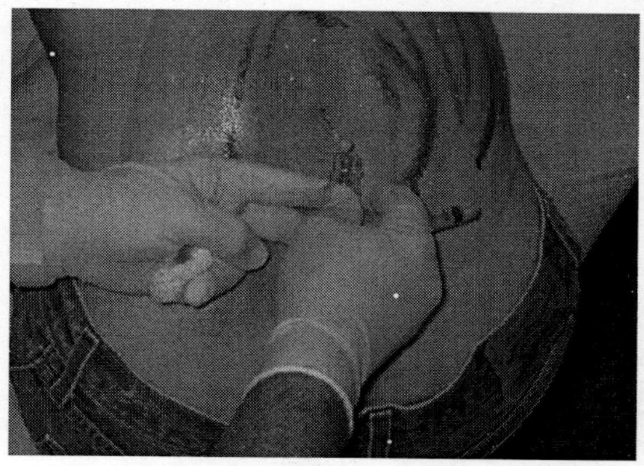

a. Ligamentum flavum b. Intervertebral disc space
c. Interspinous ligament d. Supraspinous ligament

Image shows technique of lumbar puncture.

Ans. b. Intervertebral disc space

190. Identify the cartilage labelled as 1, in figure:

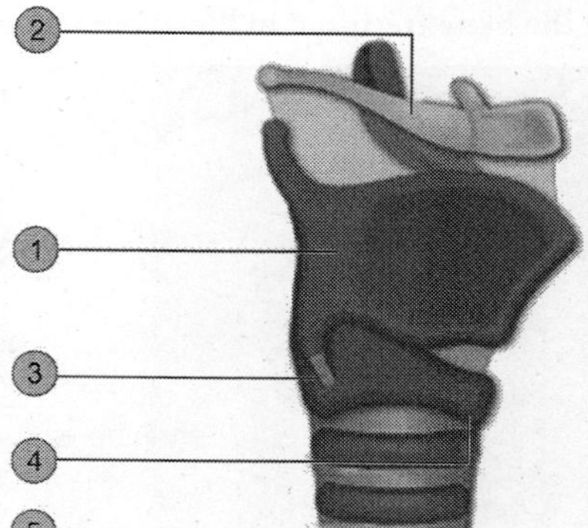

Lateral larynx

a. Cuneiform cartilage b. Arytenoid cartilage
c. Thyroid cartilage d. Corniculate cartilage

Ans. c. Thyroid cartilage

191. A patient suffering from COVID-19 infection is having a sPO_2 of 78%. Which of the following cylinder is best to provide oxygen therapy to the patient?

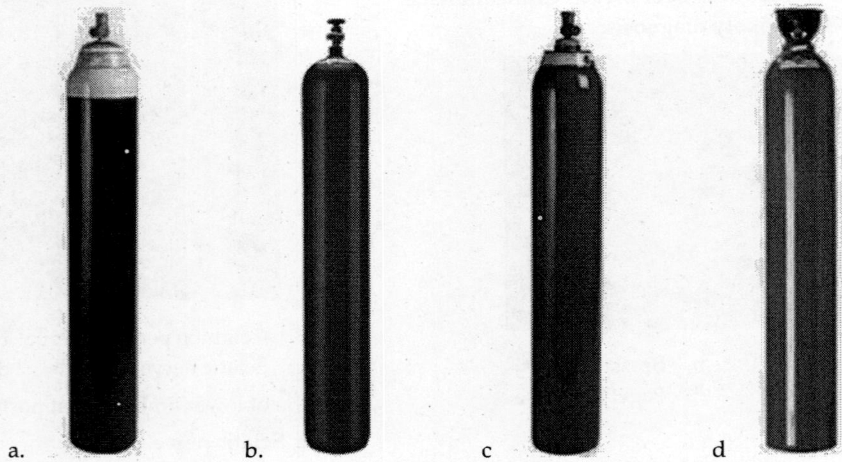

SpO_2 is low so patient needs oxygen. Oxygen cylinder has a black body and white shoulders.

Ans. a

192. Identify the virus shown in the figure:

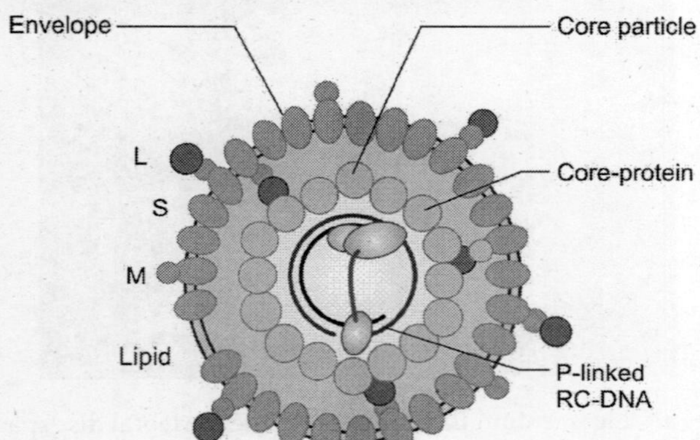

a. HBV b. EBV
c. CMV d. HIV

Ans. a. HBV

193. Identify the bone fractured in the given image:

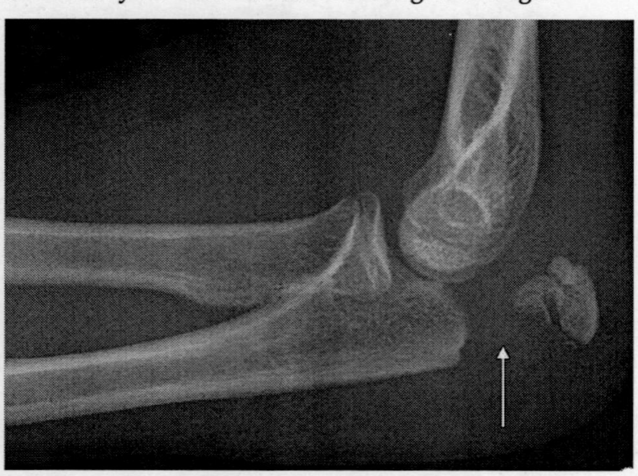

a. Head of radius b. Capitellum
c. Olecranon process d. Trochlea

Ans. c. Olecranon process

194. Identify the instrument:

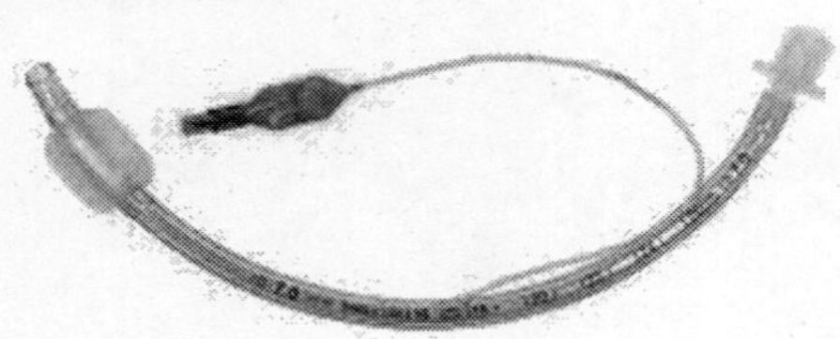

a. Double lumen endotracheal tube
b. PVC endotracheal tube
c. Laryngeal mask airway
d. AMBU bag

Ans. b. PVC endotracheal tube

195. Skull fracture shown in the figure is most likely caused by:

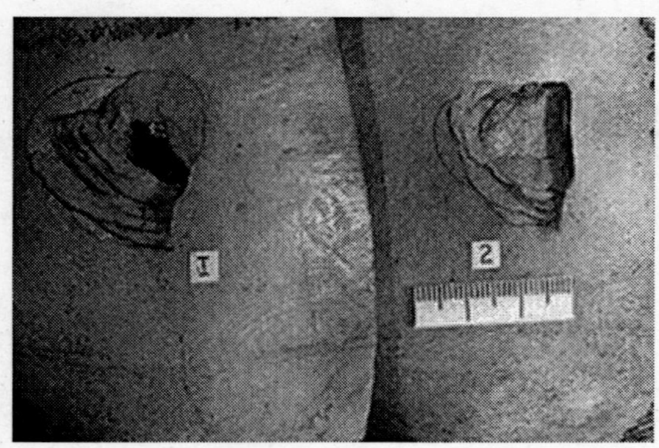

a. Fall from height b. Blunt injury
c. Road traffic accident d. Bullet

Image shows gutter fracture.

Ans. d. Bullet

Problem Based MCQs with Explanation

1 Anatomy

1. A pediatrician noted that some green coloured liquid matter is coming out from the umbilicus of a newborn baby (fecal fistula) admitted in NICU. What is the embryological basis of this condition?

a. Persistence of entire vitello-intestinal duct
b. Persistence of a portion of vitello-intestinal duct
c. Vitello-intestinal duct replaced by a fibrous band
d. Complete obliteration of vitello-intestinal duct

Occasionally the whole of the vitello-intestinal duct, or its distal part alone, may be patent. The former conditions lead to a fecal fistula at the umbilicus, where the intestinal content comes out through the umbilicus.

2. A male child presented to the Pediatric Surgery OPD with the complaints of swelling in inguinal area. On examination, it was found that there is herniation of intestinal loop along with spermatic cord reaching up to the scrotal sac. Most likely condition:

a. Direct inguinal hernia
b. Indirect inguinal hernia
c.` Femoral hernia
d. Littre's hernia

In complete (scrotal) type of indirect inguinal hernia, the sac descends to the bottom of the scrotum.

3. In anterior abdominal wall, subcostal nerve lies between:

a. External oblique muscle and internal oblique muscle
b. Internal oblique muscle and transversalis abdominis muscle
c. Transversalis abdominis and fascia transversalis
d. Fascia transversalis and parietal peritoneum

Subcostal nerve (12th intercostal nerve) runs in front of the quadratus lumborum, innervates the transversus abdominis, and passes forward between it and the abdominal internal oblique to be distributed in the same manner as the lower intercostal nerves.

4. Type of epithelium found in fallopian tube is:

a. Stratified squamous
b. Ciliated columnar
c. Transitional
d. Simple squamous

The mucous layer of the fallopian tube is thrown into longitudinal folds and is lined by single layer of tall ciliated columnar epithelium.

5. In adults, spinal cord ends at the lower border of which vertebra?

a. L1
b. L2
c. L3
d. L4

In adults, spinal cord ends at the lower border for L1 vertebra, whereas in infants, it ends at lower border of L3 vertebra.

6. All of the following are paired cartilages of larynx *except*:

a. Thyroid
b. Corniculate
c. Cuneiform
d. Arytenoid

Unpaired cartilages of larynx are epiglottis, thyroid and cricoid cartilage.

7. Abductor of vocal cord:

a. Lateral cricoarytenoid
b. Posterior cricoarytenoid
c. Thyroarytenoid
d. Cricothyroid

Posterior cricoarytenoid muscle abducts the vocal cord and is supplied by recurrent laryngeal nerve.

8. Muscle enclosed between anterior and middle lamina of thoracolumbar fascia:

a. Erector spinae
b. Psoas major
c. Quadratus lumborum
d. Psoas minor

QL forms the bulk of the posterior abdominal wall between the psoas major muscle medially and the transversus abdominis muscle laterally. It is enclosed between the anterior and middle layers of the thoracolumbar fascia.

9. If there is rupture of spongy urethra, urine will extravasate at all the places *except*:

a. Scrotum
b. Around penis
c. Superficial perineal pouch
d. Deep perineal pouch

Answers

1. a	**2.** b	**3.** b	**4.** b	**5.** a	**6.** a	**7.** b
8. c	**9.** d					

In case of rupture of spongy urethra (below the perineal membrane), urine accumulates in superficial perineal pouch, scrotum, around penis and lower part of anterior abdominal wall.

10. Decussation of corticospinal tract occurs at:

a. Upper medulla b. Lower medulla
c. Pons d. Midbrain

Main descending fibres seen at the level of pyramidal decussation are the corticospinal fibres, on their way from the cerebral cortex to the spinal cord. At this level of medulla, many of these fibres run backwards and medially to cross in the midline. These crossing fibres constitute the decussation of the pyramids. Approximately 80% of the fibres of corticospinal tract cross to opposite side (motor decussation) and 20% fibres remain uncrossed.

11. True regarding congenital diaphragmatic hernia are all *except*:

a. Absence of pleuroperitoneal membrane
b. Commonly on the right side
c. Can be diagnosed on antenatal USG
d. Associated with pulmonary hypoplasia

Hernia through foramen Bochdalek is the commonest congenital diaphragmatic hernia. It is 95% left-sided and only 5% right-sided.

12. Location of Killian's dehiscence/KD:

a. Stylopharyngeus & salpingopharyngeus
b. Palatopharyngeus & salpingopharyngeus
c. Stylopharyngeus & palatopharyngeus
d. Cricopharyngeus & thyropharyngeus

There may be gap between the thyropharyngeal and cricopharyngeal fibres. This gap is referred to as KD.

13. A 41-years-old male presented with a weak flexor pollicis longus and flexor digitorum profundus of the index finger. Which nerve could be involved?

a. Ulnar nerve
b. Median nerve
c. Posterior interosseous nerve
d. Radial nerve

Anterior interosseous nerve arises from median nerve distal to pronator teres. It supplies flexor pollicis longus, flexor digitorum profundus (lateral head) and pronator quadratus.

14. A patient complains of persistent numbness of the chin, lower lip and lower teeth. He further indicates that he had difficulty in chewing. X-ray showed a discrete mass in the infratemporal fossa. Which nerve is compressed by the mass?

a. Buccal nerve b. Lingual nerve
c. Auriculotemporal nerve d. Inferior alveolar nerve

Mental branch of inferior alveolar nerve emerges from the mental foramen and divides into branches that supply the skin over the chin, and that over the lower lip.

15. A 43-years-old woman came with a large abscess in the middle of the right posterior triangle of the neck. The physician incised and drained the abscess. Five days later, the patient noticed that she could not extend her right hand above her head to comb her hair. What is the reason?

a. Damage to scalenus medius
b. Injury to suprascapular nerve
c. Cut to spinal accessory nerve
d. Spread of infection to shoulder joint

Overhead abduction is brought about by trapezius and serratus anterior. Serratus anterior is supplied by long thoracic nerve (of Bell) and trapezius is supplied by spinal accessory nerve.

16. A patient presented with acute abdominal pain. On clinical suspicion, patient underwent cholecystectomy. On histopathological examination, the findings was normal. Gallbladder epithelium will be:

a. Squamous epithelium
b. Simple columnar with brush border
c. Simple columnar
d. Simple columnar with stereocilia

The epithelial lining of the gallbladder consists of simple columnar cells specialized for absorption, with an apical brush border of microvilli, very similar to intestinal absorptive cells.

17. A patient had a lesion in the wrist. On examination, the thumb was laterally rotated and adducted, with ape thumb deformity. Which nerve is involved?

a. Median
b. Ulnar
c. Radial
d. Posterior interosseous nerve

Ape hand deformity is a deformity in which the thumb cannot be abducted or opposed at the carpo-metacarpal joint; it remains in a position of extension (produced by the extensor pollicis longus) and adduction (produced by adductor pollicis).

18. In portal hypertension, lower end of esophagus may show dilatation of veins. Which of the following vein drains into the portal vein from the lower end of esophagus?

a. Right gastric vein b. Left gastric vein
c. Hemi-azygous vein d. Inferior phrenic vein

Answers

10. b	11. b	12. d	13. b	14. d	15. c	16. b
17. a	18. b					

The abdominal part of oesophagus is drained by left gastric veins and short gastric veins. Left gastric veins drain into portal vein.

19. Which of the following is NOT seen in oculomotor nerve palsy?

a. Medial and upward gaze b. Loss of light reflex
c. Dilatation of pupil d. Ptosis

In case of oculomotor nerve palsy, when the patient is asked to look directly forward, the affected eye is directed laterally (by the lateral rectus) and downwards (by the superior oblique).

20. Mucous membrane of cervix is lined by:

a. Simple squamous epithelium
b. Simple columnar epithelium
c. Stratified squamous epithelium
d. Ciliated columnar epithelium

The cervix consists of predominantly fibroelastic tissue and less of smooth muscle. The mucous membrane is lined by simple columnar epithelium.

21. Which type of joint is involved in looking towards right and left side?

a. Ellipsoid b. Pivot
c. Saddle d. Hinge

Being a pivot joint, the median atlanto-axial joint allows the atlas (and with it the skull) to rotate around the axis provided by the dens (the second cervical vertebra is called the axis because of this role it plays). Side-to-side movements are produced by sternocleidomastoid (of the opposite side), obliquus capitis inferior, rectus capitis posterior major and splenius capitis (of the same side).

22. Which of the following belongs to special visceral efferent nuclei?

a. Nucleus tractus solitarius
b. Nucleus ambiguus
c. Edinger-Westphal nucleus
d. Mesencephalic nucleus of trigeminal nerve

Special visceral efferent (SVE) nuclei include motor nucleus of the trigeminal nerve, nucleus of the facial nerve and the nucleus ambiguus. SVE nuclei supply striated (skeletal) muscles derived from the branchial arches.

23. Frey's syndrome is due to faulty regeneration of damaged nerve fibers of:

a. Trigeminal nerve b. Hypoglossal nerve
c. Vagus nerve d. Glossopharyngeal nerve

Frey's syndrome/auriculotemporal syndrome or gustatory sweating/perspiration, occurs post-parotid surgery. The autonomic nerve fibres supplying the parotid gland get damaged. During healing, the parasympathetic secretomotor fibres to the gland regenerate into the sheaths of the sympathetic fibres to the neighbouring sweat glands. Whenever there is salivary stimulation by taste or smell of food, the sweat gland secrete; sweating, warmth and redness of face occur. Auriculotemporal nerve is a branch of posterior division of mandibular nerve, which is a branch of trigeminal nerve.

24. Anterior 2/3rd of the tongue is demarcated from posterior 1/3rd by:

a. Circumvallate papillae b. Passavant's ridge
c. Sulcus terminalis d. Epiglottis

The sulcus terminalis divides the dorsum of tongue into an anterior larger part (pre-sulcal two-thirds) and a posterior smaller part (post-sulcal one-third).

25. Pretectal nucleus is responsible for:

a. Accommodation reflex b. Light reflex
c. Near reflex d. Conjugation reflex

In light reflex, fibres of each optic nerve enter both optic tracts as a result of partial crossing in the chiasma. Fibres from each optic tract end in both pretectal nuclei. Fibres from each pretectal nucleus reach the Edinger-Westphal nuclei of the both the sides.

26. Inferior thyroid vein drains into:

a. Internal jugular vein b. Superior vena cava
c. Brachiocephalic vein d. External jugular vein

The inferior thyroid vein forms a plexus with the fellow of the opposite side; the plexus lies in front of the upper trachea; two veins are reformed from the plexus; the left drains into the left brachiocephalic vein and the right into the right brachiocephalic vein.

27. Trigeminal nerve supplies all of the following *except*:

a. Lateral pterygoid muscle
b. Medial pterygoid muscle
c. Stylohyoid muscle
d. Tensor veli palatini muscle

Stylohyoid muscle is supplied by facial nerve.

28. All of the following are main branches of trigeminal nerve *except*:

a. Mandibular nerve b. Maxillary nerve
c. Ophthalmic nerve d. Optic nerve

Optic nerve is the second cranial nerve. Its anterior end is attached to the posterior pole of the eyeball. The attachment lies a little medial to the anteroposterior axis of the eyeball.

29. Nerve supply of supinator is similar to which of the following muscle?

a. Brachialis b. Brachioradialis
c. Biceps brachii d. Pronator quadratus

Answers

19. a	**20.** b	**21.** b	**22.** b	**23.** a	**24.** c	**25.** b
26. c	**27.** c	**28.** d	**29.** b			

Brachioradialis is supplied by radial nerve whereas supinator is supplied by posterior interosseous nerve (continuation of deep branch of radial nerve).

30. All of the following are derivatives of external oblique aponeurosis *except*:

a. Inguinal ligament b. Lacunar ligament
c. Linea semilunaris d. Pectineal ligament

On either side of the linea alba, another faint groove can be made out in some (especially muscular individuals). This is the linea seminularis (or the linea semilunare) indicating the lateral border of the rectus abdominis muscle.

31. If two buds of pancreas do not fuse, the anomaly is:

a. Ectopic pancreas
b. Pancreatic divisum
c. Annular pancreas
d. Accessory pancreas

The pancreas is derived from ventral and dorsal buds which later fuse. Most of the organ is derived from the dorsal bud. The parts derived from the two buds may remain separate resulting in divided pancreas.

32. Which is the most abundant cartilage?

a. Hyaline cartilage b. Elastic cartilage
c. Fibrocartilage d. All of the above

Hyaline cartilage is found in costal cartilages (that connect the ventral ends of the ribs to the sternum), articular cartilages (of synovial joints), skeletal framework of larynx (thyroid, cricoid), walls of trachea and large bronchi, parts of nasal septum etc.

33. First chondrosternal joint is which type of joint?

a. Fibrous joint
b. Primary cartilaginous joint
c. Secondary cartilaginous joint
d. Synovial joint

First chondrosternal joint is primary cartilaginous whereas rest of the chondrosternal joint are synovial.

34. Which of the following does NOT pass through aortic opening?

a. Aorta b. Azygous vein
c. Thoracic duct d. Phrenic nerve

Right phrenic nerve passes through vena caval orifice whereas left phrenic nerve pierces left cupola.

Answers

30. c **31.** b **32.** a **33.** b **34.** d

2 Physiology

1. A 25-years-old female was watching TV for long hours keeping her right hand under the head. Later on, she experienced tingling sensation over her right upper limb. Most likely affected nerve fibers are:

a. Type A
b. Type B
c. Type C
d. Sympathetic fibers

Type A nerve fibers are most susceptible to pressure.

2. All of the following regulates serum calcium levels *except*:

a. Parathormone
b. Vitamin D
c. Calcitonin
d. Insulin

Insulin is concerned with regulation of carbohydrate metabolism and blood glucose levels. It is also concerned with metabolism of protein and fats.

3. In an experimental laboratory, a brain structure of a man was damaged and he became fearless. Which structure is damaged?

a. Thalamus
b. Hypothalamus
c. Amygdala
d. Caudate nucleus

Stimulation of amygdala leads to fear anxiety in man. So damage of amygdala will result in a fearless character.

4. Which of the following reflex causes bradycardia and hypotension?

a. Bainbridge reflex
b. Bezold Jarisch reflex
c. Law of projection
d. Mary's reflex

Bezold-Jarisch reflex is the reflex characterized by bradycardia and hypotension, caused by stimulation of chemoreceptors present in the wall of left ventricles by substances such as alkaloids.

5. Which of the following is reabsorbed almost completely in proximal convoluted tubule?

a. Glucose
b. Urea
c. Creatinine
d. Chloride

Glucose and amino acids are reabsorbed almost 100% in proximal convoluted tubules.

6. Free hemoglobin cannot be filtered through glomerulus because of:

a. Its large size
b. Negative charge of Bowman's capsule
c. Its small size
d. Positive charge of Bowman's capsule

Glomerular filtration is called ultrafiltration because even the minute particles are filtered out. But the plasma proteins are not filtered due to their large molecular size. The protein molecules are larger than the split pores present in the endothelium of capillaries. Thus, the glomerular filtrate contains all the substances present in the plasma except the plasma proteins.

7. Effect of low dose of dopamine:

a. Renal vasodilation
b. Increased glomerular filtration
c. Increased inotropy
d. Increase in dromotropy

Dopamine is an inotropic agent that has vasodilatory effects at low doses.

8. Source of surfactant:

a. Type I pneumocytes
b. Type II pneumocytes
c. Follicular cells
d. Parafollicular cells

Pulmonary surfactant is secreted by two type of cells; type II alveolar epithelial cells (in the lungs) and Clara cells (in the bronchioles).

9. Skeletal muscle contraction ends when:

a. Sodium ion moves out of cytoplasm
b. Acetylcholine is absorbed from neuromuscular junction
c. Closure and indrawing of receptors
d. Decreased calcium outside reticulum

Relaxation of the muscle occurs when the calcium ions are pumped back into the L tubules. When calcium ions enter the L tubules, calcium content in sarcoplasm decreases leading to the release of calcium ions from the troponin. It causes detachment of myosin from actin followed by relaxation of the muscle.

Answers

1. a	**2.** d	**3.** c	**4.** b	**5.** a	**6.** a	**7.** a
8. b	**9.** d					

10. LH surge is associated with:

a. Increased estrogen and decreased progesterone
b. Increased estrogen and increased progesterone
c. Decreased estrogen and increased progesterone
d. Decreased estrogen and decreased progesterone

Estrogen secretion reaches peak during follicular phase just before ovulation. On the other hand, progesterone is virtually absent during follicular phase.

11. Which vitamin requires intrinsic factor for its absorption?

a. Riboflavin
b. Cyano-cobalamin
c. Thiamine
d. Pantothenic acid

Vitamin B_{12} (cyanocobalamin) is also known as extrinsic factor and it requires intrinsic factor (of Castle) for its absorption.

12. Weber-Fechner law is related to:

a. Number of nerve fibers
b. Number of muscle fibers
c. Quantity of stimulus
d. Intensity of stimulus

Weber-Fechner lay states that intensity of response (sensation) of a receptor is directly proportional to logarithmic increase in the intensity of the stimulus.

13. Baroreceptor reflex is which type of feedback mechanism?

a. Positive feedback
b. Negative feedback
c. Feed forward control
d. Both positive and negative feedback

Negative feedback is the one to which the system reacts in such a way as to arrest the change or reverse the direction of the change. When the arterial blood pressure rises rapidly, baroreceptors are activated to bring the arterial blood pressure back to normal level.

14. Which of the following rule explains delivery of oxygen in fetal circulation?

a. Bohr's effect
b. Halden's effect
c. Higher affinity of fetal Hb for oxygen
d. Head's paradoxical reflex

Bohr effect is the decrease in the affinity of hemoglobin for oxygen due to increased carbon dioxide tension. When carbon dioxide tension decreases, the affinity of fetal hemoglobin for oxygen is increased. All the metabolic end products including carbon dioxide are completely excreted from fetus into the maternal blood. This develops low partial pressure of carbon dioxide in fetal blood. So, the affinity of fetal hemoglobin for oxygen increases resulting in diffusion of more amount of oxygen from mother's blood into fetal blood.

15. Main role of angiotensin-II is:

a. Increases total peripheral resistance
b. Dilatation of afferent renal arteriole
c. Decrease release of aldosterone
d. Diuresis

Angiotensin-II acts in two ways to restore blood pressure. Firstly, it causes constriction of arterioles in the body so that the peripheral resistance is increased and blood pressure rises. Secondly, it stimulates the adrenal cortex to secrete aldosterone.

16. Third heart sound is heard due to:

a. Closure of atrio-ventricular valve
b. Closure of semilunar valve
c. Mid-diastolic flow in the ventricle
d. Atrial contraction

Third heart sound is a low-pitched sound that is produced during rapid filling period of the cardiac cycle. It is also known as ventricular gallop or protodiastolic gallop, as it is produced during earlier part of the diastole. It is produced by rushing of blood into ventricles and vibrations set up in the ventricular wall during rapid filling phase.

17. Effect of Bainbridge reflex:

a. Bradycardia
b. Tachycardia
c. Decreased venous return
d. Apnea

Bainbridge reflex is a cardioaccelerator reflex that increases the heart rate when venous return is increased. Since this reflex arises from right atrium, it is also called as right atrial reflex.

18. A patient was given oral rehydration solution for dehydration. What is the mechanism by which glucose is absorbed?

a. Osmosis
b. Reverse osmosis
c. Passive transport
d. Secondary active transport

Secondary active transport is the transport of a substance with sodium ion, by means of a common carrier protein. Sodium cotransport of glucose is a type of secondary active transport, where sodium cotransport of glucose occurs during absorption of glucose from the intestine.

19. A 60-years-old male presented with a vascular injury to the inferior frontal gyrus. Which function would be affected the most?

a. Vision
b. Hearing
c. Wernicke's aphasia
d. Motor speech

Broca's area lies in inferior frontal gyrus, which constitutes the motor part of speech. Lesions of the Broca's area results in motor aphasia or non-fluent aphasia.

Answers

10. a	11. b	12. d	13. b	14. a	15. a	16. c
17. b	18. d	19. d				

20. 1-alpha hydroxylation in vitamin-D metabolism takes place in:

a. Skin b. Liver
c. Kidney d. Blood

25-hydroxycholecalciferol is converted into 1,25-dihydroxy-cholecalciferol (calcitriol) in the kidney. It is the active form of vitamin D_3. This step needs the presence of parathormone.

21. Hypothalamus increases release of all hormones from anterior pituitary *except*:

a. TSH b. GSH
c. ACTH d. Prolactin

Prolactin (PrL) is a 199 amino acid chain containing polypeptide, is secreted by lactotropes (mammotrophs) of anterior pituitary/API. Hypothalamus secretes PIH (prolactin inhibiting hormone) which inhibits PrL secretion from API.

22. Which of the following is absorbed in proximal intestine?

a. Iron b. Vitamin B_{12}
c. Bile salts d. All of the above

Food iron is of two types. Heme iron and non-heme/inorganic iron. Usually, the bulk of food iron is non-heme iron (mostly inorganic). Non-heme iron is absorbed mostly from 2nd part of duodenum. These irons are in ferric (Fe^{3+}) state. Ferric iron is not absorbable. For absorption, ferric iron has to be converted into ferrous (Fe^{2+}) iron.

23. Endothelial cells synthesize which of the following?

a. Factor XII b. Factor X
c. vW factor d. Fibrinogen

vWF is a large multimeric glycoprotein present in blood plasma and produced constitutively as ultra-large vWF in endothelium (in the Weibel-Palade bodies), megakaryotes (α-granules of platelets), and subendothelial connective tissue.

24. Iodine uptake in thyroid gland is:

a. Endocytosis
b. Facilitated diffusion
c. Primary active transport
d. Secondary active transport

Secondary active transport makes use of potential energy, which are usually derived through exploitation of an electrochemical gradient. This involves pore-forming proteins that form channels across the cell membrane.

25. Secretin release is best stimulated by:

a. Water b. Food carbohydrate
c. Fatty acids d. Acid and protein

Secretin is released into circulation and/or intestinal lumen in response to low duodenal pH that ranges between 2 and 4.5 (depending on species). Also, the secretion of secretin is increased by the products of protein digestion bathing the mucosa of the upper small intestine.

26. Sensation lost on the same side in Brown-Sequard syndrome:

a. Proprioception b. Temperature
c. Touch d. Pain

Brown–Sequard syndrome is caused by damage to one half of the spinal cord, resulting in paralysis and loss of proprioception on the same (or ipsilateral) side as the injury or lesion, and loss of pain and temperature sensation on the opposite (or contralateral) side as the lesion.

27. FALSE for type-II pneumocytes:

a. Appear at 5th month intra-uterine life
b. Forms blood-air barrier
c. Mesodermal
d. Secrete surfactant

Type II pneumocytes cover a minority of the alveolar surface. Their function is to secrete surfactant, which decreases surface tension within the alveoli.

28. Which protein prevents contraction by covering binding sites on actin and myosin?

a. Troponin b. Calmodulin
c. Thymosin d. Tropomyosin

Muscle tropomyosin isoforms are involved in regulating interactions between actin and myosin in the muscle sarcomere and play a pivotal role in regulated muscle contraction. X-ray diffraction and cryoelectron microscopy suggest that tropomyosin sterically blocks the access of myosin to the actin filament.

29. Mitochondrial DNA is:

a. Linear b. Nicked circular
c. Closed circular d. Open circular

In most multicellular organisms, the mtDNA is organized as a circular, covalently closed, double-stranded DNA.

30. Transpulmonary pressure:

a. Difference between bronchus and atmospheric pressure
b. Difference between intra-alveolar and atmospheric pressure
c. Difference between intra-pleural and atmospheric pressure
d. Difference between pressure in alveoli and intra-pleural pressure

Transpulmonary pressure is the difference between the alveolar pressure and the intrapleural pressure in the lungs. During human ventilation, air flows because of pressure gradients. $P_{tp} = P_{alv} - P_{ip}$. Where P_{tp} is transpulmonary pressure, P_{alv} is alveolar pressure, and P_{ip} is intrapleural pressure.

Answers

20. c	21. d	22. a	23. c	24. d	25. d	26. d	27. b
28. d	29. c	30. d					

31. NOT a neuroglial cell of CNS:

a. Astrocytes
b. Kupffer cells
c. Microglia
d. Oligodendrocytes

Kupffer cells (KC) constitute 80–90% of the tissue macrophages present in the body. They reside within the lumen of the liver sinusoids, and are therefore constantly exposed to gut-derived bacteria, microbial debris and bacterial endotoxins, known to activate macrophages.

32. Hageman factor is involved in:

a. Extrinsic pathway
b. Intrinsic pathway
c. Fibrinolysis
d. None

Factor XII (Hageman factor) is part of the coagulation cascade and activates factor XI and prekallikrein in vitro. Factor XII itself is activated to factor XIIa by negatively charged surfaces, such as glass. This is the starting point of the intrinsic pathway.

33. Inulin clearance closely resembles:

a. PAH clearance
b. Creatinine clearance
c. Renal plasma flow
d. GFR

Inulin is uniquely treated by nephrons in that it is completely filtered at the glomerulus but neither secreted nor reabsorbed by the tubules. This property of inulin allows the clearance of inulin to be used clinically as a highly accurate measure of glomerular filtration rate (GFR)—the rate of plasma from the afferent arteriole that is filtered into Bowman's capsule measured in mL/min.

34. First site for haematopoiesis in fetus:

a. Spleen
b. Liver
c. Yolk sac
d. Bone marrow

In developing embryos, blood formation occurs in aggregates of blood cells in the yolk sac, called blood islands. As development progresses, blood formation occurs in the spleen, liver and lymph nodes. When bone marrow develops, it eventually assumes the task of forming most of the blood cells for the entire organism.

Answers

31. b	**32.** b	**33.** d	**34.** c

3 Biochemistry

1. **A 40-years-old woman presented with progressive palmoplantar pigmentation. X-ray spine shows calcification of intervertebral discs. On adding Benedict's reagent to urine, it gives greenish brown precipitate and blue-black supernatant fluid. Most likely diagnosis:**
   a. Phenylketonuria
   b. Alkaptonuria
   c. Tyrosinosis type II
   d. Arginosuccinic aciduria

   By the 3rd or 4th decade of life, patient with alkaptonuria may develop ochronosis (deposition of alkaptone bodies in intervertebral discs, cartilages of nose, pinna of ear). Diagnosis of alkaptonuria is suggested by blackish discoloration of urine, a positive Benedict's test, silver nitrate reduction and detection of elevated homogentisic acid by GC/MS (Gas chromatography/Mass spectrometry).

2. **A 6-years-old patient presented with fatigue on normal outdoor activity. In blood there was raised triglycerides, increased cholesterol, fatty acid and lactate. Blood sugar was 60 mg/dL. USG shows enlarged liver and kidney. Liver biopsy showed increased glycogen. Most likely diagnosis:**
   a. Von-Gierke's disease b. Pompe's disease
   c. Cori's disease d. McArdle's disease

   In Von-Gierke's disease, there is fasting hypoglycemia that does not respond to stimulation by adrenaline. There is hyperlipidemia, lactic acidosis and ketosis. Glycogen gets deposited in liver and massive liver enlargement can lead to cirrhosis.

3. **A patient had normal blood glucose level as estimated by Glucose-Oxidase Peroxidase method. Urine examination showed a positive Benedict's test. Most likely condition:**
   a. Fructosuria
   b. Galactosemia
   c. Denaturation of glucose
   d. Faulty tests

   Fructosuria is a benign metabolic defect due to deficiency of fructokinase. There is no abnormality other than excretion of fructose in urine. Urine gives positive Benedict's and Seliwanoff's tests.

4. **A child was found to have hypoglycemia, hepatomegaly and accumulation of highly branched glycogen called limit dextrin. Most likely diagnosis:**
   a. Cori's disease b. Von-Gierke's disease
   c. Anderson's disease d. McArdle's disease

   Cori's disease/Limit dextrinosis is characterized by accumulation of highly branched dextrin, fasting hypoglycemia, hepatomegaly and myopathy.

5. **An infant present with hepatosplenomegaly, hypoglycemia, hyperuricemia and lactic acidosis. Liver biopsy shows normal structured glycogen deposition. Which enzyme is deficient?**
   a. Debranching enzyme b. Branching enzyme
   c. Glucose-6-phosphatase d. Muscle phosphorylase

   Findings are suggestive of Von-Gierke's disease, which occurs because of deficiency of the enzyme Glucose-6-phosphatase.

6. **A person on a fat free carbohydrate rich diet continues to grow obese. Which of the following lipoprotein is likely to be elevated in his blood?**
   a. Chylomicrons b. VLDL
   c. LDL d. HDL

   The lipid abnormalities in patients who are obese include elevated serum triglyceride, VLDL, apolipoprotein B, and non-HDL-C levels. The increase in serum triglycerides is due to increased hepatic production of VLDL particles and a decrease in the clearance of triglyceride rich lipoproteins.

7. **A person was diagnosed with isolated increase in LDL. His father and brother had the same disease with increased cholesterol. Most likely diagnosis:**
   a. Familial type III hyperlipoproteinemia
   b. Abetalipoproteinemia
   c. Familial lipoprotein lipase deficiency type I
   d. LDL receptor mutation

   In type IIA hyperlipoproteinema (Primary Familial Hypercholesterolemia), there is elevation of LDL. The cause is LDL receptor defect. Receptor deficiency in liver and

Answers

1. b	**2.** a	**3.** a	**4.** a	**5.** c	**6.** b	**7.** d

peripheral tissues will result in the elevation of LDL levels in plasma, leading to hypercholesterolemia.

8. A patient with abetalipoproteinemia frequently manifests with delayed blood clotting. This is due to inability to:

a. Produce VLDL b. Synthesize fatty acids
c. Produce chylomicrons d. Synthesize clotting factors

In abeta-lipoproteinemia, there are reduced levels of VLDL, LDL, B-48 and B-100. All apo-B containing lipoproteins are reduced since microsomal triglyceride transfer protein is defective.

9. A 48-years-old lady presented with bone pain and hepatosplenomegaly. On examination of biopsy specimen from spleen, crumpled tissue paper appearance is seen. Which product is likely to have accumulated?

a. Glucocerebroside b. Sphingomyelin
c. Sulfatide d. Ganglioside

In Gaucher's disease, there is beta-glucosidase deficiency leading to accumulation of glucocerebroside. There is hepatosplenomegaly, erosion of bone and moderate anemia. Gaucher cells have the appearance of signet rings with 'wrinkled tissue paper' because the nucleus is pushed to the periphery of the cells.

10. A 7-years-old boy presented with severe abdominal pain. On examination, he has xanthomas. Blood drawn for work up has milky appearance of plasma. Which lipoprotein is increased?

a. Chylomicron b. Chylomicron remnants
c. LDL d. HDL

Lipoprotein fraction elevated in a patient with type I hyper-lipoproteinemia is chylomicron. Plasma after 24 hours shows creamy layer over clear plasma. Clinical features are eruptive xanthoma, hepatosplenomegaly and pain in abdomen.

11. In a person, LDL is highly elevated but the level of LDL receptors is normal. What could be the cause?

a. Phosphorylation of LDL receptors
b. ApoB100 mutation
c. Lipoprotein lipase deficiency
d. Cholesterol acyl CoA transferase deficiency

A mutation in apoB-100 that inhibits its binding to the LDL receptor is another genetic cause of elevations in LDL cholesterol.

12. If in a person, total cholesterol: 300 mg/dL, HDL: 25 mg/dL and triglyceride: 150 mg/dL. What would be the value of LDL?

a. 245 mg/dL b. 125 mg/dL
c. 95 mg/dL d. 55 mg/dL

LDL cholesterol = Total cholesterol – HDL cholesterol-Triglycerides

13. A 45-years-old male, blood sample gives red colour in Ehlrich's solution. The substance responsible is:

a. Urobilinogen b. Conjugated bilirubin
c. Unconjugated bilirubin d. Haemosiderin

Bilinogens (Urobilinogen and stercobilinogen) react with Ehlrich's aldehyde reagent (para-dimethyl amino benzaldehyde) to form red color.

14. If tyrosine level in blood is normal without external supplementation, deficiency of which of the following is ruled out?

a. Tryptophan b. Phenylalanine
c. Histidine d. Isoleucine

Tyrosine is formed from phenylalanine by the action of the enzyme phenylalanine hydroxylase. So if sufficient phenylalanine is supplied in diet, tyrosine level would be normal in the body.

15. Sickle cell anemia is the clinical manifestation of homozygous genes for an abnormal hemoglobin molecule. The event responsible for the mutation in the B-chain is:

a. Insertion b. Deletion
c. Non-dysjunction d. Point mutation

Sickle cell anemia is caused by point mutation. In the beta chain of the hemoglobin, the 6th amino acid normally is glutamate. In sickle-cell anemia, this is altered to valine. In the DNA, this is seen as a change from normal T replaced by abnormal A nucleotide (T to A substitution).

16. A 10-years-old child with aggressive behavior and poor concentration is brought with presenting complaints of joint pain and reduced urinary output. Mother gives history of self mutilation behavior stating that he tends to mutilate his fingers. Enzyme deficiency in such a case:

a. HGPRTase b. Adenosine deaminase
c. APRTase d. Acid maltase

Lesch-Nyhan syndrome is characterized by self-mutilation, mental retardation, excessive uric and nephrolithiasis. Gout develops in later life. There is deficiency of hypoxanthine guanine phosphoribosyl transferase.

17. A 4-years-old child diagnosed with Duchenne muscular dystrophy, an X-linked recessive disorder. Genetic analysis shows that the patient's gene for the muscle protein dystrophin contains a mutation in its promoter region. Most likely effect of this mutation:

a. Tailing of dystrophin mRNA with be defective
b. Capping of dystrophin mRNA will be defective
c. Termination of dystrophin transcription will be deficient
d. Initiation of dystrophin transcription will be deficient

Duchenne muscular dystrophy/DMD is a degenerative disease of muscle affecting only male children. The gene is

Answers

8. a	9. a	10. a	11. b	12. b	13. a	14. b
15. d	16. a	17. d				

in the middle of the short arm of X-chromosome. This gene produces a protein called dystrophin with 3700 amino acids. In DMD patients, the gene for dystrophin is mutated. These mutations affect the normal transcription of dystrophin.

18. A lady presented with fatigue and tingling sensation in both hands and legs. On examination, she is found to have a fissured red tongue, lesions at angle of mouth with a decreased RBC glutathione reductase activity. Likely vitamin deficiency:

a. Riboflavin
b. Thiamine
c. Vitamin B_{12}
d. Vitamin B_6

Manifestations of riboflavin (vitamin B_2) deficiency include glossitis, magenta colored tongue, cheilosis (redness and shiny appearance of lips), angular stomatitis (lesions at muco-cutaneous junction at corners of mouth) and cirumcorneal vascularization. Proliferation of the bulbar conjunctival capillaries is the earliest sign of riboflavin deficiency. Glutathione reductase (RBC) is an FAD (Flavin adenine dinucleotide) requiring enzyme, which is the marker for vitamin B_2 deficiency.

19. A child was weaned from breast milk on the fifth day and was given sugar cane juice. The child developed hypoglycemia and hepatomegaly. Biochemical examination showed hypophosphatasia and reducing substances in urine. Likely enzyme deficiency:

a. Aldolase B
b. Fructokinase
c. Glucose-6-phosphatase
d. Beta-galactosidase

In hereditary fructose intolerance, the defect is in aldolase-B, hence fructose-1-phosphate cannot be metabolized. This is seen when sucrose (containing fructose) is introduced in the diet of the infants, usually around 6 months of age. Accumulation of fructose-1-phosphate will inhibit glycogen phosphorylase. This leads to accumulation of glycogen in liver and associated hypoglycemia. Fructose is also excreted in urine when urine gives positive Benedict's test.

20. A 28-years-old female presented with obstructive jaundice. Which of the following type of reaction will be seen in Van Der Bergh test?

a. Direct positive
b. Indirect positive
c. Both positive
d. Biphasic

Van Der Bergh reaction is direct positive in conjugated hyperbilirubinemia. Obstructive jaundice causes conjugated hyperbilirubinemia.

21. In lead poisoning, there is inhibition of some of the enzymes of the heme biosynthetic pathway. This is reflected by the accumulation of:

a. Uroporphyrinogen III
b. Ferrochelatase
c. Porphyrobilinogen
d. Delta amino levulinic acid

Lead inhibits heme synthesis. Basophilic stippling of red cells is seen in peripheral blood and bone marrow smears. This is due to agglutination of ribosomes. Globin synthesis is adversely affected. Lead particularly inhibits delta aminolevulinic acid (ALA) synthase and ALA-dehydratase.

22. A 10-years-old boy presented with muscle weakness and fatigue with increased lead in blood. Which of the following enzyme production in liver is increased?

a. Ferrochelatase
b. PBG deaminase
c. Heme oxygenase
d. ALA synthase

Porphyria can result from lead poisoning (acquired porphyria). Most of the paints contain lead more than the permitted levels. Children suck painted toys; and they get the poison. The toxic effect of lead is due to inhibition of ferrochelatase. So, there is decreased level of heme with consequent increased activity of ALA synthase.

23. A 4-years-old boy of first-degree consanguineous couple presented with complaints of backache and bilateral knee pain. All blood investigations were normal. Urine routine microscopy is normal. However, on keeping urine outside for sometimes, it turned black. Which of the enzyme is likely to be deficient in such a patient?

a. Xanthine oxidase
b. Homogentisate oxidase
c. Tyrosinase
d. Fumaryl-acetoacetate hydroxylase

The patient is suffering from alkaptonuria, which is because of deficiency of homogentisate oxidase. Urine becomes dark on exposure to air.

24. A young male presented with pain in calves during excessive exercise without any other symptom or sign. Muscle biopsy shows increased glycogen. The enzyme deficient is:

a. Debranching enzyme
b. Muscle phosphorylase
c. Glucose-6-phosphorylase
d. Muscle phosphofructokinase

In type V glycogen storage disease (McArdle's disease), there is exercise intolerance, accumulation of glycogen in muscles and myoglobinuria. This occurs because of deficiency of the enzyme muscle phosphorylase (skeletal muscles).

25. A man complaint of diarrhea with dairy products. He must avoid all *except*:

a. Condensed milk
b. Skimmed milk
c. Yogurt
d. Ice cream

The person is suffering from lactose intolerance, which is because of deficiency of the enzyme lactase. In this condition, lactose accumulates in the gut. Irritant diarrhoea

Answers

18. a **19.** a **20.** a **21.** d **22.** d **23.** b **24.** b
25. c

and flatulence are seen. If milk is withdrawn completely, diarrhoea will be limited. Curd is an effective treatment, because the lactobacilli present in the curd contains the enzyme lactase. Lactase is abundantly seen in yeast, which could also be used for treatment.

26. A patient presents with inability to convert pyruvate to Acetyl CoA. Treatment of this condition is with the supplementation of:

a. Thiamine b. Biotin
c. Free fatty acids d. Vitamin B_6

The coenzyme form of the enzyme pyruvate dehydrogenase is TPP (thiamine pyrophosphate). This enzyme is used in oxidative decarboxylation of alpha keto acids, e.g., pyruvate dehydrogenase catalyzes the breakdown of pyruvate to acetyl CoA, and carbon dioxide.

27. After a fatty meal in a patient with lipoprotein lipase deficiency, which of the following will be raised?

a. HDL b. LDL
c. IDL d. Chylomicrons

The dietary triglycerides are transported by chylomicrons. The lipoprotein molecules are broken down by the lipoprotein lipase present on the capillary wall. Lipoprotein lipase hydrolyzes triglycerides present in chylomicrons into fatty acids and glycerol.

28. Glycine is present in all of the following *except*:

a. Creatine b. Purine
c. Glutamine d. Glutathione

Glutamine was isolated as free amino acid from beetroot by Schulze and Bosshard in 1833. Glutamine was identified as a member of all proteins by Charles Chibnall and Manayath Damodaran in 1932. The amidation of glutamic acid to glutamine is catalyzed by the enzyme glutamine synthetase.

29. Insulin increases activity of all *except*:

a. Phosphofructokinase-1
b. Glucokinase
c. Pyruvate carboxylase
d. Acetyl CoA carboxylase

During gluconeogenesis, carboxylation of pyruvate to oxaloacetate is catalyzed by a mitochondrial enzyme, pyruvate carboxylase. This enzyme needs coenzyme biotin and energy by ATP hydrolysis. Insulin inhibits gluconeogenesis, so it will not increase activity of an enzyme involved in gluconeogenesis (pyruvate carboxylase).

30. Hay's Sulphur test is used to detect:

a. Bile salts in urine b. Reducing sugars in urine
c. Ketone bodies in urine d. Urobilinogen in urine

Normally bile salts (sodium salts of taurocholic acid and glycocholic acid) are present in the bile; but are not seen in urine. Bile salts in urine are detected by Hay's test. Positive Hay's test indicates the obstruction in the biliary passages causing regurgitation of bile salts into the systemic circulation leading to excretion in urine.

31. In a person fasting overnight with carnitine deficiency, following chemical increase in blood:

a. Glucose b. Fatty acids
c. Amino acids d. Ketone bodies

Carnitine deficiency is noted in preterm infants, in whom impaired fatty acid oxidation is noticed and hence fatty acids levels would increase. Also, more glucose is utilized, resulting in episodes of hypoglycemia.

32. Vitamin B_1 is required for which reaction?

a. Transamination
b. Oxidative decarboxylation
c. Carboxylation
d. Reduction

The co-enzyme form of the enzyme pyruvate dehydrogenase is TPP (thiamine pyrophosphate). This enzyme is used in oxidative decarboxylation of alpha keto acids, e.g., pyruvate dehydrogenase catalyzes the breakdown of pyruvate to acetyl CoA, and carbon dioxide.

33. Which vitamin is synthesized in-vivo in the body by humans?

a. Folic acid
b. Niacin
c. Pantothenic acid
d. Cyano-cobalamin

The richest natural sources of niacin are dried yeast, rice polishing, liver, peanut, whole cereals, legumes, meat and fish. About half of the requirement is met by the conversion of tryptophan to niacin. About 60 mg of tryptophan will yield 1 mg of niacin.

34. Accumulation of increased amount of sphingomyelin in liver and spleen is found in:

a. Gaucher's disease
b. Niemann-Pick disease
c. Cori's disease
d. Von-Gierke's disease

Niemann- Pick disease is because of deficiency of the enzyme sphingomyelinase. As a result of this, sphingomyelin accumulates in the body. Clinical features include severe CNS damage, mental retardation, hepatosplenomegaly and Cherry red spots in macula. Death occurs by 2 years of age.

Answers

26. a	**27.** d	**28.** c	**29.** c	**30.** a	**31.** b	**32.** b
33. b	**34.** b					

4 Pathology

1. A 17-years-old boy presented with TLC of 138 × 10^9/L with 80% blasts on the peripheral smear. Chest X-ray demonstrated a large mediastinal mass. Immunotyping of this patient blasts would likely demonstrate:

a. No surface antigens (null phenotype)
b. An immature T cell phenotype (Tdt/D3/CD7 positive)
c. Myeloid markers, such as CD13, CD33 and CD15
d. B cell markers such as CD19, CD20 and CD22

Findings are consistent with the diagnosis of precursor T-cell lymphoblastic leukemia/lymphoma. Since the precursor T-cells differentiates in the thymus, this tumour often presents as mediastinal mass and pleural effusion and progresses rapidly to develop leukemia in the blood and bone marrow. On immunophenotyping, TdT (terminal deoxynucleotidyl transferase) is expressed by the nuclei of pre-T stages of differentiation of lymphoid cells. Pre-T cell type is typically positive for CD1, CD2, CD3, CD5 and CD7.

2. A 60-years-old female has history of 8 blood transfusions in past 2 years. Her Hb: 6.0 g/dL, TLC: 5800, platelets: 3.4 lakhs, MCV: 60, RBC: 2.1 lakhs/mm^3. She is having hypochromic microcytic anemia. Which investigation is NOT needed?

a. Evaluation of pulmonary hemosiderosis
b. Urinary hemosiderin
c. Bone marrow examination
d. Gastrointestinal endoscopy

The clinical presentation given above suggests deficiency of iron (normal MCV is 77-93 fL) but hemosiderosis is an iron-storage disorder in which there is excessive accumulation of iron in parenchymal cells with eventual tissue damage and functional insufficiency of organs such as liver, pancreas, heart and pituitary gland.

3. During autopsy of a patient died due to suspected myocardial infarction, the heart tissue was stained with triphenyl-tetrazolium chloride dye. What would be the color of viable myocardium?

a. Blue
b. White
c. Red
d. Dark brown

Early myocardial infarcts (3-6 hours) can be detected by histochemical staining for dehydrogenases on unfixed slice of the heart. This consists of immersing a slice of unfixed heart in the solution of triphenyltetrazolium chloride (TTC) which imparts red colour to the normal heart muscle, while the area of infarcted muscle fails to stain due to lack of dehydrogenases.

4. A 19-years-old female with short stature, wide spread nipples and primary amenorrhea, would likely to have which karyotype?

a. 47, XX+18
b. 46, XXY
c. 47, XXY
d. 45X

The clinical findings are suggestive of the diagnosis of Turner's syndrome. It is an example of monosomy (45, XO) most often due to loss of X chromosome in paternal meiosis.

5. In a 30-years-old female patient with polyarthritis, testing reveals nucleolar pattern of ANA staining. What is the likely course of this patient?

a. Malar rash, alopecia and renal failure
b. Sclerodactyly, esophageal dysmotility and Raynaud's phenomenon
c. Sjogren syndrome
d. Painful genital and oral blisters and ulcers

CREST syndrome is characterized by Calcinosis, Raynaud's phenomenon, Esophageal hypomotility, Sclerodactyly and Telangiectasia. CREST syndrome is one of the two types of scleroderma.

6. A 28-years-old female presents with recurrent abortions and pain in the calves. She is most likely suffering from a deficiency of which of the following?

a. Protein C
b. Thrombin
c. Factor XIII
d. Plasmin

Deficiency of both protein C and S are autosomal dominant disorders having either reduced amount of protein C or S, or both, or their functional defect. Clinically, both the conditions are associated with lifelong risk of thrombosis of deep leg veins (which present as calf pain).

Answers

1. b **2.** a **3.** c **4.** d **5.** b **6.** a

7. **A 55 years male presented with dry mouth and rheumatoid arthritis with high titer of anti SS-A and anti SS-B antibodies, diagnosed as a case of minor salivary gland tumour. The earliest histological finding is:**
   a. Endothelial cells b. Basophils
   c. Lymphocyte d. Eosinophils

Sjogren's syndrome is characterized by the triad of dry eyes (keratoconjunctivitis sicca), dry mouth (xerostomia), and rheumatoid arthritis. The combination of the former two symptoms is called as sicca syndrome. In early stage, the lacrimal and salivary glands show periductal infiltration by lymphocytes and plasma cells, which at times may form lymphoid follicles (pseudo-lymphoma).

8. **An undifferentiated malignant tumour on immunohistochemical stain shows cytoplasmic positivity of most of the tumour cells for cytokeratin. Most probable diagnosis of the tumour is:**
   a. Sarcoma b. Lymphoma
   c. Carcinoma d. Malignant melanoma

Immuno-stains for epithelial tumours (carcinomas) include pankeratin (fractions; high and low molecular weight keratins), epithelial membrane antigen (EMA), carcinoembryonic antigen (CEA) and neuron specific enolase (NSE).

9. **A 15-years-old girl presented with weakness for 2 months. On examination, she had pallor and icterus. Spleen was palpable. Laboratory examination showed decreased MCV, increased MCHC and reticulocytosis. Osmotic fragility test is positive. Coomb's test is negative. Most likely diagnosis:**
   a. Iron deficiency anemia
   b. Auto-immune hemolytic anemia
   c. G-6-PD deficiency
   d. Hereditary spherocytosis

Clinical features of hereditary spherocytosis include anemia (manifests as weakness and icterus), splenomegaly (a constant feature), jaundice and pigment gallstones. Laboratory findings include reticulocytosis (usually 5–20%), MCV is usually normal or slightly decreased but MCHC is increased. Osmotic fragility is increased (spheroidal nature of red cells make them lyse more readily in solutions of low salt concentration). Direct Coomb's test (antiglobulin) is negative so as to distinguish this condition from acquired spherocytosis of AIHA (autoimmune hemolytic anemia), in which it is positive.

10. **A 2-years-old child presents with scattered lesions in the skull. Biopsy revealed Langerhans giant cells. The most commonly associated marker with this condition would be:**
    a. CD1a b. CD57
    c. CD3 d. CD68

Findings are suggestive of Langerhans cell histiocytosis. Demonstration of common antigens on these Langerhans cells can be done by immune-histochemical stains for S-100 protein, CD1a and HLA-DR.

11. **One sided kidney is normal whereas the other side kidney is contracted with scar formation. Most likely diagnosis:**
    a. Chronic pyelonephritis
    b. Polycystic kidney disease
    c. Renal artery stenosis
    d. Tuberculosis of kidney

In chronic pyelonephritis, the kidney shows characteristic appearance. The kidneys are usually small and contracted (weighing less than 100 gram) showing unequal reduction, which distinguishes it from other forms of contracted kidney. The surface of the kidney is irregularly scarred; the capsule can be stripped off with difficulty due to adherence to scars.

12. **Patient with cirrhosis is HBsAg positive and has increased level of alpha fetoprotein. Most likely diagnosis:**
    a. Submassive hepatic necrosis
    b. Hepatocellular carcinoma
    c. Massive hepatic necrosis
    d. Normal

Genesis of hepatocellular carcinoma (HCC) is linked to prolonged infection with HBV. Cirrhosis of all etiologic types is more commonly associated with HCC but the most frequent association is with macronodular post-necrotic cirrhosis. Laboratory findings of HCC yield nonspecific results like anemia, markedly elevated serum alkaline phosphatase as found in cirrhosis, and high serum alpha-fetoprotein (AFP). Elevated AFP level is quite specific; very high levels of AFP (above 500 ng/mL) are observed in 70–80% cases of HCC, but lacks sensitivity since AFP is also found elevated in yolk sac tumour, cirrhosis, chronic hepatitis, massive liver necrosis and normal pregnancy.

13. **A 35-years-old male presented with history of bleeding. Peripheral smear shows platelet count: 50,000/mm^3, leucocytosis, decreased neutrophils, normal lymphocytes, blast: 20%. t(8;21) is positive. Band forms, myelocyte and metamyelocytes were also seen. Most likely diagnosis:**
    a. CLL
    b. CML
    c. AML
    d. Myelodysplastic syndrome

Acute myeloblastic leukemia has bleeding manifestations (due to thrombocytopenia; causing spontaneous bruises, petechiae, bleeding from gums etc.). The platelet count is usually moderately to severely reduced (below 50,000/microL). The total WBC count ranges from subnormal

Answers

7. c	8. c	9. d	10. a	11. a	12. b	13. c

to markedly elevated values (leucocytosis). Majority of leucocytes in the peripheral blood are blasts and there is often neutropenia due to marrow infiltration by leukemic cells. A few important examples of chromosomal mutations in AML are translocations {(t8;21)(q22q22)} and {(t15;17)(q22;q12)} and inversions {inv(16)(p13;q22)}. WHO classification for AML has revised and lowered the cut off percentage of marrow blasts to 20% (from 30% in the FAB classification) for making a diagnosis of AML.

14. A 40-years-old man presented with painless hematuria. Bimanual examination revealed a ballotable mass over the right flank. Subsequently right nephrectomy was done and the mass was seen to be composed of cells with clear cytoplasm. Areas of hemorrhage and necrosis were frequent. Cytogenetic analysis would show:

a. Abnormality of chromosome 1
b. Abnormality of chromosome 3
c. Abnormality of chromosome 11
d. Abnormality of chromosome 17

The classical clinical evidence for diagnosis of renal cell carcinoma (RCC) is the triad of gross hematuria, flank pain and abdominal mass. Clear cell type is the most common variety of RCC, histology of which shows clear cytoplasm (due to glycogen and lipid). There is homozygous loss of VHL (Von Hippel-Lindau) gene on chromosome 3 in clear cell type.

15. A lady with abdominal mass was investigated. On surgery, she was found to have bilateral ovarian masses with smooth surface. On microscopy, they revealed mucin secreting cells with signet ring shape. Most likely diagnosis:

a. Dysgerminoma
b. Krukenberg tumour
c. Mucinous adenocarcinoma of the ovaries
d. Dermoid cyst

Krukenberg tumours forms moderately large, rounded or kidney-shaped, firm, multinodular masses in both ovaries. Microscopically, it is characterised by the presence of mucin-filled signet ring cells which may lie singly or in clusters.

16. A 45-years-old patient presented with history of fever, night sweats and weight loss. On X-ray a mass in the apical lobe of lung is seen. On histopathology, it was found to have caseous necrosis. What is the likely underlying process involved?

a. Enzymatic degeneration
b. Hypersensitivity reaction with modified macrophages, lymphocytes and giant cells
c. Acute decrease in blood supply
d. Decreased supply of growth factors

Some macrophages, unable to destroy tubercle bacilli, fuse together and form multinucleated giant cells. Around the mass or cluster of epithelioid cells and a few giant cells, a zone of lymphocytes and plasma cells is formed which is further surrounded by fibroblasts. The lesion at this stage is called hard tubercle due to the absence of central necrosis. Within 10–14 days, the centre of the cellular mass begins to undergo caseation necrosis, characterised by cheesy appearance of high lipid content.

17. A patient presented with arthritis, hepatosplenomegaly, hyperpigmentation and raised serum ferritin levels. Most likely diagnosis:

a. Pseudogout
b. Hemochromatosis
c. Rheumatoid arthritis
d. Osteoarthritis

Hemochromatosis is characterised by a triad of features—micronodular pigment cirrhosis, diabetes mellitus and skin pigmentation. On the basis of last two features, the disease also has come to be termed as 'bronze diabetes.' In hemochromatosis, iron absorption goes up to 4 mg/day or more (normally around 1-1.5 mg/day), as evidenced by elevated serum iron (normal about 125 mg/dL) and increased serum transferrin saturation (normal 30%). The serum ferritin is raised in iron overload states (normal 30–250 ng/mL).

18. A 50-years-old lady, who was obese and hypertensive, came with complaints of bleeding and abdominal pain, is diagnosed to have endometrial carcinoma. Which gene is mutated?

a. JAK2
b. PTEN
c. TET
d. CFTR

Endometrial hyperplasia is a forerunner of endometroid cancer is supported by mutated PTEN gene (located on chromosome 10) seen in 20% cases of complex hyperplasia, while it is seen in 40–80% cases of endometroid carcinoma. Other gene mutations in these cases are hMLH, KRAS and beta-catenin oncogenes.

19. A female patient presented with diarrhea and abdominal pain. Small intestinal biopsy shows villous atrophy and crypt hyperplasia. Most likely diagnosis:

a. Celiac sprue
b. Tropical sprue
c. Whipple's disease
d. Hirschsprung's disease

Celiac sprue is the most important cause of malabsorption syndrome/MAS occurring in temperate climates. Clinical features of MAS include steatorrhoea (pale, bulky, foul-smelling stools), chronic diarrhoea, abdominal distension etc. In celiac sprue, there may be partial villous atrophy which is replacement of normal villous pattern by convolutions, or subtotal villous atrophy characterised by flat mucosal surface. Epithelial cells show compensatory hyperplasia, suggesting a turnover of these cells. Lamina propria shows increased number of plasma cells and lymphocytes.

Answers

14. b 15. b 16. b 17. b 18. b 19. a

20. A 40-years-old hypertensive male was admitted to the hospital with sudden onset of headache and altered sensorium. On examination, his blood pressure was observed to be 220/110 mm Hg and the patient died four hours later. Most likely pathological findings in his kidneys:

a. Small kidney with granular surface
b. Small kidney with petechial hemorrhages
c. Large kidney with waxy appearance
d. Large kidney with granular surface

Malignant nephrosclerosis is the form of renal disease that occurs in malignant or accelerated hypertension. Blood pressure is around 200/140 mm Hg or higher. Headache, dizziness and impaired vision are commonly found. Azotaemia (high blood urea nitrogen/BUN and serum creatinine) and uraemia develop soon if malignant hypertension is not treated aggressively. In a case of malignant hypertension superimposed on pre-existing benign nephrosclerosis, grossly, the kidneys are small in size, shrunken and reduced in weight and have finely granular surface.

21. A 40-years male has hemoglobin 10 gm%, MCV: 65 fL, RDW: 16% and platelet count: 4.5 lakhs/microL. What additional finding could be seen in such a patient?

a. Low serum transferrin
b. Raised iron binding capacity
c. Increased HbA_2
d. Increased serum copper

Features of iron deficiency anemia include a fall in haemoglobin concentration, diminished MCV (normal is 77–93 fL), increased red cell distribution width (normal up to 14.5% in males), platelet count is usually normal (1.5-4 lakhs/microL) but may be slightly to moderately elevated in patients who have recent bleeding and total iron binding capacity/TIBC is high (normal 250–450 microgram/dL).

22. Arterial biopsy of elderly male shows fragmentation of elastic lamina, lymphocyte infiltration and giant cells. Most likely diagnosis:

a. Temporal arteritis
b. Takayasu disease
c. Polyarteritis nodosa
d. Kawasaki disease

Histologically in temporal (giant cell) arteritis, the internal elastic lamina of artery is fragmented, non-specific inflammatory cell infiltrate consisting of neutrophils, lymphocytes and eosinophils is found throughout the arterial wall and giant cells of foreign body or Langerhan's are found (in two-third of cases).

23. A 55-years-old, chronic smoker underwent mass resection from bronchus. Most useful immuno-histochemical marker to make a proper diagnosis would be:

a. Cytokeratin
b. Vimentin
c. Desmin
d. Leucocyte common antigen

Immuno-stains for epithelial tumours (carcinomas) include pankeratin (fractions; high and low molecular weight keratins), epithelial membrane antigen (EMA), carcinoembryonic antigen (CEA) and neuron specific enolase (NSE).

24. Kinky hair disease/Menkes disease is a disorder where an affected child has peculiar white stubby hair, growth is retarded, brain degeneration is seen and dies by the age of 2 years. Mrs. 'X' is hesitant about having children because her 2 sisters had sons who died from Kinky hair disease. Her mother's brother also died of the same condition. Possible mode of inheritance:

a. X-linked recessive
b. X-linked dominant
c. Autosomal recessive
d. Autosomal dominant

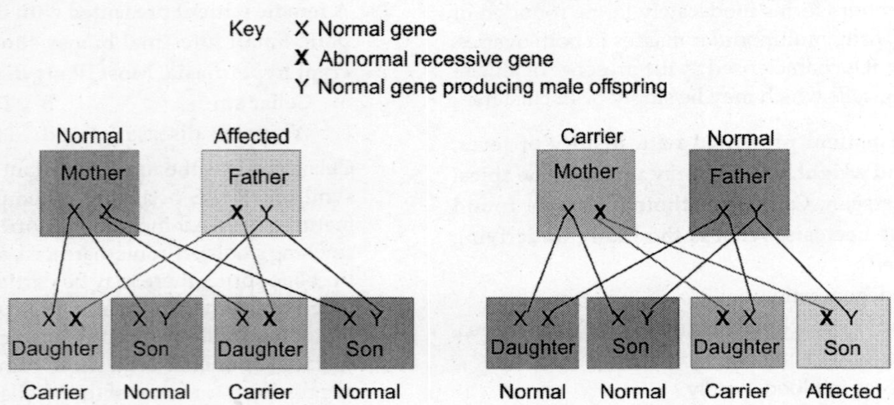

Answers

20. a 21. b 22. a 23. a 24. a

X-linked genetic disorders are conditions caused by a non-working gene on the X-chromosome and manifest in males. Females that have a non-working gene present on one of their X-chromosomes are carriers for that disorder. Carrier females usually do not display symptoms because females have two X-chromosomes and only one carries the non-working gene. However, since males have one X-chromosome, inherited from the mother, if a male inherits an X-chromosome harbouring a non-working gene, he will develop the disease (in question, it is mentioned that all the males died because of the disease). Female carriers of an X-linked disorder have a 50% chance to have a son affected with the disease and a 50% chance of an unaffected son. There is a 50% chance with each pregnancy to have asymptomatic "carrier" daughter like themselves, and a 50% chance to have a non-carrier daughter. If a male with an X-linked disorder is able to reproduce, he will pass the non-working gene to all of his daughters who will be carriers. A male cannot pass an X-linked gene to his sons because males always pass their Y-chromosome instead of their X-chromosome to male offspring.

25. A 30-years-old lady presents with an erythematous butterfly rash on her cheeks. Which antibody should be assayed initially for her suspected condition?

a. Anti-Ds DNA
b. Anti-Ro
c. Anti-centromere
d. Anti-mitochondrial

Cutaneous lesions (erythematous eruptions) in systemic lupus erythematosus/SLE include butterfly area on nose and cheek. Antibodies to double-stranded DNA (anti-dsDNA) is the most specific antibodies for SLE, especially in high titres, and is present in 70% cases.

26. A child is born with a single functional copy of a tumour suppressor gene. At the age of 5 years, the remaining normal allele is lost through mutation. As a result, the ability to control the transition from G-1 to S phase of the cell cycle is lost. This mechanism can result in which neoplasm?

a. Retinoblastoma
b. Breast carcinoma
c. Adenocarcinoma of colon
d. Cerebral astrocytoma

Retinoblastoma (RB) gene has been identified as 14 band on the long arm of chromosome 13 (13q 14) and is a 'cancer suppressor' or 'antioncogenic' gene. Deletion or inactivation of both the normal alleles of this protective gene by two mutations (Knudson's two hit hypothesis, 1971) results in occurrence of retinoblastoma.

27. A patient presented with anemia. Peripheral smear of a patient showed feature of thalassemia. Family history is also positive. Investigation needed to establish the diagnosis would be:

a. ESR estimation
b. Blood spherocyte estimation
c. Bone marrow aspiration
d. Hemoglobin electrophoresis

Haemoglobin electrophoresis is confirmatory for the diagnosis of thalassemia and shows increased amounts of HbF, increased amount of HbA_2, and almost complete absence or presence of variable amounts of HbA. The increased level of HbA_2 has not been found in any other haemoglobin abnormality except beta-thalassemia.

28. A 45-years-old female presented with painless supra-clavicular lymphadenopathy. Biopsy revealed binucleated eosinophilic owl eye appearance with floating lymphocytes in empty space, which was CD15 and CD30 positive. Most likely diagnosis:

a. Lymphocyte predominant Hodgkin disease (HD)
b. Nodular sclerosis HD
c. Mixed cellularity HD
d. Lymphocytic depleted HD

Nodular sclerosis is the most frequent type of HD, seen more commonly in women than in men. It is characterised by bands of collagen and lacunar type Reid Sternberg (RS) cells (there is distinctive pericellular halo; cells appear lacunar due to the shrinkage of cytoplasm in formalin-fixed tissue). The nodules between the fibrous septa consist predominantly of lymphocytes and macrophages. RS cells are CD15+ and CD30+.

29. A renal biopsy from a 56-years-old woman with progressive renal failure for the past 3 years shows glomerular and vascular deposition of pink amorphous material. It shows apple green birefringence under polarized light after Congo red staining. These deposits are positive for lambda light chains. Diagnosis:

a. Rheumatoid arthritis
b. Tuberculosis
c. Systemic lupus erythematosus
d. Multiple myeloma

In multiple myeloma, renal failure occurs in about 25% of patients, while renal pathology occurs in 50% of cases. Causes of renal failure in myeloma are hypercalcemia, glomerular deposits of amyloid, hyperuricemia and infiltration of the kidney by myeloma cells. Amyloid deposition occurs primarily in the glomeruli. Amyloid tissue when, stained with Congo red stain and viewed in polarized light, the amyloid tissue characteristically shows apple-green birefringence due to cross-beta-pleated sheet configuration of amyloid fibril.

Answers

25. a **26.** a **27.** d **28.** b **29.** d

30. A 20-years-old female is diagnosed with granulosa cell tumor of the ovary. Which biomarker would be most useful for follow-up of patient?

a. CA 19-9 b. CA-50
c. Inhibin d. Neuron-specific enolase

Granulosa-cell tumors produce inhibin. Since serum inhibin levels reflect the size of the tumor, measurements of inhibin can be used as a marker for primary as well as recurrent disease.

31. A 50-years-old male presented with skin rash and glomerulonephritis. What could be the next investigation?

a. c-ANCA b. HBsAg
c. Anti-HBs d. Anti-HCV

Focal or diffuse necrotizing glomerulonephritis is one of the essential features of clinicopathologic triad of Wegener's granulomatosis. There can be involvement of skin as well. The serum of these patient shows c-ANCA positivity.

32. A 50-years-old patient presented with a lesion in the midline involving the sacrum. It is found to be osteolytic. Most likely diagnosis:

a. Metastatic b. Chordoma
c. Osteosarcoma d. Chondrosarcoma

Chordoma is a slow growing malignant tumour arising from remnants of notochord. Notochord is the primitive axial skeleton which subsequently develops into spine. Chordomas thus occur in the axial skeleton, particularly sacrum and coccyx (50%), spheno-occipital region (35%) and less often in the spine (15%). Radiographically, the tumour usually appears as an osteolytic lesion.

33. There are electron dense deposits in the region of hyalinosis and sclerosis with diffuse loss of foot process seen in electron microscopy, suggest the diagnosis of:

a. Minimal change disease
b. Membranous glomerulonephritis
c. Membrano-proliferative glomerulonephritis
d. Focal segmental glomerulosclerosis

Electron microscopy of focal segmental glomerulosclerosis (focal sclerosis/focal hyalinosis) shows diffuse loss of foot processes as seen in minimal change disease, but, in addition, there are electron-dense deposits in the region of hyalinosis and sclerosis which are believed to be immune complexes.

34. A 20-years-old patient presented with a small firm nodular swelling in wrist joint since 2 years. Swelling was mobile only in one direction. Biopsy of nodule performed showed presence of spindle cells with Verocay bodies. Most likely diagnosis:

a. Lipoma b. Schwannoma
c. Neurilemmoma d. Neuroma

Characteristic Verocay bodies may be seen in schwannoma. These consist of parallel columns of elongated nuclei on either side of a homogenous acellular material.

Answers

30. c **31.** a **32.** b **33.** d **34.** b

5 Pharmacology

1. **A patient on anti-tubercular drug therapy developed tingling sensation on lower limb. Which of the following drug should be used for management?**
   a. Thiamine
   b. Folic acid
   c. Pyridoxine
   d. Vitamin B_{12}

   Isoniazid/INH interferes with the utilization of pyridoxine and increases its urinary excretion, causing pyridoxine deficiency, which manifests as peripheral neuritis and variety of neurological manifestations (paresthesia, numbness, mental disturbances), accounting for most important dose dependent toxic effects of INH.

2. **Which of the following is WRONGLY matched regarding mechanism of action of anti-fungal drugs?**
   a. Azoles inhibit lanosterol-alpha-demethylase thereby preventing ergosterol synthesis
   b. Flucytosine inhibit microtubule synthesis thus preventing mitosis
   c. Echinocandins act by inhibiting beta-1, 3 glucan synthesis
   d. Amphotericin-B binds with ergosterol resulting in disruption of cell membrane

   Flucytosine is a pyrimidine antimetabolite which is inactive as such. After uptake into fungal cells, it is converted into 5-fluorouracil and then to 5-fluorodeoxyuridic acid which is an inhibitor of thymidylate synthesis.

3. **ACE inhibitors are the primary pharmacological treatment for all of the following conditions *except*:**
   a. Congestive heart failure
   b. Hypertension
   c. Diabetic nephropathy
   d. Myocardial infarction

   Though ACE inhibitors may be given after MI to reduce the incidence of heart failure, but ACE inhibitors are not the first drug of choice for MI.

4. **An obese diabetic patient was on metformin monotherapy, but his sugar levels were not well-controlled. He is allergic to sulpha drugs and does not comply to injectables. He has history of pancreatitis and family history of bladder carcinoma. In view of the raised glucose levels, which other anti-diabetic drug should be added?**
   a. Liraglutide
   b. Sitagliptin
   c. Canagliflozin
   d. Pioglitazone

   Practically all the glucose filtered at the glomerulus is reabsorbed in the proximal tubules. The major transporter which accomplishes this is SGLT2, whose inhibition induces glucosuria and lowers blood glucose in type 2 DM, as well causes weight loss. Members of this group are dapagliflozin and canagliflozin.

5. **A medical student presented with protracted vomiting. For this, he was given an anti-emetic following which he developed abnormal posturing. Which drug is responsible?**
   a. Metoclopramide
   b. Ondansetron
   c. Domperidone
   d. Pantoprazole

   Extrapyramidal side effects of metoclopramide include dystonia. This is because of blockade of central D2 receptors.

6. **A patient with infertility was prescribed bromocriptine by the gynecologist. What could be the cause?**
   a. Hypogonadotropic hypogonadism
   b. Premature ovarian failure
   c. Hyperprolactinemia
   d. Polycystic ovarian syndrome

   Bromocriptine and cabergoline are the first line of drug for most cases of hyperprolactinemia (due to microprolactinoma) presenting as galactorrhoea, amenorrhoea and infertility in women; gynecomastia, impotence and sterility in men.

7. **Which of the following drug is NOT used in detoxification of chronic alcoholics?**
   a. Flumazenil
   b. Disulfiram
   c. Acamprosate
   d. Naltrexone

   Therapeutic effects of flumazenil include benzodiazepine overdose and reversal of effects of benzodiazepines.

Answers

1. c	2. b	3. d	4. c	5. a	6. c	7. a

8. Which of the following is commonly used in the treatment of cancer-associated thrombo-embolism?

a. Low molecular weight heparin
b. Antithrombin III inhibitors
c. Direct Xa inhibitors
d. Warfarin

Heparin is used for immediate anticoagulation for MI, deep venous thrombosis, stroke and pulmonary thrombo-embolism. Low molecular weight heparin is more commonly used instead of unfractionated heparin, because it inhibits only factor Xa.

9. A patient is on indinavir, lamivudine and ketoconazole. He developed breast hypertrophy, nephrolithiasis, hyper-lipidemia and central obesity. Identify the responsible drug:

a. Lamivudine
b. Indinavir
c. Ketoconazole
d. Nevirapine

Adverse effects of indinavir include nephrolithiasis and cholelithiasis.

10. Manufacturer of a drug company labels that the drug contains 500 mg of paracetamol. On analysis, it was found to contain only 200 mg of drug. Such a drug is known as:

a. Orphan drug
b. Counterfeit drug
c. Spurious drug
d. Unethical drug

A counterfeit medicine is one which is deliberately and fraudently mislabeled with respect to identity and/or source. Counterfeiting can apply to both branded and generic products and counterfeit products and may include products with the correct ingredients, wrong ingredients, without active ingredients, with insufficient quantity of active ingredients or with fake packaging.

11. A patient developed acute biliary colic for which an analgesic was given. But this drug increased the severity of the pain. Which analgesic drug was administered?

a. Nefopam
b. Morphine
c. Diclofenac
d. Paracetamol

Morphine can worsen the biliary colic as it causes spasm of sphincter of Oddi (biliary sphincter) and can cause acute rise in intra-biliary pressure. So, morphine should be used cautiously in patients with gallbladder and biliary tract dysfunction.

12. A boy was planning to travel by a bus, but he is a known case of motion sickness. Which drug can be given to prevent an episode of motion sickness?

a. Fexofenadine
b. Promethazine
c. Levocetrizine
d. Sumatriptan

Anticholinergic and H_1 antihistaminic drugs are more effective in motion sickness as vestibular apparatus send impulses to brain via cholinergic muscarinic and H_1 histaminic receptors. Among antihistaminics, first generation/old antihistaminics (promethazine) are preferred over second generation antihistaminics (levocetrizine, fexofenadine etc.).

13. A patient on lithium therapy developed hypertension. He was started on thiazides to control hypertension. After few days, he developed coarse tremors and other features indicating lithium toxicity. Most likely mechanism of such a toxicity:

a. Thiazides increase tubular reabsorption of lithium
b. Thiazides potentiated action of lithium
c. Thiazides inhibited metabolism of lithium
d. Thiazides and lithium acts on same receptors

Thiazides (diuretics) promote proximal tubular reabsorption of lithium, as they cause loss of sodium ions. By promoting lithium reabsorption, thiazide may precipitate lithium toxicity.

14. Imipenem, a newer antibiotic with a broad antibacterial spectrum is co-administered with cilastatin. Best reason for combination is:

a. Combination of antibiotics is synergistic against pseudomonas species
b. Cilastatin promotes gastrointestinal absorption of imipenem
c. Cilastatin inhibits beta-lactamase enzyme which degrades imipenem
d. Cilastatin inhibits an enzyme in kidney, which degrades imipenem

Imipenem is hydrolyzed quickly in the brush borders of the proximal convoluted tubule of kidney by the enzyme dehydropeptidase. Since cilastatin inhibits dehydropeptidase, so it is combined with imipenem.

15. Regardless of the symptoms, antiretrovial therapy should be initiated in a HIV patient, if the CD_4 count falls below:

a. 100
b. 200
c. 300
d. 400

When the CD_4 count is below 200 cells/mm^3, it is an urgency to initiate anti-retroviral therapy.

16. Which of the following is helpful in obtaining variation in sensitivity of response to different doses of a drug in different individuals?

a. Phase I of clinical trials
b. Bioavailability
c. Dose-response curve
d. Therapeutic window phenomenon

Dose response curve (DRC) in studying the linear relationship between the dose and the response.

Answers

8. a	9. b	10. b	11. b	12. b	13. a	14. d
15. b	16. c					

17. **Which of the following anti-retroviral drug is antagonist of both CC-chemokine receptor type 2 (CCR2) and CC-chemokine receptor type 5 (CCR5)?**

a. Maraviroc b. Cenicriviroc
c. Zidovudine d. Nevirapine

Cenicriviroc, an anti-HIV drug, acts as an entry inhibitor (prevents entry of virus into a human cell) by inhibiting both CCR2 and CCR5 receptors. It is an experimental drug.

18. **Which antibiotic acts by inhibiting protein synthesis by acting at translocation step?**

a. Penicillin b. Erythromycin
c. Aminoglycosides d. Ciprofloxacin

Different steps in protein synthesis include initiation of protein synthesis, elongation and termination of protein synthesis. Elongation of polypeptide chain comprises of formation of peptide bond and translocation. Translocation is inhibited by clindamycin and erythromycin.

19. **Drug which should NEVER be given along with sildenafil:**

a. Danazol b. Dopamine
c. Vasoconstrictors d. Vasodilators

Phospho-di-esterase-5 inhibitors (sildenafil, todafil, vardenafil) should not be taken with vasodilators (like nitrates) as they potentiate the vasodilator action of nitric acid and may cause severe hypotension.

20. **Hyperprolactinemia is maximally caused by which atypical antipsychotic?**

a. Clozapine b. Haloperidol
c. Risperidone d. Olanzapine

Risperidone belongs to the class of atypical antipsychotics. It acts by blocking D_2 activity (dopaminergic). Because of this feature, it has marked extrapyramidal effects. It can also cause hyperprolactinemia.

21. **A known case of schizophrenia is responding well to haloperidol, but later on, he developed symptoms of parkinsonism. Drug of choice to treat this complication:**

a. Anticholinergic b. Bromocriptine
c. Levodopa d. Tolcapone

Haloperidol has high tendency to cause extra-pyramidal effects (drug-induced parkinsonism). Central anti-cholinergics are the only effective drugs for this complication. They act by reducing unbalanced cholinergic activity. Trihexyphenidyl is the usually given drug.

22. **Deficiency of which enzyme results in 5-fluoro-uracil induced mucositis, myelo-suppression and neuro-psychiatric manifestations?**

a. CYP2D7
b. Dihydro-folate reductase
c. Tetra-hydro-folate reductase
d. Dihydro-pyrimidine dehydrogenase

Patients with dihydro-pyrimidine-dehydrogenase deficiency are at increased risk of developing 5-fluoro-uracil related toxicity as this enzyme is the rate limiting step (and initial step) in the breakdown of 5-fluoro-uracil.

23. **Oxybutynin, which is used for urinary incontinence in neurogenic bladder acts on which class of cholinergic receptors?**

a. M_1 cholinergic receptor b. M_2 cholinergic receptor
c. M_3 cholinergic receptor d. M_4 cholinergic receptor

Increased micturition occurs because of cholinergic system mediated relaxation of trigone and stimulation of detrusor muscle. This effect is mediated through M_3 cholinergic receptors. So selective M_3 receptor blockers (in urinary bladder) are valuable in managing urinary incontinence (drugs like oxybutynin, solifenacin etc.)

24. **A known case of chronic asthma is on theophylline. Which antimicrobial drug should NEVER be avoided?**

a. Amoxycillin b. Co-trimoxazole
c. Cefotaxime d. Erythromycin

Metabolism of theophylline is inhibited by enzyme inhibitors like erythromycin and hence toxic level is increased. Thus, the dose of theophylline should be decreased with concomitant use of enzyme inhibitors.

25. **A known case of COPD and type II diabetes underwent a surgery. Postoperatively, he developed urinary retention. Drug used for short-term relief in such a patient:**

a. Tamsulosin b. Bethanecol
c. Methacholine d. Atropine

Because of the presence of chronic obstructive pulmonary disease, case of postoperative urinary retention should be managed with tamsulosin. Postoperative urinary retention is better managed by bethanechol (M_3 muscarinic agonist) but it can result in bronchoconstriction as well because of stimulation of M_3 muscarinic receptors in respiratory system, so it is avoided in a patient with COPD.

26. **During surgery, a patient was administered a nicotinic receptor acting competitive neuromuscular blocker drug. Which drug is indicated to reverse the effect of this drug at the end of operation?**

a. Carbachol b. Physostigmine
c. Neostigmine d. Suxamethonium

Neostigmine is the commonly used drug for reversal of non-depolarizing/competitive neuromuscular drug (physostigmine can also be used) because it increases the concentration of acetylcholine by inhibiting its breakdown by the enzyme cholinesterase. So it antagonizes competitive blockers action.

Answers

17. b	**18.** b	**19.** d	**20.** c	**21.** a	**22.** d	**23.** c
24. d	**25.** a	**26.** d				

27. A known case of rheumatoid arthritis was started on some drug, but he developed blurring of vision and corneal opacity after 2 years of use. Which drug the patient was taking?

a. Methotrexate
b. Amiodarone
c. Chloroquine
d. Sulfasalazine

Corneal deposits and visual loss are few commoner side effects of chloroquine (CQ). Prolonged use of CQ causes retinal damage (Bull's eye retinopathy) and may cause visual loss.

28. A known case of bipolar disorder was taking lithium since 6 months. After keeping fast for few days, she developed seizures, coarse tremors, weakness of limbs and confusion. What investigation should be done?

a. MRI of brain
b. EEG
c. Estimation of serum lithium levels
d. Serum electrolytes estimation

Any factor which causes reduction in glomerular filtration rate (GFR) with cause lithium toxicity, which manifests as seizures, confusion, coarse tremors and weakness of limbs. Reduction in GFR may result from dehydration as seen in fasting conditions.

29. A patient developed tremors, rigidity, bradykinesia and sialorrhea on taking fluphenazine for few weeks. Such a patient is best managed by:

a. Haloperidol
b. Trihexyphenidyl
c. Clozapine
d. Atropine

Fluphenazine use can cause drug-induced parkinsonism which manifests as tremors, bradykinesia, excessive salivation (sialorrhoea) and rigidity. Drug-induced parkinsonism is best managed by central anticholinergics like benzhexol (trihexiphenidyl), benztropine etc.

30. A 50-years-old male with renal failure under renal transplant surgery and was prescribed a nucleotide derivative. Which is the drug of therapeutic importance in this case?

a. Cytarabine
b. Azathioprine
c. Methotrexate
d. 5-fluorouracil

Azathioprine primarily suppresses cell mediated immunity (CMI) and is used mainly in auto-immune disease (rheumatoid arthritis, ulcerative colitis) as well as in organ transplantation.

31. A 54-years-old chronic smoker, who use to smoke around 50 packs per years, presented with lesions suggestive of oral leukoplakia. Which drug can regress the lesions?

a. Alpha-tocopherol
b. Isotretinoin
c. Beta-carotene
d. Selenium

Isotretinoin causes dramatic improvement in acne. It is also effective in the prevention and treatment of skin cancers. Oral leukoplakia, actinic keratoses and other premalignant lesions can be treated, but benefit-risk ratio is not clear.

32. A newborn is having cleft lip, cleft palate and inter-atrial septal defect. Mother took some drug during pregnancy. Which drug it could be?

a. Erythromycin
b. Paracetamol
c. Chloroquine
d. Isotretinoin

Isotretinoin is highly teratogenic; up to 25% exposed fetuses had birth defects—craniofacial, heart and CNS abnormalities (Accutane embryopathy).

33. A patient who was given primaquine, developed dark coloured urine. Likely cause is:

a. Glcose-6-phosphatase deficiency
b. Glucose-6-phosphate-dehydrogenase deficiency
c. Galactose-6-phosphatase deficiency
d. Galactose-6-phosphate dehydrogenase deficiency

The most important toxic potential is dose-related haemolysis, methemoglobinemia, tachypnoea and cyanosis. These are due to the oxidant property of primaquine. Its metabolites are more potent in this regard. However, in normal individual doses <60 mg (base) produces little haemolysis. Those with G-6-PD deficiency are highly sensitive and haemolytic anemia can occur with 15–30 mg/day.

34. A girl on sulphonamides developed abdominal pain and presented to the emergency with seizures. Most likely diagnosis:

a. Acute intermittent porphyria
b. Congenital erythropoietic porphyria
c. Infectious mononucleosis
d. Anaphylaxis

Drugs that lead to increased activity of the hepatic P450 system, such as phenobarbital, sulfonamides, estrogens, and alcohol, are associated with acute intermittent porphyria.

Answers

27. c 28. c 29. b 30. b 31. b 32. d 33. b
34. a

6 Microbiology

1. **A gardener has multiple vesicles on hand and multiple eruptions along the lymphatics. Fungus responsible for such a presentation:**
   a. Sporothrix schenckii
   b. Cladosporium
   c. Histoplasma
   d. Candida

   Sporotrichosis/Rose Gardner's disease is a chronic subcutaneous pyogranulomatous disease caused by a thermally dimorphic fungus, Sporothrix schenkii. Lymphocutaneous type is the most common type of sporotrichosis (80%) and is characterized by nodulo-ulcerative lesions (painless) occurring along the lymphatics.

2. **A 25-years-old male presented with diarrhea for 6 months. On examination, the causative agent was found to be acid fast with 12 micrometer diameter. Most likely agent is:**
   a. Cryptosporidium
   b. Isospora
   c. Cyclospora
   d. Giardia

   Cyclospora Cayetanensis causes prolonged diarrhea with abdominal pain, low-grade fever, and fatigue. The oocytes can be stained by Zeihl-Neelson stain. Oocysts of Cyclospora are acid fast and stain red in color. The oocyst is a non-refractile sphere, measuring 8–10 micrometer in diameter.

3. **A resident doctor sustained a needlestick injury while sampling blood of a patient who is HIV positive. A decision was taken to offer him post-exposure prophylaxis. Which one is the best recommendation?**
   a. Zidovudine + Lamivudine for 4 weeks
   b. Zidovudine + Lamivudine + Nevirapine for 4 weeks
   c. Zidovudine + Lamivudine + Indinavir for 4 weeks
   d. Zidovudine + Stavudine + Nevirapine for 4 weeks

   Expanded regimen (NACO guidelines for post-exposure prophylaxis) is given for 4 weeks. 3 drugs are given (2 NRTI's + 1PI); Zidovudine (300 mg twice a day), Lamivudine (300 mg twice a day) and Indinavir (800 mg thrice a day)/Nelfinavir (750 mg thrice a day).

4. **A 30-years-old patient with CSF leak is presenting with neck rigidity, fever and seizures. What could be the probable infective agent?**
   a. Streptococcus pneumoniae
   b. N. meningitidis
   c. Listeria monocytogenes
   d. E. coli

   Neck rigidity/stiffness, fever and seizures suggest the diagnosis of meningitis. Streptococcus pneumoniae is the leading cause of meningitis in all ages (except in neonates).

5. **When an antigen is administered for the first time to an animal or a human being who has never been exposed to it, the first antibody to develop is:**
   a. IgG type
   b. IgM type
   c. IgA type
   d. IgE type

   IgM is the first antibody to be produced following an infection; represents acute or recent infection. It is also called as primary immune response antibody.

6. **A teacher presents with profuse bloody diarrhoea and fever of 104°F. Many children studying in the same school had similar episodes. Possible organism is:**
   a. Shigella dysenteriae
   b. Staphylococcus aureus
   c. Yersinia
   d. Entamoeba histolytica

   Dysentery phase of shigellosis is characterized by frequent passage of bloody mucopurulent stools with increased tenesmus and abdominal cramps. It is preceded by fever, malaise, anorexia and vomiting. Risk factors for shigellosis include overcrowding, poor hygiene and children less than 5 years. It tends to occur as epidemics in developing countries such as Indian subcontinent and sub-Saharan Africa.

7. **A 14-years-old boy is admitted with history of fever, icterus, conjunctival suffusion and hematuria for 20 days. Which serological test can be of diagnostic utility?**
   a. Widal test
   b. Microscopic agglutination test
   c. Paul Bunnell test
   d. Weil Felix test

   High-grade fever, jaundice and raised liver enzymes, hemorrhages (pulmonary hemorrhage, petechiae and

Answers

1. a **2.** c **3.** c **4.** a **5.** b **6.** a **7.** b

purpura, conjunctival hemorrhage) and raised urea - creatinine suggest the diagnosis of Weil's disease/Hepato-renal-hemorrhagic syndrome. It is caused by Leptospira interrogans. MAT (microscopic agglutination test) detects antibodies against specific serovars of L. interrogans. It is the gold standard method and the reference test for the diagnosis of leptospirosis.

8. A 30-years-old patient presented with history of jaundice for 10 days. His liver function tests showed bilirubin of 10 mg/dL. SGOT/SGPT: 1100/1450 and serum alkaline phosphatase: 240 IU. He was positive for HBsAg. Confirmatory test to establish acute Hepatitis B virus infection:

a. IgM anti-HBc antibody
b. HBeAg
c. HBV DNA PCR
d. HBcAg

Anti-HBc IgM is the first antibody to be elevated following infection. It appears within 1–2 weeks after the appearance of HBsAg and lasts for 3–6 months. Its presence indicates acute hepatitis B infection.

9. A 36-years-old IT professional had a business trip to China where he ate crab. Now after coming back to India, he is having dyspnea, high-grade fever, cough and rusty sputum. Sputum is negative for mycobacterium tuberculosis. Most likely causative organism is:

a. Fasciola hepatica
b. Fasciola buskii
c. Paragonismus westermanii
d. Clonorchis sinensis

Paragonismus westermani is endemic in the Far East – Japan, Korea, Taiwan, China etc. Man acquires infection by eating undercooked crab or cray fish containing metacercariae. Patient presents with cough, chest pain, and hemoptysis. The viscous sputum is speckled with the golden-brown eggs. Chronic cases may resemble pulmonary tuberculosis.

10. A child is presenting with constipation, dilated pupil and ptosis after eating outside food. Most probable cause of food poisoning:

a. Cl. tetani
b. Cl. septicum
c. Cl. perfringenes
d. Cl. botulinum

The manifestations of botulism are due to decreased acetylcholine in cranial nerve and parasympathetic nerve terminals. Common symptoms include diplopia, dysphasia, dysarthria, descending symmetric flaccid paralysis of voluntary muscles, decreased deep tendon reflexes, constipation etc. Food-borne botulism results from consumption of foods contaminated with preformed botulinum toxin (home-made canned food).

11. A diabetic presented with bloody nasal discharge, orbital swelling and pain. Culture of periorbital pus showed broad aseptate hyphae. Which is the most probable organism?

a. Mucor
b. Candida
c. Aspergillus
d. Rhizopus

Diabetic ketoacidosis is the most important risk factor for development of mucormycosis. Acidosis causes release of iron from the sequestered proteins in serum. Most common form of mucormycosis is rhinocerebral mucormycosis; starts as eye and facial pain, may progress to cause orbital cellulitis, proptosis and vision loss. Histopathological staining of tissue biopsies shows broad aseptate hyaline hyphae with wide angle branching.

12. A 24-years-old AIDS patient develops chronic abdominal pain, low-grade fever, diarrhoea and malabsorption. Oocysts were demonstrated in stool. Likely cause of his diarrhea:

a. E. histolytica
b. G. lamblia
c. Microsporodia
d. Isospora belli

Infection with Isospora belli results in abdominal discomfort, mild fever, diarrhoea, and malabsorption. The diarrhoea is usually watery and does not contain blood or pus and is self-limiting. However, protracted diarrhoea, lasting for several years can be seen in immunocompromised persons, particularly in the human immunodeficiency virus (HIV) infected. The staining technique used are modified Ziehl-Neelsen stain or Kinyoun acid fast staining of stool smear. In these methods, pink colored acid-fast large oocyst (>25 micrometers) can be demonstrated.

13. A patient presented to the hospital with severe hydrophobia. You suspect rabies and obtain corneal scrapings from the patient. What test should be done on this specimen for diagnosing rabies?

a. RT-PCR for rabies virus
b. Negri bodies
c. Antibodies to rabies virus
d. Indirect immunofluorescence

Reverse transcription-polymerase chain reaction (RT-PCR) can be used to amplify genes of rabies virus RNA from the brain tissue. It is the most sensitive and specific assay available at present for the diagnosis of rabies.

14. A 48-years-old woman develops fever and focal neurological signs. MRI shows a left temporal lobe lesion. Most appropriate test that can be used to confirm the diagnosis of HSV encephalitis in this patient is:

a. Brain biopsy
b. Tzanck smear
c. PCR assay for viral DNA in CSF
d. Serum IgM antibody detection

Answers

8. a **9.** c **10.** d **11.** a **12.** d **13.** a **14.** c

Polymerase chain reaction (PCR) is the most sensitive test for detecting HSV infections and can be used to differentiate between HSV-1 AND HSV-2.

15. Serological testing of patient shows HBsAg, IgM anti-HBc and HBeAg positive. The patient has:

a. Chronic hepatitis B with low infectivity
b. Acute hepatitis B infection with high infectivity
c. Chronic hepatitis with high infectivity
d. Acute on chronic hepatitis B infection

Acute hepatitis B infection with high infectivity is indicated by HBsAg positive, IgM anti-HBc positive and HBeAg positive tests.

16. A 25-years-old sexually active woman presented with purulent vaginal discharge and dysuria for 7 days after an unprotected sexual intercourse with a new partner. Most sensitive investigation to determine the etiological agent:

a. A polymerase chain reaction for nucleic acids
b. An enzyme immunoassay
c. Gram stain
d. Culture on selective medium

Non-gonococcal urethritis/NGU is characterized by mucopurulent discharge followed by dysuria and urethral irritation. Chlamydia trachomatis is the most common cause of NGU, responsible for 30–50% of cases of NGU. Nucleic acid amplification test (NAAT) has revolutionized the diagnosis of chlamydial infections. Various methods available (for NAAT) are polymerase chain reaction (PCR), ligase chain reaction (LCR), transcription mediated amplification (TMA) and strand displacement assay (SDA).

17. A patient of acute lymphocytic leukemia with fever and neutropenia develops diarrhea after administration of amoxicillin therapy. Likely causative organism:

a. Salmonella typhii
b. Clostridium difficile
c. Clostridium perfringens
d. Shigella flexneri

Clostridium difficile is responsible for a unique colonic disease – pseudomembranous colitis. Clostridium difficile infection is associated with prolonged antimicrobial use. This can result in disruption of the normal colonic flora, which enhances the susceptibility to Clostridium difficile infection. Cephalosporins (e.g., ceftriaxone) are frequently responsible for this condition. Other antibiotics, such as clindamycin, ampicillin and fluoroquinolones (ciprofloxacin) are also implicated in hospital outbreaks.

18. The mechanism by which specific information encoded in a nucleic acid chain in a virus is transferred to mRNA is known as?

a. Transcription
b. Transversion
c. Transformation
d. Transduction

Transcription is the process of making a RNA copy of a gene sequence. This copy, called a messenger RNA (mRNA) molecule, leaves the cell nucleus and enters the cytoplasm, where it directs the synthesis of the protein, which it encodes.

19. A chest physician performs bronchoscopy in the procedure room of the out-patient department. To make the instrument safe for use in the next patient waiting outside, the most appropriate method to disinfect the endoscope is by:

a. 70% alcohol for 5 minutes
b. 2% glutaraldehyde for 20 minutes
c. 2% formaldehyde for 10 minutes
d. 1% sodium hypochlorite for 15 minutes

Glutaraldehyde is less toxic, less irritant and less corrosive; hence is best used to sterilize hospital and laboratory equipment, such as endoscopes and cystoscopes. It is used as 2% concentration (2% Cidex). It usually disinfects objects within 20 minutes but may require as long as 12 hours to kill spores.

20. In tuberculosis, the cytokine playing major role in the conversion of tissue macrophages into epithelioid cells is:

a. Interferon gamma
b. Tumour necrosis factor
c. Interleukin 12
d. Macrophage chemoattractant protein

Interferon-gamma activates the resting alveolar macrophages into activated macrophages which are capable of killing and digesting tubercle bacilli. These activated macrophages aggregate around the center of the lesion and form characteristic granuloma called tubercles.

21. A 22-years-old male presented with history of fever, sore throat and enlarged neck lymph nodes. He was ordered a Paul-Bunnell test with a suspicion of infectious mononucleosis. What is the immunological basis behind the use of this test?

a. Heterophile antibody test
b. Complement mediated agglutination reaction
c. Homophile antibody test
d. Latex agglutination test

Paul-Bunnell test (for infectious mononucleosis) is a tube agglutination test that uses RBCs sheep to detect heterophile antibodies in patient's serum.

22. A person presents with pneumonia. His sputum was sent for culture. The bacterium obtained was gram-positive cocci in chains and alpha hemolytic colonies on sheep agar. Antibiotic utilized for confirming diagnosis:

a. Novobiocin
b. Optochin
c. Bacitracin
d. Oxacillin

Answers

15. b **16.** a **17.** b **18.** a **19.** b **20.** a **21.** a
22. b

Streptococcus pneumoniae (commonly referred to as pneumococcus; a gram-positive cocci) is the leading cause of lobar pneumonia, otitis media in children and meningitis in all ages. They are alpha hemolytic and may present as commensals in human upper respiratory tract. They differ from alpha hemolytic viridans streptococci in many ways such as their shape (lanceolate-shaped diplococci), bile solubility, optochin sensitivity and presence of polysaccharide capsule.

23. A 20-years-old male presents to the STD clinic with a genital ulcer. The gram stain of the smear from ulcer shows gram-negative coccobacilli. Most appropriate media for culture would be:

a. Thayer-Martin media
b. Blood agar with X & V factors
c. Chocolate agar with isovitalex
d. Tellurite blood agar

Hemophilus ducreyi is a pleomorphic gram-negative coccobacillus; occurs in groups or in parallel chains. It is an etiologic agent of chancroid (or soft chancre), a sexually transmitted disease characterized by painful genital ulceration that bleeds easily. H. ducreyi requires factor X (hemin), but not factor V for its growth. Primary isolation is difficult. It can be grown on rabbit blood agar or chocolate agar enriched with 1% isovitalex and made selective by adding vancomycin.

24. A farmer presenting with fever off and on for the past 4 years was diagnosed to be suffering from chronic brucellosis. Which of the following serological test would NOT help in making a diagnosis?

a. Standard agglutination test
b. 2-Mercapto-ethanol test
c. Complement fixation test
d. Coomb's test

As isolation of Brucella is difficult, serological tests are of paramount importance in diagnosis of brucellosis. Several tests have been developed, such as standard agglutination test, 2-mercaptoethanol (2ME) agglutination test, complement fixation test and ELISA.

25. A patient is having pneumonia. Sputum examination is showing gram-positive branched organism which is strict aerobe and partial acid fast. Most likely organism:

a. Nocardia
b. Actinomycetes
c. Mycobacterium tuberculosis
d. Pneumococcus

Nocardia species (named after Edmond Nocard, 1898) are gram-positive branching filamentous bacilli similar to Actinomyces; however, they differ from the later by being aerobic and acid fast. Lobar pneumonia is the most common form of pulmonary nocardiosis, characterized by subacute onset of cough with thick, purulent sputum.

26. A 15-years-old girl was admitted to the infectious disease hospital with a provisional diagnosis of rabies. The most suitable clinical sample that can confirm the antemortem diagnosis is:

a. Serum for anti-rabies IgG antibody
b. Corneal impression smear for immunofluorescence
c. CSF sample for viral culture
d. Giemsa stain on smear prepared from salivary secretions

Direct immunofluorescence test (direct-IF) can be performed to detect rabies nucleoprotein antigens in specimens by using specific monoclonal antibodies tagged with fluorescein dye. The best specimen is hair follicle of nape of neck (most sensitive). Corneal impression smear can also be used. It is usually positive in late stage with a sensitivity of 30%.

27. Gonococci can be differentiated by meningococci by following sugar fermentation test:

a. Glucose
b. Sucrose
c. Mannitol
d. Maltose

Neisseria meningitidis ferment both glucose and maltose whereas Neisseria gonorrhoeae ferments only glucose.

28. A 30-years-old male presented with subcutaneous itchy nodules over the left iliac crest. On examination, they are firm, non-tender and mobile. Skin scrapings contains microfilariae and adult worms of:

a. Loa loa
b. Onchocerca volvulus
c. Brugia malayi
d. Mansonella persutans

The subcutaneous nodule or onchocercoma is a circumscribed, firm, non-tender tumor, formed as a result of fibroblastic reaction around the worms. They tend to occur over anatomical sites where the bones are superficial, such as scalp, scapulae, ribs, elbows, iliac crest, sacrum, and knees. The nodules are painless and cause no trouble except for their unsightly appearance.

29. Gram-stained peri-orbital exudates in a severe pan-ophthalmitis with cellulitis in an elderly diabetic shows irregular branching, aseptate and broad hyphae. Most likely diagnosis:

a. Candida
b. Aspergillus
c. Penicillium
d. Apophysomyces species

Apophysomyces elegans and Apophysomyces trapeziformis are able to cause mucormycosis, in humans, which is often fatal but very rare. Most common form of mucormycosis is rhinocerebral mucormycosis; starts as eye and facial pain, may progress to cause orbital cellulitis, proptosis and vision loss. Histopathological staining of tissue biopsies shows broad aseptate hyaline hyphae with wide angle branching.

Answers

23. c 24. d 25. a 26. b 27. d 28. b 29. d

30. A Veterinary doctor had pyrexia of unknown origin. His blood culture in special laboratory media was positive for gram-negative short bacilli which was oxidase positive. Most likely organism grown in culture is:

a. Pasteurella species
b. Francisella species
c. Bartonella species
d. Brucella species

Brucella is an obligate aerobic, fastidious, non-sporing, non-motile, non-capsulated small gram-negative coccobacillus, responsible for highly contagious febrile illness called brucellosis. Classic triad of brucellosis include fever with profuse sweats, arthralgia/arthritis and hepatosplenomegaly. Brucella do not ferment carbohydrates, is catalase positive and oxidase positive (except some strains of Bacillus abortus, Bacillus neotomae and Brucella ovis).

31. A person returns to Delhi from Bangladesh. After 2 days he had diarrhea. Stool examination shows RBC's in stools. Likely causative organism:

a. Enteropathogenic E. coli
b. Enterotoxigenic E. coli
c. Salmonella typhi
d. Shigella dysenteriae

Dysentery phase of shigellosis is characterized by frequent passage of bloody mucopurulent stools with increased tenesmus and abdominal cramps. It is preceded by fever, malaise, anorexia and vomiting. Risk factors for shigellosis include overcrowding, poor hygiene and children less than 5 years. It tends to occur as epidemics in developing countries such as Indian subcontinent and sub-Saharan Africa. Wet mount preparation of feces shows large number of pus cells, erythrocytes and macrophages.

32. During the window period of patient with AIDS, best diagnostic test is:

a. ELISA
b. Western Blot
c. Rapid test
d. RT-PCR

Polymerase chain reaction detecting proviral DNA is extremely useful for diagnosing of paediatric HIV and to differentiate latent HIV infection from active viral transcription. It is also useful during the window period, viral estimation (real time PCR) and detection of genotypes.

33. A 50-years-old male has fever for the past 1 week with abdominal distension and loss of appetite. It is not responding to antibiotics and antimalarials. Widal test is negative but RK39 dipstick test is positive. Which drug can be used in such a patient?

a. Bedaquilline
b. Linezolid
c. Fluconazole
d. Liposomal Amphotericin-B

The onset of Kala-azar is insidious. The clinical illness begins with fever, splenomegaly and hepatomegaly. A specific rapid immune-chromatographic dipstick (ICT) method for antibody has been developed using a recombinant leishmania antigen rk39 consisting of 39 amino acids conserved in kinesin region of Leishmania infantum. The sensitivity of the test is 98% and specificity of 90%. Liposomal amphotericin-B has been developed and used extensively to treat visceral leishmaniasis in all parts of the world.

34. A patient comes to your clinic with complaints of multiple episodes of loose watery stool for 3 days. On probing, you discover that these episodes starting after ingestion of shellfish in a restaurant, 3 days back. Other people who had food from that restaurant had similar symptoms. Most common cause of such viral diarrhea:

a. Adenovirus
b. Calcivirus
c. Rotavirus
d. Norovirus

Ingestion of shellfish that have not been sufficiently heated—under 75°C (167°F)—poses a high risk for norovirus infection. Norovirus infection is characterized by nausea, vomiting, watery diarrhoea, abdominal pain, and in some cases, loss of taste. A person usually develops symptoms of gastroenteritis 12 to 48 hours after being exposed to norovirus.

Answers

30. d 31. d 32. d 33. d 34. d

7 Forensic Medicine

1. **A MBBS doctor referred a patient to a radiologist for chest X-ray. In turn, MBBS doctor received a cheque from radiologist. This is referred to as:**
   a. Medical dichotomy
   b. Conduct money
   c. Vicarious liability
   d. Criminal negligence

   Dichotomy is an unethical act. It defines that a physician shall not give solicit, or receive nor shall he offer to give, solicit or receive any gift, gratuity, commission or bonus in consideration of, or return for the referring, recommending or procuring any patient for medical, surgical or other treatment.

2. **Excessive sexual desire in male is known as:**
   a. Sadism b. Transvestism
   c. Nymphomania d. Satyriasis

   Lack of sexual power is common in those suffering from paranoia, tabes dorsalis and general paralysis of the insane. Occasionally, the reverse effect, i.e., satyriasis or excessive sexual desire is seen.

3. **King cobra venom is:**
   a. Hemolytic b. Neurotoxic
   c. Myotoxic d. Cardiotoxic

   Ptosis is the earliest neuro-paralytic manifestation of cobra venom, followed by ophthalmoplegia. There may be extraocular muscle weakness and strabismus. Weakness of the muscles increases, and develops into paralysis of the lower limbs.

4. **Lucid interval is seen in:**
   a. Extradural hemorrhage
   b. Subdural hemorrhage
   c. Subarachnoid hemorrhage
   d. Pontine hemorrhage

   Immediate unconsciousness occurs due to concussion, then the person slowly recovers consciousness and again loses consciousness gradually due to compression. A so called 'lucid interval' thus intervenes between the two stages of unconsciousness.

5. **A young male farmer presented with the complain of excessive sweating following consumption of some unknown poison. On examination, there is bradycardia and hypotension. Treatment is by:**
   a. Acetylcholine
   b. Atropine
   c. Edrophonium
   d. Dexamethasone

   Clinical findings suggest the diagnosis of organophosphate poisoning. Atropine sulfate is given, which arrests the muscarinic effects of post-ganglionic parasympathetic (peripheral) activity (muscarinic receptor antagonist) and arrests CNS effects. Edrophonium, physostigmine and succinylcholine are avoided.

6. **Headache, behavioural changes, schizophrenia like psychosis, visual hallucination and paranoid symptoms are seen in intoxication of:**
   a. Cocaine b. Alcohol
   c. Amphetamines d. Cannabis

   Acute intoxication of amphetamine causes paranoid hallucinatory syndrome which closely mimics paranoid schizophrenia. There may be auditory or visual hallucinations in a setting of clear consciousness.

7. **A verbal statement recorded by the magistrate without any oath, by an assaulted person narrating the sequence of events responsible for his/ her condition is known as:**
   a. Dying declaration
   b. Dying deposition
   c. Summon
   d. Inquest

   Dying declaration can be recorded by anyone (doctor, police, magistrate etc.). Oath is not administered as it is believed that a dying person would not lie.

8. **A 45-years-old lady attended the skin OPD with photosensitive lesion on malar area of the face. The type of consent given for examination of face, in such a case is:**
   a. Informed consent b. Implied consent
   c. Expressed content d. Written consent

Answers

1. a	**2.** d	**3.** b	**4.** a	**5.** b	**6.** c	**7.** a
8. b						

Implied consent means consent is presumed be there. If a patient has come to the doctor for treatment, it is presumed that he has given consent for routine physical examination (inspection, palpation, percussion and auscultation).

9. **A child complains of pain in the anal region after being sodomized. Anal swabs were taken and treated with a card to obtain yellow crystals. Such a test is known as:**
   a. Hensley test b. Acid phosphatase test
   c. Barberio's test d. Florence test

   In Barberio's test, yellow needle-shaped rhombic crystals of spermine picrate are formed, when a saturated aqueous or alcoholic solution of picric acid is added to spermatic fluid.

10. **A patient is dependent on cocaine. He is consistently scratching skin and have scratch marks on skin. This phenomenon is known as:**
    a. Withdrawl phenomenon b. Locard's principle
    c. Uthoff phenomenon d. Magnan's phenomenon

    A patient with chronic overuse of cocaine presents with persecutory delusions and tactile hallucinations (formication). Tactile hallucinations are manifested as bugs crawling under the skin (cocaine bugs/ Magnan's symptoms).

11. **A person was brought for autopsy. His relatives said that he has tattoo marks but no tattoo marks were visible. Which site should be explored to confirm the presence of tattoo?**
    a. Spleen b. Lymph nodes
    c. Brain d. Liver

    Lymph nodes near tattoo marks shows pigment deposition as the pigment from tattoo goes to the draining lymph node of that area, where tattoo was made. So microscopic examination of lymph node would help in detection of tattoo pigment.

12. **In the court of law, willful utterance of falsehood while under oath, the witness is liable to be persecuted for perjury, with extension of imprisonment up to 7 years. Which IPC defines this:**
    a. IPC 191 b. IPC 192
    c. IPC 193 d. IPC 194

    Section 193 IPC defines the punishment for false evidence (perjury), which includes fine and imprisonment up to 7 years.

13. **Nothing is an offence, which is done by a person who, at the time of doing it, by reason of unsoundness of mind, is incapable of knowing the nature of the act, or that he is doing, what is either wrong or contrary to law. This is defined as:**
    a. Durham's law b. McNaughten's law
    c. Curren's law d. Locard's principle

    Section 84, IPC states that an accused person is not legally responsible for that act, if it is clearly proved that at the time of committing the act, the person has such an abnormality of the mind, that he did not know the nature and quality of the act he was doing, or that what ever he is doing, is wrong.

14. **A 14-years-old rape victim with 22 weeks of gestation comes to the hospital. All of the following can be done *except*:**
    a. No need to collect vaginal swab
    b. Male doctor can examine her with a female attendant
    c. Urine pregnancy test not required
    d. Doctor can abort the fetus if the patient request so

    In case of minor (<18 years of age), written consent of guardian is required before performing abortion. Minor's consent holds no validity.

15. **An adult came to casualty with complaints of rapid heart rate. On examination, everything else was normal except for episodic tachycardia and occasional extra-systole and amblyopia. What could be the reason?**
    a. Cannabis b. Nicotine
    c. Atropine d. Cocaine

    Features of chronic nicotine poisoning include amblyopia, blindness, irregularity of the heart rate with extra-systoles etc.

16. **A 70-years-old male presents with amblyopia, external chest pain, episodic tachycardia and extra-systoles on ECG. What is the cause?**
    a. Cocaine poisoning
    b. Arsenophagia
    c. Cannabis ingestion
    d. Chronic nicotine poisoning

    In chronic nicotine poisoning, there may be occasional attacks of chest pain suggestive angina pectoris.

17. **A 19-years-old patient presented to the emergency with altered sensorium. A non-contrast CT revealed hydrocephalus, requiring urgent neurosurgical intervention. But there was no attendant with the patient. Neurosurgeon can perform surgery without taking informed consent from a guarding as per:**
    a. Sec 302 IPC b. Sec 193 IPC
    c. Sec 87 IPC d. Sec 92 IPC

    Section 92 IPC states that any harm caused to a person in good faith, even without the person's consent is not an offence if the circumstances were such that it was impossible

Answers

9. c	10. d	11. b	12. c	13. b	14. d	15. b
16. d	17. d					

to obtain consent of the person or his lawful guardian at the time, that thing has to be done for the benefit of the patient.

18. A doctor gave some injection to a HIV patient. The same needle was used again in another patient, resulting in HIV infection in that patient too. Doctor is punishable for negligence under:

a. Sec 302 IPC
b. Sec 195 IPC
c. Sec 307 IPC
d. Sec 269 IPC

Section 269 IPC deals with negligent act likely to spread the infection or disease so as to endanger life.

19. A 40-years-old female presented to the emergency with extensive burns. Patient had grade III burns on face, neck, back, upper arms and forearms with singeing of hairs. Which is NOT a proof of inhalational burns?

a. Black colored soot deposition on posterior part of the tongue
b. Hoarseness and stridor of voice
c. Singeing of eyebrows and facial hairs
d. Yellow coloured sputum

In cases of burn injury, there is no yellow-coloured sputum production. Blackish coal particles are embedded in frothy mucus which covers the congested mucosa.

20. A patient presented to the emergency with overdose of some drug. There was increased salivation and increased bronchial secretions. On examination, the blood pressure was 80/60 mm Hg. RBC cholinesterase level is <50% of normal. What should be used in management?

a. Physostigmine
b. Neostigmine
c. Protamine sulphate
d. Atropine

Muscarinic manifestations of organophosphate poisoning include salivation, lacrimation, urination, defecation, gastrointestinal distress and emesis (SLUDGE). There is also increased bronchial secretions. RBC cholinesterase level of less than 50% of normal suggest organophosphate poisoning. Atropine is the drug of choice in organophosphate poisoning and it should be continued until the tracheobronchial tree is cleared of secretions and most secretions are dried.

Answers

18. d	19. d	20. d

8 Preventive and Social Medicine

1. **The sequence of events leading to disability and handicap is:**
   a. Disease → Disability → Impairment → Handicap
   b. Disease → Impairment → Disability → Handicap
   c. Disease → Handicap → Impairment → Disability
   d. Disease → Disability → Handicap → Impairment

   Sequence of events leading to disability and handicap: Disease → Impairment → Disability → Handicap

2. **Which one of the following statements is NOT true for taking a decision on screening for disease?**
   a. Disease prevalence should be high
   b. Disease is lethal
   c. Proportion of false negatives is high
   d. Sensitivity and specificity are high

   In a screening test, a proportion of false positive is tolerable but not false negatives.

3. **In a case-control study, 300 women aged 20–45 years suffering from breast cancer were compared with age-matched 300 women without breast cancer. It was observed that 120 women among cases and 60 women among controls were obese. The odds ratio of developing breast cancer among obese women is:**
   a. 9/5
   b. 11/5
   c. 8/3
   d. 11/3

   Odd's ratio:

Obesity (Exposure)	Cases	Controls
Yes	120 (a)	60 (b)
No	180 (c)	240 (d)
Total	300 (a+c)	300 (b+d)

   Odd's ratio (Cross product ratio): ad/bc
   120 × 240/60 × 180 = 8/3

4. **In a family of six (2 parents and 4 children), the youngest child catches measles infection. The parents are immune to the infection. On 3rd and 5th day of the infection of the first child, the two other children also suffer from measles. The secondary attack rate (SAR) of measles is:**
   a. 33.3%
   b. 40%
   c. 50%
   d. 66.6%

   SAR: Number of exposed persons developing the disease × 100/Total number of exposed/susceptible persons.

   In this case, 2 children had developed the disease out of the total number of exposed/susceptible 3 children. The one child, who have the disease would not be counted in numerator or denominator. Parents are immune so they are not susceptible. So, SAR would be: 2 × 100/3

5. **What is the relative risk of developing pulmonary embolism in users of oral contraceptives as per the information given below?**

Women using OCs	Pulmonary embolism: Yes	Pulmonary embolism: No	Total
Yes	120 (a)	80 (b)	200 (a+b)
No	10 (c)	70 (d)	80 (c+d)
Total	130	150	280

   a. 0.48
   b. 4.80
   c. 2.40
   d. 0.24

   Incidence among exposed: a/a + b = 120/200 = 600
   Incidence among non-exposed: c/c + d = 10/80 = 125
   Relative risk: Incidence among exposed/Incidence among nonexposed = 600/125 = 4.80

6. **Which one of the following epidemiologic methods can be used to identify risk factors and estimate the degree of risk?**
   a. Cohort study and Randomized control trial
   b. Case control and Cross-sectional studies
   c. Case control and Cohort studies
   d. Cohort study and Ecological studies

   From case-control study and cohort study, one can show whether any association exists between the suspected factor and the disease of the hypothesis. If so, what is the strength

Answers

1. b **2.** c **3.** c **4.** d **5.** b **6.** c

of the association between the suspected factor and the disease under study.

7. **In a population of 5000, there are 19% eligible couples. To achieve a couple protection rate (CPR) of 60%, how many of these should be covered for family planning services?**
   a. 530 b. 550
   c. 570 d. 590

In this MCQ, 19% (eligible couple) of total population (5000) is 950. 60% (Couple protection rate) of the total eligible couples (950) comes out to be 570.

8. **An adult weighs 73 kg and has a height of 1.75 meter. For the purpose of classification of overweight and obesity as per WHO recommendation, this person will be classified as:**
   a. Underweight b. Normal
   c. Pre-obese d. Overweight

BMI = Weight in kilograms/(height in meter)^2 = 73/(1.75)^2 = 23.85. Normal BMI is 18.5 to 24.9

9. **A village 'X' has a population of 5000 with a birth rate of 25 per thousand. In any given month, how many pregnancies should be registered with the ANM of this village?**
   a. 66 b. 67
   c. 68 d. 69

Birth rate = 25/1000 population
Population = 5000
Therefore, expected number of live births = Birth rate × Population/1000 = (25 × 5000)/1000 = 125 births
Correction factor (pregnancy wastage) = 10% of expected number of live births = 10% of 125 (i.e. [10/100] × 125) = 13
As a thumb rule, in any given month, approximately half the number of pregnancies estimated above should be in ANMs records.
Therefore, total no. of expected pregnancies in a year = 125 + 13 = 138
The ANM should have about 69 pregnancies registered with her

10. **In India, for providing HIV treatment services Link ART Centres are situated at:**
    a. Select medical colleges
    b. Medical colleges and district level hospitals
    c. Sub-district level hospitals and Community Health Centres
    d. Primary Health Centres

The ART (anti-retroviral therapy) services are presently being rolled out through ART centres located mainly in medical colleges, tertiary hospitals and district hospitals. As the antiretroviral treatment is a lifelong therapy and drugs are generally provided once in a month, the frequent visits lead to inconvenience, long travel distance and cost to the patients. This may lead to sub-optimal drug adherence and risk of early drug resistance. Hence, in order to make the treatment services easily accessible to PLHIV (people living with HIV), it was decided to set up Link ART centres at ICTCs (Integrated Counselling and Testing Centers) in the district/sub-district level hospitals/CHCs nearer to the patient's residence. These centers are linked to a Nodal ART centre and function as its outreach units.

11. **Which one of the following statements regarding predictive value of a positive test is true?**
    a. It does not tell about diagnostic power of test
    b. The more prevalent the disease, the less accurate the test is
    c. It tells the probability that a patient with positive test has the disease in question
    d. It tells the probability that a patient with positive test does not have the disease in question

Positive predictive value is the probability that subjects with a positive screening test truly have the disease. Negative predictive value is the probability that subjects with a negative screening test truly do not have the disease.

12. **Flattening of the growth curve in the growth chart signifies:**
    a. Child is on a healthy path
    b. Child is severely malnourished
    c. Child is showing signs of growth failure
    d. Child does not need special care

Abnormal flattening or falling of child weight's curve signals growth failure which is an early indicator of PEM (protein energy malnutrition).

13. **What is the relative risk of developing tuberculosis among tobacco users as per the information given below?**

	Tuberculosis		
Tobacco user	*Yes*	*No*	*Total*
Yes	40	80	120
No	10	70	80
Total	50	150	200

    a. 0.48 b. 1.33
    c. 2.67 d. 3.90

Relative risk/risk ratio is the ratio of incidence of the disease among exposed and the incidence of the disease among unexposed (RR = IE/IO)
IE is calculated as number of subjects developing the disease out of the total exposed.
IE = 40/120 = 0.333
IO is calculated as number of subjects developing the disease out of the total un-exposed.

Answers

7. c	8. b	9. d	10. c	11. c	12. c	13. c

IO = 10/80 = 0.125
RR = 0.333/0.125 = 2.664

14. What is the attributable risk of tobacco for developing tuberculosis as per the information given below?

	Tuberculosis		
Tobacco users	*Present*	*Absent*	*Total*
Yes	40	80	120
No	10	70	80
Total	50	150	200

a. 50.5%
b. 62.5%
c. 70.6%
d. 80.6%

Attributable risk (AR) is the ratio of risk difference (RD) and the incidence of the disease among exposed, often expressed as percentage.

AR = RD/IE

RD = IE – IO

IE (Incidence in exposed) is calculated as number of subjects developing the disease out of the total exposed.
IE = 40/120 = 0.333

IO (Incidence in unexposed) is calculated as number of subjects developing the disease out of the total unexposed.

IO = 10/80 = 0.125

RD = IE – IO = 0.208

AR = 0.208/0.333 = 62.46%

15. What is the sensitivity of EEG for detecting brain tumours as per the information given below:

	Brain tumour	
EEG result	Absent	Present
Positive	54,000	36
Negative	3,06,000	4
	3,60,000	40

a. 90%
b. 85%
c. 0.07%
d. 99.99%

Sensitivity is the ability of a test to correctly identify those having the disease, i.e., true positives (% of the disease persons, showing the test result positive).

Sensitivity = a × 100/a+c

Where a is number of patients showing positive test in the presence of disease and c is number of patients showing test negative in the presence of disease (so a + c is the total number of the subjects with disease).

Sensitivity = 36000/40 = 90%

16. A cohort study was conducted among 200 men aged 20–30 years in Rampur village. Out of 200, 120 men were tobacco users and rest 80 did not take any form of tobacco. At the end of one year, 40 men among tobacco users and 10 men among non-tobacco users developed tuberculosis. The incidence of tuberculosis among tobacco users is:

a. 12.5 per 100 men/year
b. 25.0 per 100 men/year
c. 30.0 per 100 men/year
d. 33.3 per 100 men/year

Incidence rate of the disease among exposed =

Number of persons developing the disease after exposure a × 1000/Total number of persons exposed/at risk (a + b)

Incidence among tobacco users = 40 × 1000/120 = 33.3 per 100 men/year

17. What constitutes the denominator in 'Total Dependency Ratio'?

a. Population 15–45 years of age
b. Mid-year population
c. Population 15–64 years of age
d. Population less than 14 and more than 65 years of age

The dependency ratio is an age-population ratio of those typically not in the labor force (the dependent part ages 0 to 14 and 65+) and those typically in the labor force (the productive part ages 15 to 64).

18. By which one of the following studies can relative risk be best calculated?

a. Cohort study
b. Correlation study
c. Case-control study
d. Randomised control trial

In cohort study, strength of association is estimated by relative risk and attributable risk.

19. Orthotolidine (OT) test is done for determining residual free chlorine quantitatively and qualitatively. What is the colour of the solution after adding OT which indicates presence of free chlorine:

a. Red
b. Yellow
c. Blue
d. Green

Orthotolidine (OT) test enables total, free and combined chlorine in water to be determined with speed and accuracy. The reagent is 'analytical grade Orthotolidine', dissolved in 10% solution of HCl. When this reagent is added to the water containing chlorine, it turns yellow.

20. The most important indicator for assessment of impact in Salt Iodization Programme is:

a. Testing Iodine content of salt at consumer level
b. Testing Iodine content of salt at production level
c. Testing median urinary Iodine excretion
d. Testing serum Iodine levels

Answers

14. b **15.** a **16.** d **17.** c **18.** a **19.** b **20.** c

The iodization of salt used in households and food processing is the most effective and sustainable strategy for IDD (iodine deficiency disorder) control. The impact of salt iodization programmes is best assessed through the measurement of urinary iodine concentrations (UIC) in populations.

21. These toxic effects like abdominal colic, obstinate constipation, loss of appetite, anaemia, stippling of red cells and blue line on gums are due to exposure to:

a. Carbon monoxide
b. Asbestos
c. Lead
d. Radiation

Chronic lead poisoning usually presents with symptoms affecting multiple systems, but is associated with three main types of symptoms: gastrointestinal, neuromuscular, and neurological. A blue line along the gum with bluish black edging to the teeth, known as a Burton line, is important indication of chronic lead poisoning.

22. As per Biomedical Waste Management Rule 2016 the metallic body implants should be discarded in which of the following?

a. Yellow colored non-chlorinated plastic bag
b. Red colored non-chlorinated plastic bag
c. Card board box with blue colored marking
d. Separate collection system

Categories of biomedical waste schedule – I

Category	*Type of waste*	*Type of bag or container to be used*	*Treatment and disposal option*
Blue	**Glassware**: Broken or discarded and contaminated glass including medicine vials and ampoules except those contaminated with cytotoxic wastes	Cardboard boxes with blue colored marking	Disinfection (by soaking the washed glass waste after cleaning with detergent and Sodium Hypochlorite treatment) or through autoclaving or microwaving or hydro-claving and then sent for recycling.
	Metallic Body Implants		

23. The appropriate statistical test to find out obesity as a significant risk factor for breast cancer is:

a. Student's paired 't' test
b. Student's unpaired 't' test
c. Chi-square test
d. Wilcoxon's signed rank test

The chi-squared test is used to determine whether there is a significant difference between the expected frequencies and the observed frequencies in one or more categories.

24. In a case control study, confounding factors can be minimized by the following *except:*

a. Matching of variables such as age and sex
b. Randomization during selection
c. Stratification during analysis
d. Increasing sample size for cases and controls

Confounding factors can be prevented by use of randomization, restriction, or matching. Confounding can also be controlled by adjusting for it after completion of a study using stratification or multivariate analysis.

25. Which one of the following is FALSE regarding confounding factor in epidemiological studies?

a. Associated both with exposure and disease
b. Distributed equally between study and control groups
c. Independent risk factor for disease in question
d. Source of bias is interpretation

Confounding factor can be defined as one which is associated both with exposure and disease, and is distributed unequally in study and control groups.

26. A well of contaminated water resulting in an epidemic of acute watery diarrhoea is a typical example for:

a. Common source, single exposure epidemic
b. Common source, continuous exposure epidemic
c. Slow epidemic
d. Propagated epidemic

In common source, single exposure epidemic, exposure is brief and simultaneous. All cases develop with one incubation period. There is no secondary wave. For example, Bhopal gas tragedy in India.

27. Which of the following statements is NOT correct regarding case fatality rate?

a. Very useful indicator for both acute and chronic diseases
b. One of the measures related to virulence
c. It is the ratio of deaths to cases expressed as percentage
d. Variation can occur for the same disease because of changes in the agent factors

Case fatality rate, also called case fatality ratio, is the proportion of people who die from a specified disease among all individuals diagnosed with the disease over a certain period of time. It is used typically in acute diseases. In chronic diseases, it has a limited role because period from onset of disease and death is variable.

Answers

21. c **22.** c **23.** c **24.** d **25.** b **26.** b **27.** a

28. Suraksha Clinics are conducted under the aegis of which National Health Programme?

a. Revised National Tuberculosis Control Programme
b. Iodine Deficiency Disorders Programme
c. National AIDS Control Programme
d. Reproductive and Child Health Programme

Suraksha Clinic (formerly Designated STI/RTI Clinics) are a chain of STI/RTI Clinics. These clinics are established by National AIDS Control Organization for the better health services and for the prevention of HIV/AIDS in India.

29. Which of the following tests is NOT used for checking quality of pasteurization of milk?

a. Phosphatase test b. Standard Plate count
c. Coliform count d. Orthotolidine test

Orthotolidine (OT) test enables total, free and combined chlorine in water to be determined with speed and accuracy.

30. Tetanus spores can only be killed by:

a. Large doses of penicillin b. Anti tetanus serum
c. Tetanus toxoid d. Gamma irradiation

Endospores are resistant to most agents that would normally kill the vegetative cells they formed from. Prolonged exposure to ionizing radiation, such as X-rays and gamma rays, will also kill most endospores.

31. Due to a measles outbreak in a community, a medical officer decided to immunize a child aged seven months with measles vaccine. When should the next measles vaccine be administered?

a. Not required
b. After four weeks
c. When the child completes nine months of age
d. When the child completes fifteen months of age

After one dose of measles, 85% of children nine months of age and 95% over twelve months of age are immune. Nearly all of those who do not develop immunity after a single dose develop it after a second dose. When rates of vaccination within a population are greater than ~92% outbreaks of measles typically no longer occur; however, they may occur again if rates of vaccination decrease. The vaccine's effectiveness lasts many years. The vaccine may also protect against measles if given within a couple of days of exposure to measles.

32. Retrospective cohort studies have the following features *except:*

a. Outcomes have occurred before the start of the study
b. Generally, more expensive than prospective studies
c. Results are obtained more quickly
d. Investigator goes back in time to select study groups

Retrospective cohort study is more economical and less time taking than prospective cohort study. The association between the angiosarcoma of the liver (a very rare disease) in relation to polyvinyl chloride was picked up only because of retrospective cohort study.

33. The maternal and child health care indicator that gives a good indicator of the extent of pregnancy wastage as well as the quantity and quality of health care available to the mother and newborn is:

a. Maternal Mortality Rate b. Still Birth Rate
c. Infant Mortality Rate d. Perinatal Mortality Rate

Perinatal mortality rate gives a good indication of the extent of pregnancy wastage as well as the quality and quantity of the health care available to the mother and the newborn. It reflects the maternity care more clearly than the neonatal death rate.

34. For a child aged four years, an Anganwadi Worker detects that the weight is lower than expected. What should the Anganwadi Worker do first regarding the malnutrition detected in the child?

a. Refer the child to the nearby health centre
b. Refer the child a nearby nutritional rehabilitation centre
c. Give nutritional counselling to the mother
d. Start fortnightly deworming

Nutrition and health education and counselling to the mothers is done by AWW when she notices that in growth chart, there is grade I malnutrition and the growth line is between first and second growth curve.

35. A pregnant woman visits a medical officer for an antenatal check-up. The woman mentions that she had received two doses of Tetanus Toxoid vaccine three years ago. Which of the following steps should the medical officer take with regard to administration of Tetanus Toxoid vaccine as per the Government of India recommended schedule?

a. Tetanus Immunoglobulin should be administered in the third trimester of pregnancy
b. Two doses of Tetanus Toxoid vaccine should be administered with an interval of four weeks between the two doses
c. Only one dose of Tetanus Toxoid vaccine is required
d. No Tetanus Toxoid vaccine is required

To maximize the maternal antibody response and passive antibody transfer to the infant, the national immunization schedule in India recommends the 2 doses of tetanus toxoid (TT) for unknown immunization status of pregnant women i.e. the first dose of tetanus toxoid should be administered as soon as pregnancy is detected, second dose of tetanus toxoid is administered after 4 weeks and if a mother received 2 TT

Answers

28. c	29. d	30. d	31. c	32. b	33. d	34. c	35. c

doses in the last pregnancy and mother gets again pregnant with in 3 years than only one dose of TT is recommended and that dose is called booster dose.

36. At the end of an immunization session, you found that a reconstituted BCG vaccine vial has around two doses left in it. What should be done in such a situation?

a. Can reuse the remaining two doses during the next immunization session
b. Discard the vial in a black coloured bin
c. Discard the vial in a red coloured bin
d. Take decision depending upon the Vaccine Vial Monitor (VVM) status

Reconstituted BCG vaccine is very unstable and must be discarded within six hours of reconstitution. Segregation and storage of the plastic portion of the cut syringes and unbroken (but discarded) vials should be done in red bag/ containers.

37. The two important values necessary for describing the variation in a series of observations are:

a. Mean and standard deviation
b. Mean and range
c. Median and range
d. Median and standard deviation

Variation in a series of observations include mean and standard deviation. The sample mean is the average and is computed as the sum of all the observed outcomes from the sample divided by the total number of events. The standard deviation is a summary measure of the differences of each observation from the mean.

38. In the estimation of statistical probability, Z score is applicable to:

a. Normal distribution
b. Skewed distribution
c. Binomial distribution
d. Poisson distribution

A Z-score is also known as a standard score and it can be placed on a normal distribution curve.

39. A rapid mass screening method that can be employed by a paramedical worker for detecting malnutrition in pre-school (age: 1 to 5 years) children is:

a. Weight for age
b. Height for age
c. Mid-arm circumference
d. Body Mass Index

Mid-Upper Arm Circumference (MUAC) is the circumference of the left upper arm, measured at the mid-point between the tip of the shoulder and the tip of the elbow (olecranon process and the acromion). MUAC is used for the assessment of nutritional status from 1–5 years. The modified tape (Shakir's tape) can be used easily by a village health worker simply by visualizing and he need not be very educative to screen correctly.

40. Districts are classified into different categories regarding neonatal tetanus/NT risk. Which one of the following correctly describes 'Neonatal Tetanus Elimination' status?

a. Incidence rate more than 2/1000 births, two doses of TT vaccine coverage less than 70%, attended deliveries between 60% and 70%
b. Incidence rate between 1 to 2/1000 births, three doses of TT vaccine coverage 70%, attended deliveries more than 75%
c. Incidence rate 0.5 to 1/1000 births, three doses of TT vaccine coverage between 70 and 80%, attended deliveries between 65 and 70%
d. Incidence rate less than 0.1/1000 births, two doses of TT vaccine coverage more than 90%, attended deliveries more than 75%

Category	*NT incidence rates*	*Immunization coverage levels*	*Proportion of clean deliveries by trained professionals*
NT High risk	>1/1000 live births	TT2 coverage <70%	Attended deliveries <50%
NT	<1/1000 live births	TT2 coverage >70%	Attended deliveries >50%
NT elimination	<0.1/1000 live births	TT2 coverage >90%	Attended deliveries >75%

41. With reference to International Certificate of Vaccination for Yellow Fever, the validity of the certificate begins how many days after the vaccination?

a. 5 days
b. 10 days
c. 14 days
d. 20 days

Protective efficacy of yellow fever vaccine starts from 10th day of vaccination and lasts for lifetime.

42. What is the window period for HIV infection?

a. 3–15 days
b. 6–24 weeks
c. 6–8 months
d. None of these

The window period is time between potential exposure to HIV infection and the point when the test will give an accurate result. During the window period a person can be infected with HIV and be very infectious but still test

Answers

36. c 37. a 38. a 39. c 40. d 41. b 42. d

HIV negative. The window period can be from 10 days to 3 months, depending on the person's body and on the HIV test that is used.

43. Among the following foodstuffs, which one has the highest protein content per 100 gm?

a. Black gram b. Egg
c. Ragi d. Wheat

Foodstuff	Protein content (per 100 gram)
Egg	6.0 g
Ragi	7.3 g
Wheat	6.8 g
Black gram	17.1 g

44. A new drug does NOT prevent a disease from occurring, does not cure that disease fully, but reduce death due to that disease. Which of the following is true?

a. It will increase the incidence and prevalence
b. It will decrease the incidence and prevalence
c. Prevalence is increased
d. Incidence is increased

Prevalence refers to the number of cases of a disease that are present in a particular population at a given time (new cases plus old cases), whereas incidence refers to the number of new cases that develop in a given period of time. If a new drug prevents death without curing, it will increase the total number of cases (prevalence) as new cases are also adding to the total number of cases.

45. Incubation period of plasmodium vivax:

a. 1–7 days b. 7–10 days
c. 10–14 days d. 15–30 days

Species	Incubation period
Plasmodium falciparum	12 days
Plasmodium malariae	28 days
Plasmodium ovale	17 days
Plasmodium vivax	14 days

46. The number of live births per 1000 women in the reproductive age group in a year refers to:

a. Gross reproduction rate b. Total fertility rate
c. Net reproduction rate d. General fertility rate

The general fertility rate (GFR) is the total number of live births per 1,000 women of reproductive age (ages 15 to 49 years) in a population

47. Protein quality indicator adopted by ICMR in recommending dietary protein requirement is:

a. Protein efficiency ratio b. Biological value
c. Net protein utilization d. Amino acid score

The net protein utilization, or NPU, is the ratio of amino acid converted to proteins to the ratio of amino acids supplied. This figure is somewhat affected by the salvage of essential amino acids within the body, but is profoundly affected by the level of limiting amino acids within a foodstuff.

48. Preferred bacteriological indicator of faecal contamination of water:

a. Faecal streptococci b. Cl. perfringens
c. Faecal staphylococci d. E. coli

Number of coliforms	Interpretation
No coliforms in 100 cc of water	Excellent water
1–3 coliforms in 100 cc of water	Satisfactory water
4–10 coliforms in 100 cc of water	Suspicious water
More than 10 coliforms in 100 cc of water	Unsatisfactory water

49. All of the following are duties of a health worker female/ HWF *except*:

a. Detect malpresentation b. Detect oligohydramnios
c. Diagnose renal diseases d. Detect anemia

Primary responsibilities health workers female/HWF (now designated as multipurpose worker/MPW) may include treating minor illnesses, looking after pregnant women (detect malpresentation, oligohydramnios and anemia) and caring for children. Additional duties may involve family planning services, promotion of sanitation and hygiene, screening for communicable diseases, performing health education activities, collecting statistics, maintaining records and providing health care referrals. Diagnosing renal diseases is not a duty of HWF.

50. Cluster testing is helpful in detecting cases of:

a. Measles b. Diabetes
c. Cancer d. STD

In a sense, "cluster testing" is really an extension of contact tracing for sexually transmitted illnesses. It was long ago noted that certain patients, when approached by the venereal disease investigator or the clinician, would offer the suggestion that: "You ought to have a look at Sam Jones, too. He's got a bad rash just like mine." Sometimes the health worker, on one pretext or another, did "have a look at Sam Jones, too." Sometimes Sam had scabies. But sometimes Sam had secondary syphilis.

51. Under the National Polio Eradication Programme, a case of Acute Flaccid Paralysis is confirmed as polio, under the following circumstances *except*:

a. If a case is lost to follow-up
b. If a case could not be confirmed because the patient dies before that
c. If a wild strain of polio virus is isolated from stools
d. If a patient develops paralysis within 30 days diagnosis of AFP

Answers

43. a **44.** c **45.** c **46.** d **47.** c **48.** d **49.** c **50.** d
51. d

Compatible case (of AFP) is reviewed for 60 days by an expert committee, consisting of a pediatrician, a virologist and a neurologist, to decide whether to confirm or discard the given case as polio case.

52. Strength of sewage is expressed in terms of:
a. Biological oxygen demand
b. Chemical oxygen demand
c. Suspended solids
d. E. coli count

Biochemical oxygen demand (BOD) is the amount of dissolved oxygen needed (i. e., demanded) by aerobic biological organisms to break down organic material present in a given water sample at certain temperature over a specific time period. The BOD value is most commonly expressed in milligrams of oxygen consumed per litre of sample during 5 days of incubation at 20°C and is often used as a surrogate of the degree of organic pollution of water. BOD can be used as a gauge of the effectiveness of wastewater treatment plants.

53. Perinatal death includes death:
a. After 28 weeks of pregnancy
b. 7 days after birth
c. Both
d. None

Perinatal mortality is the sum of the number of resident fetal deaths of 28 or more weeks gestation plus the number of resident newborns dying under 7 days of age in a specified geographic area (country, state, county, etc.).

54. Vector for Yellow fever is:
a. Aedes b. Culex
c. Anopheles d. Mansonoides

Some species of Aedes genus transmit serious diseases, including dengue fever, yellow fever, the Zika virus, and chikungunya.

55. All are true statements about filariasis *except*:
a. Extrinsic incubation period of 10–14 days
b. Man is the intermediate host
c. Adults live in the lymphatics of host
d. No multiplication in the mosquito

Human filarial nematode worms have complicated lifecycles, which primarily consists of five stages. After the male and female worms mate, the female gives birth to live microfilariae by the thousands. The microfilariae are taken up by the vector insect/mosquito (intermediate host) during a blood meal. In the intermediate host, the microfilariae molt and develop into third-stage (infective) larvae. Upon taking another blood meal, the vector insect injects the infectious larvae into the dermis layer of the skin. After about one year, the larvae molt through two more stages, maturing into the adult worms. Man is a definitive host.

56. Malarial parasite ABSENT in India:
a. P. malariae b. P. ovale
c. P. falciparum d. P. vivax

P. ovale is primarily concentrated in sub-Saharan Africa and islands in the western Pacific.

57. Use of which of the following vaccine is CONTRA-INDICATED in pregnancy?
a. Yellow fever b. Rabies
c. Cholera d. Hepatitis-B

Pregnancy is a precaution for yellow fever vaccine administration. The safety of yellow fever vaccination during pregnancy has not been studied in a large prospective trial. However, a recent study of women who were vaccinated with yellow fever vaccine early in their pregnancies found no major malformations in their infants. A slight increased risk was noted for minor, mostly skin, malformations in infants. A higher rate of spontaneous abortions in pregnant women receiving the vaccine was reported but not substantiated. So theoretically it is contraindicated, but can be given under special circumstances.

58. The installation and usage of sanitary latrines by general public constitutes which level of prevention?
a. Health promotion
b. Specific protection
c. Early diagnosis and treatment
d. Disability limitation and rehabilitation

The primary means of health promotion occur through developing healthy public policy that addresses the prerequisites of health such as income, housing, food security, employment, and quality working conditions.

59. True statement for confounding factors:
a. Associated with either the exposure or the disease
b. Confounding can be eliminated by selecting a small group
c. It is a risk factor for the disease
d. Found equally between study and the control groups

A confounding variable is a variable (say, pollution) that can cause the disease under study (cancer) and is also associated with the exposure of interest (smoking).

60. Which of the following is secondary level of prevention?
a. Prophylactic drug administration
b. Admitting disabled child in special schools
c. Vaccination
d. Cervical pap smear checking

An example of secondary level of prevention is the Pap test to screen for cancer of the cervix, or a PSA blood test for prostate cancer; other instances include teaching people about the early signs of disease that they should watch for, and what type of treatment to seek.

Answers

52. a 53. c 54. a 55. b 56. b 57. a 58. a 59. c
60. d

61. All are true regarding killed polio vaccine *except*:
a. Produces circulatory antibody
b. Does NOT require stringent refrigeration
c. Immunity against paralytic and wild strains
d. NOT effective in an epidemic

IPV (Inactivated Polio Vaccine) prevents the disease but does not prevent the re-infection of the gut by wild polio virus.

62. Man is dead-end for:
a. Rabies, tetanus
b. Tetanus, yellow fever
c. Measles, yellow fever
d. Tetanus, measles

A dead-end host or incidental host is an intermediate host that does generally not allow transmission to the definitive host, thereby preventing the parasite from completing its development. For example, humans are dead-end hosts for *Echinococcus canine* tapeworms, tetanus, rabies etc.

63. As per WHO, anemia is considered to exist in pregnancy, if the hemoglobin level is below:
a. 11 gm%
b. 14 gm%
c. 12 gm%
d. 13 gm%

Age group	Cut-off values of Hb in venous blood
Adult male	13 g/dL
Adult woman (non-pregnant)	12 g/dL
Adult woman (pregnant)	11 g/dL
Child above 6 years	12 g/dL
Child below 6 years	11 g/dL

64. Deficiency seen in a child exclusively fed on cow milk:
a. Thiamine
b. Vitamin A
c. Riboflavin
d. Iron

Cow's milk consumption has long been associated with iron deficiency and iron deficiency anemia in children. Because cow's milk is a staple in the diet of most toddlers, they are at particular risk for these conditions.

65. Value of free residual chlorine should be:
a. 0.2 mg/L
b. 0.3 mg/L
c. 0.4 mg/L
d. 0.5 mg/L

A free chlorine level of 0.5 mg/L of free chlorine will be enough residual to maintain the quality of water through the distribution network, but is most likely not adequate to maintain the quality of the water when this water is stored in the home in a bucket or jerry can for 24 hours.

66. Each community development block consists of:
a. 100 villages and a population of ten thousand
b. 100 villages and a population of one lakh
c. 1000 villages and a population of ten thousand
d. 1000 villages and a population of one lakh

The Community development block (CD Block) is a rural area earmarked for administration and development in India. The area is administered by a Block Development Officer. A community development block covers several gram panchayats, local administrative unit at the village level. Currently, CD Blocks are administrative units of 3rd level in some states of India (equal to tehsils in other states). Under Community development program, the rural India has been organised into community development blocks, each block comprising of 100 villages, covering a population of about 1 lakh (80,000 – 1,20,000 population).

67. There were 50 patients in a ward (20 females and 30 males). 10 females and 20 males require surgery. Probability of each patient selected for surgery is:
a. 1/6
b. 2/6
c. 3/5
d. 6/25

Total patients: 50
Patients requiring surgery: 30 (10 females and 20 males)
So, probability of selection: 30/50 = 3/5

68. Outdated drugs and cytotoxic drugs are disposed of by:
a. Incineration
b. Store for month and burial
c. Destruction and disposal in landfill
d. Dumping

Many cytotoxic drugs can be disposed of by chemical destruction or disposition in secured landfill.

69. True regarding comparison values of cow and human milk are all *except*:
a. Human milk has comparatively less of protein
b. Human milk has comparatively less of calcium
c. Human milk has comparatively less of minerals
d. Human milk has comparatively less of lactose

Lactose is the primary carbohydrate found in human milk. Milk is the only natural source of lactose.

70. Life cycle of filaria is:
a. Cyclo-developmental
b. Cyclo-propagative
c. Propagative
d. Transovarian

Cyclo-developmental transmission of an arthropod transmitted disease wherein the causal organism undergoes cyclical changes but does not multiply in the body of the arthropod. It is seen in filariasis.

Answers

61. c **62.** a **63.** a **64.** d **65.** d **66.** b **67.** c **68.** c
69. d **70.** a

9 Ear, Nose and Throat

1. Which is the most pulsatile condition found in the external auditory meatus, which bleeds on touch:

a. CSOM
b. Chronic adhesive otitis media
c. Acute otitis media
d. Glomus tumour

On increasing the ear canal pressure with Siegle's speculum, glomus tumour pulsates vigorously and then blanches. Reverse happens with release of pressure (Brown's sign).

2. A patient with history of head injury developed unilateral conducting hearing loss. On examination, tympanic membrane is normal and mobile. The cause for deafness could be:

a. Collection of fluid in the middle ear
b. Osteoma
c. Dislocation of the incudostapedial joint
d. ASOM

Conductive Hearing Loss (CHL) with normal TM can be seen in temporal bone fracture, congenital fixity of ossicles, otosclerosis, congenital cholesteatoma or glomus tumour.

3. A child with otitis media, not responding to ampicillin presents with bulging membrane with dull look. Treatment of choice is:

a. Ciprofloxacin
b. Mastoidectomy
c. Myringotomy
d. Grommet insertion

Indications of myringotomy in ASOM: (i) Bulging eardrum (ii) Acute excruciating pain (iii) Unresponsiveness to antibiotics (iv) Complications like facial paralysis, labyrinthitis or meningitis with bulging tympanic membrane.

4. A patient presented with high fever and signs of raised intracranial tension. There is past history of CSOM. Likely diagnosis is:

a. Brain abscess
b. Pyogenic meningitis
c. Acute subarachnoid hemorrhage
d. Acute osteomyelitis of the skull

Fifty percent cases of brain abscesses in adults and 25% in children are otogenic. In adults, cholesteatoma and in children AOM are the most common causes. Cerebral abscess occurs more frequently than cerebellar abscess.

5. A patient is having scanty, foul-smelling discharge from the ear and hearing loss. Treatment of choice in such a case:

a. Radical mastoidectomy
b. Modified radical mastoidectomy
c. Suction clearance
d. Cautery with trichloroacetic acid

Modified radical mastoidectomy eradicates diseases from the attic and mastoid and exteriorizes both into EAC by removal of the posterior meatal and lateral attic walls. The remnant of tympanic membrane, functioning ossicles and the reversible mucosa and function of the Eustachian tube, which are necessary to reconstruct hearing mechanism, are preserved.

6. Unilateral nasal obstruction with blood-stained discharge in a child is commonly due to:

a. Foreign body
b. Choanal atresia
c. Polyps
d. Fungal infection

Causes of unilateral blood-stained discharge include forgotten foreign body nose, rhinolith and sequestra, nasal diphtheria, nasal myiasis (maggots), acute and chronic unilateral sinusitis and malignancy of nose and paranasal sinuses

7. All of the following statements about nasopharyngeal carcinoma are true *except*:

a. Bimodal age distribution
b. Nasopharyngectomy with radical neck dissection is the treatment of choice
c. IgA antibody to EBV is observed
d. Squamous cell carcinoma is the most common histological subtype

Irradiation is the primary treatment of choice for nasopharyngeal carcinoma. External radiation or intracavitary implants (brachytherapy) or both are used.

Answers

1. d **2.** c **3.** c **4.** a **5.** b **6.** a **7.** b

8. **All of the following are true regarding tracheostomy tube *except*:**
   a. Double lumen tube
   b. Made of titanium silver alloy
   c. Cuffed tube prevents aspiration of pharyngeal secretions
   d. Ideally should be changed every 3rd day

Inner cannula is removed, and cleaned regularly for the first 3 days to prevent respiratory distress. Outer tube is changed daily after 3-4 days of tracheostomy when a track is formed that facilitates easy tube placement.

9. **A patient who had undergone tooth extraction for dental caries, presents with swelling in posterior part of middle 1/3rd of sternomastoid and tonsil is pushed medially. The diagnosis is:**
   a. Retropharyngeal abscess b. Parapharyngeal abscess
   c. Ludwig's angina d. Vincent's angina

The parapharyngeal abscess collects medial to the medial pterygoid muscle. The otogenic parapharyngeal abscess is caused by petrositis. In other instances, it occurs due to caries/extraction of molar tooth. Patient develops trismus, fever and swelling that pushes the tonsil medially and spreads laterally posterior to sternocleidomastoid.

10. **Which of the following bone does NOT contribute in the formation of nasal septum?**
   a. Nasal bones b. Frontal bone
   c. Maxilla d. Lacrimal

Septum proper has very small contribution from crest of nasal bones, nasal spine of frontal bone, rostrum of sphenoid, crests of palatine and maxilla and the anterior nasal spine of maxilla.

11. **A child presents with unilateral, foul smelling nasal discharge. Most probable cause could be:**
   a. Acute sinusitis
   b. Foreign body
   c. Rhinolith
   d. Nasal synechiae

A unilateral foul smelling purulent nasal discharge in a child is mostly due to forgotten foreign body nose.

12. **A 31-years-old female patient complains of bilateral impairment of hearing for the past 5 years. On examination, tympanic membrane is normal and audiogram shows a bilateral conductive deafness. Acoustic reflexes are absent. All constitute part of treatment *except*:**
   a. Hearing aid b. Stapectomy
   c. Sodium fluoride d. Gentamycin

In aminoglycoside antibiotics group, streptomycin, gentamycin and tobramycin are primarily vestibulotoxic. So patients presents with dizziness/vertigo. In large doses, they can damage the cochlea also.

13. **The most common clinical presentation of acoustic neuroma is feature of:**
   a. Brainstem involvement
   b. Cerebellar involvement
   c. Facial nerve involvement
   d. Cochleovestibular symptoms

Progressive unilateral SNHL, which is often accompanied by tinnitus, is the most common presenting symptom.

14. **In sinus X-rays pictures, Water's view (Occipito-mental) provides good visualization of the following *except*:**
   a. Maxillary sinus
   b. Orbito-frontal sinus
   c. Frontal sinus
   d. Sphenoid sinus

Anterior and posterior extents of sphenoid sinus are best seen on lateral view (also seen in frontal and maxillary sinuses, sella turcica, ethmoid sinuses, alveolar process, condyles and neck of mandible).

15. **An adult patient presented with headache, epiphora and nasal obstruction, but there was NO fever. Condition could be:**
   a. Meningitis
   b. Foreign body obstruction
   c. Cavernous sinus thrombosis
   d. Carcinoma of maxillary sinus

Late features of maxillary carcinoma appear when tumour spreads and destroys the bony confines and involves surrounding structures. Medial spread towards nasal cavity result in nasal obstruction, discharge and epistaxis. Superior spread towards orbit result in facial paresthesia/anesthesia, proptosis, diplopia, ocular pain and epiphora.

16. **NOT a component of Trotter's triad:**
   a. Ipsilateral soft palate immobility
   b. VII nerve palsy
   c. Trigeminal neuralgia
   d. Conduction deafness

Trotter's triad of NPC includes conductive deafness, ipsilateral temporo-parietal neuralgia (CN V) and palatal paralysis (CN X).

17. **FALSE regarding nasolabial cyst:**
   a. Usually seen in adults
   b. Bilateral
   c. Presents submucosally in anterior nasal floor
   d. Arises from odontoid epithelium

Answers

8. d	9. b	10. d	11. b	12. d	13. d	14. d
15. d	16. b	17. d				

Nasolabial/nasoalveolar/Klestadt's cyst is a squamous epithelium-lined cyst which arises from the epithelial rests situated at the junction of globular, lateral nasal and maxillary processes.

18. Which of the following does NOT drain into middle meatus?

a. Ethmoidal sinus
b. Maxillary sinus
c. Lacrimal duct
d. Frontal sinus

Nasolacrimal duct opens in the anterior part of inferior meatus.

19. NOT an attachment of quadrilateral cartilage:

a. Maxilla
b. Sphenoid
c. Vomer
d. Ethmoid

Septal cartilage is a large quadrilateral septal cartilage wedged between vomer and ethmoid bone. It rests anteriorly on anterior nasal spine of maxilla.

20. Nasal septal perforation is NOT seen in:

a. Trauma
b. Rhinophyma
c. Septal abscess
d. Leprosy

Rhinophyma is a slow growing benign tumour occurring due to the hypertrophy of sebaceous glands in the region of nasal tip.

21. A child presented with ear pain and markedly congested tympanic membrane. Diagnosis is:

a. ASOM
b. CSOM
c. Serous otitis media
d. Otosclerosis

In stage of pre-suppuration, patient presented with marked throbbing ear pain, which can awake the child from sleep in night. On examination, pars tensa is congested and bulging out with cart-wheel appearance (leash of blood vessels along the handle of malleus and at the periphery of tympanic membrane) and loss of light reflex.

22. An infant with a past history of ear infection is suspected to have meningitis. Organism commonly responsible for such a presentation would be:

a. Mycobacterium
b. Moraxella catarrhalis
c. Pseudomonas
d. Streptococcus pneumoniae

Meningitis is the MC (most common) intracranial complication of SOM (suppurative otitis media). In infants and children, meningitis is often the complication of AOM (acute otitis media), while in adults it occurs due to cholesteatoma. The one-third cases of meningitis are otogenic in origin. Major pathogens are Hemophilus influenza and Streptococcus pneumoniae.

23. NOT a component of Gradenigo's syndrome:

a. Otorrhoea
b. VII cranial nerve palsy
c. VI cranial nerve palsy
d. V cranial nerve palsy

Gradenigo's triad consists of otorrhea, abducens palsy and retrobulbar pain, and is the classic presentation of petrous apicitis.

24. A patient hears better in noise. The diagnosis is:

a. Hyperacusis
b. Hypoacusis
c. Presbycusis
d. Paracusis

In paracusis willisii the patient's hearing improves in noisy background.

25. Which is NOT seen in Meniere's disease?

a. Tinnitus
b. Hearing loss
c. Loss of consciousness
d. Vertigo

Patient with Meniere's disease may have occasional sudden unexplained falls without loss of consciousness or associated vertigo. Patient feels pushing or moving during this short-lived spells (drop attacks/otolithic crises of Tumarkin).

26. Stylalgia may present with ear pain. Which nerve may refer the pain?

a. Auriculotemporal nerve
b. Posterior auricular nerve
c. Occipital nerve
d. Glossopharyngeal nerve

Elongated styloid process (Eagle's syndrome) or calcification of stylohyoid ligament can cause pain in tonsillar fossa and upper neck. Pain radiates to ear and gets aggravated on swallowing. The ear pain is secondary to stretching and irritation of glossopharyngeal nerve from elongated styloid process.

27. Hyperacusis is seen in all of the following *except*:

a. Exposure to loud sounds
b. Otosclerosis
c. Meniere's disease
d. Severe head injury

Otosclerosis is characterized by gradually progressive conductive hearing loss with normal tympanic membrane. In paracusis Willisii, the patient's hearing improves in noisy background.

28. True regarding Weber test in conductive deafness:

a. Sound louder in normal ear
b. Sound louder in diseased ear
c. Heard with intensity in both the ear
d. Inconclusive test

In conductive hearing loss, Weber test is lateralized toward the affected ear. If both the ears have CHL, Weber is lateralized to worst ear.

Answers

18. c	19. b	20. b	21. a	22. d	23. b	24. d
25. c	26. d	27. b	28. b			

29. Rinne test is positive in:

a. Normal ear
b. Otomycosis
c. CSOM
d. Wax in ear

Rinne test is said to be positive when AC is longer or louder than BC. The positive Rinne (AC > BC) is seen in cases of normal hearing or SNHL.

30. The most effective means of identifying site of sensorineural deafness is:

a. Stapedial reflex
b. Audiometry
c. BERA
d. CT scan

BERA finds out the threshold of hearing in infants, which are in high-risk groups. It aids in the diagnosis of retrocochlear lesions.

Answers

29. a **30.** c

10 Ophthalmology

1. **Microscopy of corneal ulcer showed branching septate hyphae. The probable diagnosis is:**
   a. Candida
   b. Mucormycosis
   c. Aspergillus
   d. Histoplasma

   Aspergillus and many other species have septate hyphae.

2. **A 28-years-old male complains of glare in both eyes. Examination of cornea showed whorl like opacities of epithelium. There is a past history of Amiodarone therapy. Most likely diagnosis is:**
   a. Arcus senilis
   b. Band-shaped keratopathy
   c. Cornea verticillata
   d. Terrain's marginal degeneration

   Cornea verticillata, also called Fleischer vortex, Vortex keratopathy or Whorl keratopathy, is a condition characterized by corneal deposits at the level of the basal epithelium forming a faint golden-brown whorl pattern. It is seen in Fabry disease or in case of prolonged amiodarone intake.

3. **In a child with retinoblastoma, which of the following is NOT a common finding in the X-ray?**
   a. Intraorbital calcification
   b. Intracerebral calcification
   c. Multiple cranial deposits
   d. Widening of optic foramen

   In areas of the world where ultrasonography and computerized tomography are not available, X-ray studies may be the only means of identifying intraocular (NOT intracerebral) calcium in patients with opaque media.

4. **Lesions of the visual cortex with homonymous hemianopia may be seen in occlusion of:**
   a. Basilar artery
   b. Middle cerebral artery
   c. Posterior cerebral artery
   d. Anterior cerebral artery

   Vascular and neoplastic (malignant or benign tumours) lesions from the optic tract, to visual cortex can cause a contralateral homonymous hemianopsia. Injury to the right side of the brain will affect the left visual fields of each eye. The more posterior the cerebral lesion, the more symmetric (congruous) the homonymous hemianopsia will be. For example, a person who has a lesion of the right optic tract will no longer see objects. Homonymous hemianopsia secondary to posterior cerebral artery occlusion—may result in syndromes of memory impairment, opposite visual field loss (homonymous hemianopsia), and sometimes hemisensory deficits. The PCA supplies the occipital lobe and the medial portion of the temporal lobe.

5. **A person has inability to look downward and laterally. The nerve injured is:**
   a. Occulomotor
   b. Trochlear
   c. Abducent
   d. Trigeminal

   The primary (main) action of the superior oblique muscle is intorsion (internal rotation), the secondary action is depression (primarily in the adducted position) and the tertiary action is abduction (lateral rotation).

6. **True about keratoconus are all of the following *except*:**
   a. Can be seen in Down's syndrome
   b. It manifests just after birth
   c. Munsen sign is characteristic
   d. Corneal transplantation is needed in severe cases

   Keratoconus (conical cornea) is a noninflammatory bilateral (85%) ectatic condition of cornea in its axial part. It usually starts at puberty and progresses slowly.

7. **True about indirect gonioscopy are all *except*:**
   a. Done under local anesthesia
   b. A contact lens is inserted between the lids
   c. Single mirror gonioscopes allows examination of 360°C of the angle
   d. Better visualization of the anterior chamber angle

   Indirect gonioscopy is more frequently used in the clinician's office. Indirect gonioscopy also eliminates the total internal reflection at the surface of the cornea. Light reflected from the chamber angle passes into the indirect gonioscopy lens and is reflected by a mirror within the lens. Indirect

Answers

1. c	**2.** c	**3.** b	**4.** c	**5.** b	**6.** b	**7.** c

gonioscopy may be used with the patient in an upright position, with illumination and magnification provided by a slit lamp. A *goniolens*, which contains a mirror or mirrors, yields an inverted and slightly foreshortened image of the opposite angle. Although the image is inverted with an indirect goniolens, the right–left orientation of a horizontal mirror and the up–down orientation of a vertical mirror remain unchanged. The foreshortening, combined with the upright position of the patient, makes the angle appear a little shallower than it does with direct gonioscopy systems.

8. The following structure is NOT derived from surface ectoderm:

a. Crystalline lens
b. Sclera
c. Corneal epithelium
d. Epithelium of lacrimal glands

Ocular structures which are mesodermal in origin are extraocular muscles, endothelial lining of blood vessels of the eye, blood vessels in sclera and choroid, sclera and choroid, vitreous, suspensory fibres and Bowman's membrane and stroma (of cornea).

9. Fincham test is used to differentiate:

a. Acute congestive glaucoma and chronic simple glaucoma
b. Chronic simple glaucoma and iridocyclitis
c. Acute congestive glaucoma and cataract
d. Simple glaucoma and cataract

The coloured halos in glaucoma must be differentiated from those found in acute purulent conjunctivitis and early cataractous changes. In conjunctivitis, the halos can be eliminated by irrigating the discharge. The halos of glaucoma and immature cataract may be differentiated by Fincham's test in which a stenopaeic slit is passed across the pupil. During this test glaucomatous halo remains intact, while a halo due to cataract is broken up into segments. Emsley-Fincham stenopaeic-slit test demonstrating breaking up of halos due to immature cataract into different segments.

10. True for chalazion:

a. Acute inflammation of Zeis gland
b. Acute inflammation of meibomian gland
c. Chronic inflammation of meibomian gland
d. Chronic inflammation of Zeis gland

A chalazion, also known as a meibomian gland lipogranuloma, is a cyst in the eyelid that is caused by inflammation of a blocked meibomian gland, usually on the upper eyelid. Chalazia differ from styes (hordeola) in that they are subacute and usually painless nodules. They may become acutely inflamed, but unlike a stye, chalazia usually sit inside the lid rather than on the lid margin.

11. Visual field defect in pituitary tumour with supracellular extension is:

a. Bitemporal hemianopia
b. Binasal hemianopia
c. Homonymous hemianopia
d. Pie in the sky vision

Bitemporal hemianopsia (bitemporal heteronymous hemianopsia or bitemporal hemianopia) is a type of partial blindness where vision is missing in the outer half of both the right and left visual field. It is usually associated with lesions of the optic chiasm, the area where the nasal fibers of optic nerves from the right and left eyes cross near the pituitary gland.

12. True regarding buphthalmos are all *except*:

a. Developmental anomaly of the angle of the anterior chamber
b. Bull-like eyes
c. Unilateral
d. Photophobia is the initial sign

In most cases buphthalmos affects both eyes (i.e., it is bilateral), but the effect is not necessarily the same on each eye.

13. Which of the following statement is true regarding Acanthamoeba keratitis?

a. For the isolation of the causative agent, corneal scraping should be cultured on a nutrient agar plate
b. The causative agent, Acanthamoeba is a helminth whose normal habitat is soil
c. Keratitis due to Acanthamoeba is NOT seen in the immunocompromised patient
d. Acanthamoeba does NOT depend upon a human host for the completion of its life-cycle

Species within the genus Acanthamoeba are generally free-living trophozoites. These trophozoites are relatively ubiquitous and can live in, but are not restricted to, tap water, freshwater lakes/rivers and soil.

14. True about Fuchs, endothelial dystrophy are all *except*:

a. Commonly seen in the elderly female
b. Symmetrical and unilateral condition
c. Cornea guttatae is characteristic
d. Patient typically complains of seeing halos in the morning

Fuchs, endothelial dystrophy is characterized by an asymmetrical, bilateral, slowly progressive edema of the cornea in elderly patients.

15. NOT a feature of trachoma:

a. Corneal opacity
b. Chalazion
c. Herbert's pits
d. Ectropion

The later structural changes of trachoma are referred to as "cicatricial trachoma". These include scarring in the eyelid (tarsal conjunctiva) that leads to distortion of the eyelid

Answers

8. b **9.** c **10.** c **11.** a **12.** c **13.** d **14.** b
15. d

with buckling of the lid (tarsus) so the lashes rub on the eye (trichiasis). These lashes will lead to corneal opacities and scarring and then to blindness. There is also entropion, tylosis (thickening of lid margins), ptosis, madarosis and ankyloblepharon.

16. Polymorphic infiltration is NOT seen in:

a. Acute bacterial conjunctivitis
b. Allergic conjunctivitis
c. Angular bacterial conjunctivitis
d. Hyperacute bacterial conjunctivitis

The ocular allergic response (in allergic conjunctivitis) is a cascade of events that is coordinated by mast cells. Beta chemokines such as eotaxin and MIP-1 alpha have been implicated in the priming and activation of mast cells in the ocular surface. When a particular allergen is present, sensitization takes place and prepares the system to launch an antigen specific response. TH2 differentiated T cells release cytokines, which promote the production of antigen specific immunoglobulin E (IgE). IgE then binds to IgE receptors on the surface of mast cells. Then, mast cells release histamine, which then leads to the release of cytokines, prostaglandins, and platelet-activating factor. Mast cell intermediaries cause an allergic inflammation and symptoms through the activation of inflammatory cells.

17. Conjunctival xerosis is seen in all of the following *except*:

a. Steven-Johnson syndrome
b. Keratoconjunctivitis sicca
c. Vitamin A deficiency
d. Sarcoidosis

Sarcoidosis is a disorder resulting in noncaseating granulomas in one or more organs and tissues; etiology is unknown. The lungs and lymphatic system are most often affected, but sarcoidosis may affect any organ. Pulmonary symptoms range from none to exertional dyspnea and, rarely, lung or other organ failure.

18. One percent atropine is given in uveitis to:

a. Cause mydriasis and prevent formation of anterior synechiae
b. Cause miosis and prevent formation of posterior synechiae
c. Cause mydriasis and prevent formation of posterior synechiae
d. Cause miosis and prevent formation of posterior synechiae

A long-acting cycloplegic agent, such as cyclopentolate, homatropine, scopolamine, or even atropine, should be used to help relieve both pain and photophobia and to prevent the formation of posterior synechiae in acute symptomatic anterior uveitis.

19. NOT an antiglaucoma drug:

a. Brimonidine b. Prednisolone
c. Dorzolamide d. Timolol

Prednisolone is a synthetic glucocorticoid, a derivative of cortisol, used to treat a variety of inflammatory and autoimmune conditions and some cancers. It is the active metabolite of the drug prednisone.

20. True regarding retinoscopy, are all of the following *except*:

a. Helps in estimating the condition of the refraction
b. Usually performed at 1 m distance
c. Consists of a plane and a concave mirror
d. Hyperopes display an "against" movement

Static retinoscopy is a type of retinoscopy used in determining a patient's refractive error. It relies on Foucault's principle, which states that the examiner should simulate optical infinity to obtain the correct refractive power. Hence, a power corresponding to the working distance is subtracted from the gross retinoscopy value to give the patient's refractive condition, the working distance lens being one which has a focal length of the examiner's distance from the patient (e.g., +1.50 dioptre lens for a 67 cm working distance). Myopes display an "against" reflex, which means that the direction of movement of light observed from the retina is a different direction to that in which the light beam is swept. Hyperopes, on the other hand, display a "with" movement, which means that the direction of movement of light observed from the retina is the same as that in which the light beam is swept.

21. All are true regarding direct ophthalmoscopy *except*:

a. Image is erect
b. Magnification is more than indirect ophthalmoscopy
c. Wide area of fundus with least magnification can be seen in hypermetropics
d. It has a large field of view

Binocular indirect ophthalmoscopy technique allows for viewing the fundus at a wider angle which allows examination of the peripheral retina and also a better view through lens opacities as well.

22. Which of the following is known as dangerous zone of the eye?

a. Sclera b. Retina
c. Optic nerve d. Ciliary body

Owing to the extensive destruction which is apt to follow septic infection of the ciliary region, it has been termed the dangerous area of the eye.

23. Placido disc is useful detecting:

a. Microcornea b. Megalocornea
c. Corneal scars d. Keratoconus

Answers

16. b	17. d	18. c	19. b	20. d	21. d	22. d
23. c						

A keratoscope, sometimes known as *Placido's disk*, is an ophthalmic instrument used to assess the shape of the anterior surface of the cornea. A series of concentric rings is projected onto the cornea and their reflection viewed by the examiner through a small hole in the centre of the disk. A regular-shaped cornea should show equally spaced symmetric reflections. If the patient is suffering from astigmatism or from a corneal dystrophy, the rings will be distorted.

24. Important in Herpes simplex involvement of the eye are all *except*:

a. Type of lesion b. Corneal anaesthesia
c. Iridocyclitis d. Purulent discharge

Herpes infection begins with infection of epithelial cells on the surface of the eye and retrograde infection of nerves serving the cornea. Primary infection typically presents as swelling of the conjunctiva and eyelids (blepharoconjunctivitis), accompanied by small white itchy lesions on the corneal surface. The effect of the lesions varies, from minor damage to the epithelium (superficial punctate keratitis), to more serious consequences such as the formation of dendritic ulcers. Infection is unilateral, affecting one eye at a time. Subsequent recurrences may be more severe, with infected epithelial cells showing larger dendritic ulceration, and lesions forming white plaques. The epithelial layer is sloughed off as the dendritic ulcer grows, and mild inflammation (iritis) may occur in the underlying stroma of iris. Sensation loss occurs in lesional areas, producing generalized corneal anaesthesia with repeated recurrences.

25. Rubeosis iridis is NOT seen in:

a. Neovascularization b. Diabetic retinopathy
c. CRAO d. CRVO

Rubeosis iridis is a condition of the iris of the eye in which new abnormal blood vessels (i.e., neovascularization) are found on the surface of the iris. This condition is often associated with diabetes in advanced proliferative diabetic retinopathy. Other conditions causing rubeosis iridis include central retinal vein occlusion, ocular ischemic syndrome, and chronic retinal detachment.

26. Constantly changing refractive error is seen in:

a. Traumatic cataract b. Diabetic cataract
c. Morgagnian cataract d. Intumescent cataract

Diabetic cataract formation follows an increase in sugars in the lens. The excess sugar within the lens is reduced by aldose reductase to its alcohol, but the lens capsule is relatively impermeable to sugar alcohols. Because of the excess sugar alcohol (polyol), the lens imbibes water, causing osmotic imbalance. Eventually, increased sodium and decreased potassium levels and decreased glutathione levels lead to cataract formation.

27. Which of the following is NOT an eyelid gland?

a. Zeis b. Lacrimal
c. Meibomian d. Moll

The lacrimal glands are paired almond-shaped glands, one for each eye, that secrete the aqueous layer of the tear film. They are situated in the upper, outer portion of each orbit, in the lacrimal fossa of the orbit formed by the frontal bone.

28. All of the following are done for retinal function examination *except*:

a. Visual acuity
b. Visual field
c. Swinging flash light test
d. Contrast sensitivity test

Swinging flash light test check pupillary reaction on exposure to light.

29. Which condition represents fat like nodules, bilaterally on nasal side of conjunctiva?

a. Pterygium b. Pinguecula
c. Chalazion d. Hordeolum

Pinguecula is seen as a yellow-white deposit on the conjunctiva adjacent to the limbus (the junction between the cornea and sclera). It is to be distinguished clinically from pterygium, which is a wedge-shaped area of fibrosis that appears to grow into the cornea. It usually does not cause any symptoms. It is most prevalent in tropical climates and is in direct correlation with UV exposure.

30. NOT a feature of keratoconus:

a. Progressive vision loss
b. KF rings
c. Scissoring reflex in retinoscopy
d. Munsen sign positive

Kayser Fleischer ring are seen in Wilson disease (Fleischer's ring is seen in keratoconus).

Answers

24. d **25.** c **26.** b **27.** b **28.** c **29.** b **30.** b

11 Medicine

1. A 40-years-old male is admitted with acute inferior wall myocardial infarction. Half an hour later his BP is 80/50 mm Hg and heart rate is 40/minute with sinus rhythm. The *most appropriate* step in the management of this patient would be:

a. Administration of normal saline 300 mL over 15 minutes
b. Immediate insertion of temporary pacemaker
c. Intravenous administration of atropine sulfate
d. Intravenous administration of iso-prenaline 50 μg/minute

Bradycardia is defined as any rhythm disorder with a heart rate less than 60 beats per minute. There are 3 medications that are used in the Bradycardia ACLS Algorithm. They are atropine, dopamine (infusion), and epinephrine (infusion).

2. A patient of cirrhosis develops oliguria and worsening azotemia. Urinary sediment is normal. Urinary sodium concentration is 5 mEq/L. The most likely cause could be:

a. Interstitial nephritis
b. Acute tubular necrosis
c. Acute glomerulonephritis
d. Hepatorenal syndrome

Hepatorenal syndrome (often abbreviated HRS) is a life-threatening medical condition that consists of rapid deterioration in kidney functions in individuals with cirrhosis or fulminant liver failure. Type 2 HRS is slower in onset and progression. It is defined by an increase in serum creatinine level to >133 μmol/L (1.5 mg/dL) or a creatinine clearance of less than 40 mL/min, and a urine sodium < 10 μmol/L.

3. A 55-years-old man, non-smoker presents with sudden onset of shortness of breath. On examination, pulse rate is 110/minute and BP 180/110 mm Hg. Patient is restless and anxious. Examination of chest shows bilateral rhonchi and crepitation. S3 gallop is heard on auscultation of precordium. There is no history of chronic bronchitis. The most likely diagnosis is:

a. Bronchial asthma
b. Acute LVF
c. Pneumothorax
d. Acute exacerbation of COPD

Features of left ventricular failure include increased rate of breathing (tachypnea) and increased *work* of breathing (non-specific signs of respiratory distress); rales or crackles or crepitations, heard initially in the lung bases, and when severe, throughout the lung fields suggest the development of pulmonary edema (fluid in the alveoli); cyanosis which suggests severe low blood oxygen, is a late sign of extremely severe pulmonary edema; laterally displaced apex beat (which occurs if the heart is enlarged) and a gallop rhythm (additional heart sounds) may be heard as a marker of increased blood flow or increased intracardiac pressure.

4. A 60-years-old patient presents with gradually increasing dysphagia to solids for 3 months with significant loss of weight. The most probable diagnosis is:

a. Stricture oesophagus
b. Carcinoma oesophagus
c. Reflux oesophagitis
d. Neurogenic oesophagus

The first and the most common symptom of carcinoma esophagus is usually difficulty in swallowing, which is often experienced first with solid foods and later with softer foods and liquids. Pain while swallowing is less usual at first. Weight loss is often an initial symptom in cases of squamous-cell carcinoma, though not usually in cases of adenocarcinoma. Eventual weight loss due to reduced appetite and undernutrition is common.

5. In a patient with lacerated injury foot who is not actively immunized against tetanus, which one of the following is indicated for tetanus prophylaxis?

a. Penicillin
b. Tetanus toxoid
c. Tetanus immunoglobulin
d. Triple vaccine

Anti-tetanus immunoglobulin, also known as tetanus immune globulin (TIG) and tetanus antitoxin, is made up of antibodies against the tetanus toxin. It is used to prevent

Answers

1. c **2.** d **3.** b **4.** b **5.** c

tetanus in those who have a wound that is at high risk and have not been fully vaccinated with tetanus toxoid. It is also used to treat tetanus along with antibiotics and muscle relaxants.

6. **A 16-years-old boy presents with exertional dyspnea, haemoptysis and occasionally paroxysmal nocturnal dyspnea. There was history of joint pains five years back. The most probable diagnosis is:**
   a. Aortic regurgitation
   b. Mitral stenosis
   c. Tricuspid stenosis
   d. Aortic stenosis

   Signs and symptoms of mitral stenosis include heart failure symptoms, such as dyspnea on exertion, orthopnea and paroxysmal nocturnal dyspnea (PND); palpitations; chest pain; hemoptysis and thromboembolism in later stages when the left atrial volume is increased (i.e., dilation). The latter leads to increase risk of atrial fibrillation, which increases the risk of blood stasis (motionless). This increases the risk of coagulation. History of joint pain five years back suggests the episode of acute rheumatic fever (migrating polyarthritis).

7. **A patient presents with breathlessness and occasional dry cough. On physical examination, he is found to have bilateral basal crepitations. His pulmonary function tests reveal a decrease in total lung capacity and vital capacity (VC), with normal FEV1/FVC ratio. He is most likely suffering from:**
   a. Chronic bronchitis
   b. Idiopathic pulmonary fibrosis
   c. Cystic fibrosis
   d. Allergic bronchopulmonary aspergillosis

   Most common clinical features of idiopathic pulmonary fibrosis include age over 50 years; dry, non-productive cough on exertion; progressive exertional dyspnea (shortness of breath with exercise); dry, inspiratory bibasilar "velcro-like" crackles on auscultation (a crackling sound in the lungs during inhalation similar to Velcro being torn apart slowly, heard with a stethoscope) and clubbing of the digits, a disfigurement of the finger tips or toes. Abnormal pulmonary function test results, with evidence of restriction and impaired gas exchange. Spirometry classically reveals a reduction in the vital capacity (VC) with either a proportionate reduction in airflow, or increased airflow for the observed vital capacity. The latter finding reflects the increased lung stiffness (reduced lung compliance) associated with pulmonary fibrosis, which leads to increased lung elastic recoil.

8. **A 45-years-old hypertensive male patient presented to the casualty with 3 hours history of sudden onset severe headache associated with nausea and vomiting. On clinical examination, patient had right-sided ptosis and neck stiffness. Rest of the neurological examination was normal. The most likely diagnosis in this case is:**
   a. Hypertensive brain damage
   b. Migraine
   c. Aneurysmal subarachnoid bleed
   d. Acute pyogenic meningitis

   Subarachnoid hemorrhage (SAH) is bleeding into the subarachnoid space—the area between the arachnoid membrane and the pia mater surrounding the brain. Symptoms may include a severe headache of rapid onset, vomiting, decreased level of consciousness, fever, and sometimes seizures. Neck stiffness or neck pain are also relatively common. In about a quarter of people a small bleed with resolving symptoms occurs within a month of a larger bleed. SAH may occur as a result of a head injury or spontaneously, usually from a ruptured cerebral aneurysm.

9. **A 60-years-old male with Marfan's syndrome comes to emergency department with severe generalized tearing pain localized to chest anteriorly and inter-scapular region, sweating and weakness. On examination, his BP is 200/140 mm Hg. X-ray chest shows widening of superior mediastinum. ECG shows sinus tachycardia. What is the most likely diagnosis?**
   a. Acute pulmonary embolism
   b. Dissection of aorta
   c. Acute myocardial infraction
   d. Acute pericarditis

   Aortic dissection is more common in those with a history of high blood pressure, a number of connective tissues disorder that affect blood vessel wall strength such as Marfan's syndrome, a bicuspid aortic valve, and previous heart surgery.

10. **A patient underwent hip replacement surgery. On fourth postoperative day, he had dyspnoea, pleuritic pain and haemoptysis. Most likely diagnosis is:**
    a. Pulmonary embolism
    b. Pneumonia
    c. Pulmonary oedema
    d. Pericarditis

    Symptoms of pulmonary embolism are typically sudden in onset and may include one or many of the following: dyspnea (shortness of breath), tachypnea (rapid breathing), chest pain of a "pleuritic" nature (worsened by breathing), cough and hemoptysis (coughing up blood). More severe cases can include signs such as cyanosis (blue discoloration, usually of the lips and fingers), collapse, and circulatory instability because of decreased blood flow through the lungs and into the left side of the heart. About 15% of all cases of sudden death are attributable to PE.

Answers

6. b **7.** b **8.** c **9.** b **10.** a

11. A 55-years-old male with a history of chronic obstructive pulmonary disease was rushed to emergency department with increasing shortness of breath, fever and a productive cough with yellow green sputum. He has difficulty in communicating because of his inability to complete a sentence. Measurement of arterial blood gas shows pH: 7.3, $PaCO_2$: 68 mmHg, HCO_3: 28 mmol/L, and PaO_2: 60 mmHg. How would you interpret this?

a. Respiratory acidosis, uncompensated
b. Respiratory alkalosis, uncompensated
c. Respiratory acidosis, partially compensated
d. Respiratory alkalosis, partially compensated

Normal pH: 7.35–7.45; Normal $PaCO_2$: 4.7–6 and Normal HCO_3: 22–24. Respiratory acidosis means pH is less and $PaCO_2$ is more. Partial compensation means there is slight increase in HCO_3.

12. A 40-years-old woman presents with hematuria, ecchymoses and menorrhagia of six months duration. What is the most likely diagnosis?

a. Haemophilia A
b. Haemophilia B
c. Idiopathic thrombocytopaenic purpura
d. Henoch–Schonlein purpura

Signs of idiopathic thrombocytopenic purpura/ITP include the spontaneous formation of bruises (purpura) and petechiae (tiny bruises), especially on the extremities, bleeding from the nostrils and/or gums, and menorrhagia (excessive menstrual bleeding), any of which may occur if the platelet count is below 20,000 per μL. A very low count (<10,000 per μL) may result in the spontaneous formation of hematomas (blood masses) in the mouth or on other mucous membranes.

13. A 45-years-old female comes to you with dysphagia. She is found to have anaemia and koilonychia. Most likely diagnosis is:

a. Plummer–Vinson syndrome
b. Boerhaave syndrome
c. Carcinoma oesophagus
d. Reflux oesophagitis

Plummer–Vinson syndrome (PVS), also called Paterson–Brown–Kelly syndrome or sideropenic dysphagia, is a rare disease characterized by difficulty in swallowing, iron-deficiency anemia, glossitis, cheilosis and esophageal webs. Treatment with iron supplementation and mechanical widening of the esophagus generally provides an excellent outcome.

14. A patient develops skin necrosis 3 days after being started on warfarin for deep vein thrombosis. What is the most likely cause?

a. Antiphospholipid antibody syndrome
b. Protein C deficiency
c. Disseminated intravascular coagulation
d. Thrombotic thrombocytopaenic purpura

Protein C is vitamin K-dependent. Patients with Protein C deficiency are at an increased risk of developing skin necrosis while on warfarin. Protein C has a short half-life (8 hour) compared with other vitamin K-dependent factors and therefore is rapidly depleted with warfarin initiation, resulting in a transient hypercoagulable state.

15. A 15-years-old boy is brought to emergency with two days history of headache, vomiting and altered sensorium. His BP is 70 mmHg systolic and he has ecchymoses on his skin. Most likely organism causing his condition is:

a. *Haemophilus influenzae*
b. *Listeria monocytogenes*
c. *Neisseria meningitidis*
d. *Streptococcus pneumoniae*

Waterhouse–Friderichsen syndrome can be caused by a number of different organisms. When caused by *Neisseria meningitidis*, WFS is considered the most severe form of meningococcal sepsis. The onset of the illness is nonspecific with fever, rigors, vomiting, and headache. Soon a rash appears; first macular, not much different from the rose spots of typhoid, and rapidly becoming petechial and purpuric with a dusky gray color. Low blood pressure (hypotension) develops and rapidly leads to septic shock. The cyanosis of extremities can be extreme and the patient is very prostrated or comatose. In this form of meningococcal disease, meningitis generally does not occur.

16. A child presents with episode of hematuria soon after respiratory tract infection. What is the most likely diagnosis?

a. IgA nephropathy
b. Wegener granulomatosis
c. Post-streptococcal glomerulonephritis
d. Churg–Strauss syndrome

The classic presentation (in 40–50% of the cases) of IgA nephropathy is episodic hematuria, which usually starts within a day or two of a non-specific upper respiratory tract infection (hence *synpharyngitic*), as opposed to post-streptococcal glomerulonephritis, which occurs sometime (weeks) after initial infection. Less commonly gastrointestinal or urinary infection can be the inciting agent.

17. Widespread concave ST segment elevation and PR depression in most leads except aVR lead favours the diagnosis of:

a. Acute myocardial infarction
b. Pericarditis
c. Digoxin toxicity
d. Hypertrophic obstructive cardiomyopathy

Answers

11. c 12. c 13. a 14. b 15. c 16. a 17. b

The preferred initial diagnostic testing in a suspected case of pericarditis is the ECG, which may demonstrate a 12-lead electrocardiogram with diffuse, non-specific, concave ("saddle-shaped"), ST-segment elevations in all leads except aVR and V1 and PR-segment depression possible in any lead *except aVR*; sinus tachycardia, and low-voltage QRS complexes can also be seen if there is subsymptomatic levels of pericardial effusion. The PR depression is often seen early in the process as the thin atria are affected more easily than the ventricles by the inflammatory process of the pericardium.

18. A known case of lepromatous leprosy was initiated on treatment. She developed painful erythematous papules with fever and lymphadenopathy. What is the likely reactional state?

a. Type 1 lepra reaction b. Type 2 lepra reaction
c. Lucio's phenomenon d. Lupus pernio

Erythema nodosum (EN), also known as subacute migratory panniculitis of Vilanova and Piñol, is an inflammatory condition characterized by inflammation of the fat cells under the skin, resulting in tender red nodules or lumps that are usually seen on both shins. EN may also be due to excessive antibody production in lepromatous leprosy leading to deposition of immune complexes.

19. A 20-years-old male walked into outpatient department with high-grade fever, cough and chest pain for one day. Chest X-ray showed consolidation of left upper zone. His respiratory rate is 22/minute, pulse rate 96/minute, BP systolic 120 mmHg and blood urea 18 mg/dL. What is his CURB score?

a. 0 b. 1
c. 2 d. 3

CURB-65	
Symptom	*Points*
Confusion	1
BUN >7 mmol/L	1
Respiratory rate ≥30	1
SBP <90 mmHg, DBP ≤ 60 mmHg	1
Age ≥65	1

20. A 55-years-old patient on treatment for pulmonary tuberculosis with Rifampicin, Isoniazid, Pyrazinamide and Ethambutol complain of pain in large and small joints. Which one of the following investigations will you order?

a. Serum creatinine b. Serum amylase
c. SGOT/SGPT d. Serum uric acid

Gout is a form of inflammatory arthritis characterized by recurrent attacks of a red, tender, hot, and swollen joint. Pain typically comes on rapidly in less than twelve hours. The joint at the base of big toe is affected in about half of cases. It may also result in tophi, kidney stones, or urate nephropathy.

21. A middle-aged male known smoker presented with recurrent sinusitis, haemoptysis, haematuria, arthralgia and palpable purpura. What is the most likely diagnosis?

a. Wegener granulomatosis
b. Goodpasture syndrome
c. Polyarteritis nodosa
d. Systemic lupus erythematosus

Initial signs of Wegener granulomatosis/Granulomatosis with polyangiitis (GPA) are extremely variable, and diagnosis can be severely delayed due to the nonspecific nature of the symptoms. In general, rhinitis is the first sign in most people. Lungs signs include pulmonary nodules (referred to as "coin lesions"), infiltrates (often interpreted as pneumonia), cavitary lesions, pulmonary hemorrhage causing hemoptysis, and rarely bronchial stenosis. Kidney signs include rapidly progressive glomerulonephritis (75%), leading to chronic renal failure. Arthritis is also seen, with pain or swelling (60%), often initially diagnosed as rheumatoid arthritis. Skin signs include subcutaneous nodules (granulomas) on the elbow, purpura etc.

22. A patient presents with diarrhoea, steatorrhea and weight loss. Which of the following disease is LEAST possible?

a. Whipple disease b. Tropical sprue
c. Celiac disease d. Menetrier disease

Individuals with the Menetrier disease present with upper abdominal pain (epigastric), at times accompanied by nausea, vomiting, loss of appetite, edema, and weight loss. A small amount of gastrointestinal bleeding may occur, which is typically due to superficial mucosal erosions; large volume bleeding is rare. 20% to 100% of patients, depending on time of presentation, develop a protein-losing gastropathy accompanied by low blood albumin and edema.

23. A patient with long-term implantable cardioverter defibrillator device developed neck and facial swelling, hoarseness of voice, nasal congestion, dysphagia and haemoptysis. The facial swelling increased on supine position. This patient most likely developed:

a. Cardiac tamponade
b. Intracardiac thrombosis
c. Superior vena cava obstruction
d. Pulmonary thromboembolism

Superior vena cava/SVC syndrome occurs due to partial or complete obstruction of the SVC. One of the causes is deep venous thrombosis due to pacemaker/defibrillator leads. Features of superior vena cava syndrome include shortness of breath is the most common symptom, followed by face or arm swelling, difficulty breathing, headache, facial swelling,

Answers

18. b **19.** a **20.** d **21.** a **22.** d **23.** c

venous distention in the neck and distended veins in the upper chest and arms, upper limb edema, light headedness, cough and edema (swelling) of the neck, called the *collar of Stokes*.

24. A patient of AIDS developed ophthalmoplegia, ataxia and global confusion. He is likely to have the deficiency of:

a. Biotin
b. Niacin
c. Pyridoxine
d. Thiamine

Wernicke encephalopathy (WE) also Wernicke's encephalopathy is the presence of neurological symptoms caused by biochemical lesions of the central nervous system after exhaustion of B-vitamin reserves, in particular thiamine (vitamin B1). Classically, Wernicke encephalopathy is characterized by the triad—ophthalmoplegia, ataxia, and confusion. However, only 10% of patients exhibit all three features, and other symptoms may also be present.

25. An elderly male presents with persistent productive cough with large volume purulent sputum production. He has had several episodes in the past. He also had digital clubbing. He is a case of:

a. Empyema
b. Bronchiectasis
c. Bronchopneumonia
d. Necrotising pneumonia

Some people with bronchiectasis may have a cough productive of frequent green/yellow mucus (sputum), up to 240 mL (8 oz) daily. Bronchiectasis may also present with coughing up blood (hemoptysis) in the absence of sputum, called "dry bronchiectasis". Sputum production may also occur without coloration. People with bronchiectasis may have bad breath indicative of active infection. Frequent bronchial infections and breathlessness are two possible indicators of bronchiectasis. Crepitations and expiratory rhonchi may be heard on auscultation. Nail clubbing is rare.

26. A chemical factory worker has acute onset dyspnoea with fever, chills, and malaise, following a few hours of exposure to a new chemical. These symptoms resolve in four to five days after removal from exposure. He is likely to have:

a. Hypersensitivity pneumonitis
b. Atypical pneumonia
c. Cryptogenic organizing pneumonia
d. Non-specific interstitial pneumonia

Hypersensitivity pneumonitis [(HP; also called allergic alveolitis, bagpipe lung, or extrinsic allergic alveolitis (EAA)] is an inflammation of the alveoli within the lung caused by hypersensitivity to inhaled organic dusts. Sufferers are commonly exposed to the dust by their occupation or hobbies. In the acute form of HP, symptoms may develop 4–6 hours following heavy exposure to the provoking antigen. Symptoms include fever, chills, malaise, cough, chest tightness, dyspnea, rash, swelling and headache. Symptoms resolve within 12 hours to several days upon cessation of exposure.

27. A 25-years-old man presents with nausea, vomiting and diarrhoea with crampy abdominal pain. He gives history of consumption of rice preparation in his last meal. What is the likely organism causing the above complaints?

a. *Clostridium perfringens*
b. *Bacillus cereus*
c. *Staphylococcus aureus*
d. *Campylobacter jejuni*

The 'emetic' form of Bacillus foodborne illness is commonly caused by rice cooked for a time and temperature insufficient to kill any spores present, then improperly refrigerated. It can produce a *toxin, cereulide*, which is not inactivated by later reheating. This form leads to nausea and vomiting one to five hours after consumption. It can be difficult to distinguish from other short-term bacterial foodborne intoxications such as by *Staphylococcus aureus*.

28. A 70-years-old man reports to the emergency with acute chest pain. ECG shows inferior wall Myocardial Infarction (MI). He has recently been discharged 7 days back following thrombolysis with streptokinase for acute anterior wall MI. What will be the appropriate management?

a. Aspirin, sublingual nitroglycerin, clopidogrel, primary PCI
b. Aspirin, sublingual nitroglycerin, clopidogrel, streptokinase
c. Aspirin, sublingual nitroglycerin, clopidogrel, heparin
d. Aspirin, sublingual nitroglycerin, clopidogrel, beta blockers

Best management of such a case would be aspirin, sublingual nitroglycerin, clopidogrel and primary PCI. For people who have already had a heart attack or stroke, taking aspirin daily for two years prevented 1 in 50 from having a cardiovascular problem (heart attack, stroke, or death), but also caused non-fatal bleeding problems to occur in 1 of 400 people. Improved myocardial oxygen demand vs oxygen delivery ratio (on administering sublingual nitroglycerine) leads to the following therapeutic effects during episodes of angina pectoris—subsiding of chest pain, decrease of blood pressure, increase of heart rate, and orthostatic hypotension. Clopidogrel is used to prevent heart attack and stroke in people who are at high-risk of these events, including those with a history of myocardial infarction and other forms of acute coronary syndrome, stroke, and those with peripheral artery disease. Percutaneous coronary intervention (PCI) may be appropriate for patients with stable coronary artery disease if they meet certain criteria, such as having any coronary stenosis greater than 50 percent or having angina symptoms that are unresponsive to medical therapy.

Answers

24. d 25. b 26. a 27. b 28. a

29. A 64-years-old man presents with chest pain of 24 hours duration. His ECG reveals ST elevation, anterior wall myocardial infarction. The preferred treatment modality for him is:

a. Primary percutaneous coronary intervention
b. Thrombolysis with alteplase
c. Thrombolysis with streptokinase
d. Nitroglycerin infusion, aspirin and beta blockers

Management of anterior wall MI include aspirin is given straightaway in a dose of 325 mg to be chewed. It is the first line drug in the initial management of AMI and all other forms of ischemic heart disease. In acute MI with angina, congestive heart failure, persistent angina or hypertension, nitrates are given for the first 24–48 hours. Beta-blockers, when used in the early hours of infarction, they limit infarct size, reduce the incidence of ventricular arrhythmias, atrial fibrillation and cardiac arrest.

30. The treatment of choice for a 32-years-old male patient of severe mitral stenosis (Rheumatic) with thickened and calcified valves on echocardiography is:

a. Balloon mitral valvuloplasty (BMV)
b. Mitral valve replacement (MVR)
c. Medical management only
d. Mitral valvotomy (MV)

MVR is an accepted procedure for patients who are not candidates for surgical commissurotomy or BMV. When there is associated MR or when the valve is rigid and calcified, MVR is indicated.

31. An adult with fever and right-sided chest pain is found to have a moderate right-sided pleural effusion. Chest X-ray (PA view) also shows a moderate pleural effusion. A diagnostic thoracocentesis reveals straw coloured exudates with 50 mg% of sugar and lymphocytic pleocytosis. ADA levels are borderline. What investigation would be most likely to confirm a diagnosis of tuberculosis?

a. Needle biopsy of the pleura
b. Pleural fluid Xpert MTB/RIF assay
c. Pleural fluid AFB smear
d. Pleural fluid AFB-culture

Tubercle bacilli are difficult to demonstrate in serous effusion by conventional methods. Needle biopsy is helpful, but this is not required in the ordinary case.

32. A 26-years-old woman presents with fever, arthralgia and erythema nodosum. Her chest X-ray reveals bilateral hilar lymphadenopathy. Her mantoux test is negative. The most likely diagnosis is:

a. Tuberculosis
b. Allergic bronchopulmonary aspergillosis
c. Sarcoidosis
d. Pulmonary thromboembolism

The commonest presentation of sarcoidosis is as bilateral hilar lymphadenopathy with associated fever and erythema nodosum.

33. A middle-aged patient with chronic liver disease presents with pain abdomen and distension. He also has diarrhoea and fever since one day. On examination, he is hemodynamically stable with fever of 100°F. There is jaundice, pallor, pedal edema and ascites. A diagnostic paracentesis is done. Ascitic fluid protein is 0.8 gm%, sugar 100 mg%, total count 500/mm³ of which 85% are polymorphonuclear leukocytes and 15% lymphocytes. Most likely diagnosis is:

a. Spontaneous bacterial peritonitis
b. Secondary bacterial peritonitis
c. Perforation peritonitis
d. TB peritonitis

Spontaneous bacterial peritonitis is diagnosed if the fluid contains neutrophils at greater than 250 cells per mm³ (equals a cell count of 250 × 10^6/L) fluid in the absence of another reason for this (such as inflammation of one of the internal organs or a perforation). The crux of this algorithm is *Runyon's Criteria* for secondary bacterial peritonitis, which requires two of these three features: total protein >1 g/dL, glucose <50 mg/dL (2.8 mM), and lactate dehydrogenase above the upper limit of normal for serum.

34. A young male comes to the OPD with history of jaundice since many years. He has noted that the jaundice may fluctuate but is often aggravated when he is fasting. There is no history of hospitalization, no drug use, alcoholism or blood transfusion. Family history is not significant. Clinical examination is unremarkable except for mild scleral icterus. What is the likely diagnosis?

a. Dubin-Johnson syndrome
b. Crigler–Najjar syndrome type-I
c. Gilbert's syndrome
d. Rotor syndrome

Gilbert's syndrome (GS) is a mild liver disorder in which the liver does not properly process bilirubin. Many people never have symptoms. Occasionally a slight yellowish color of the skin or sclera may occur. Episodes of jaundice may be triggered by stress such as exercise, menstruation, or not eating.

35. A right handed 70-years-old man has a brain scan which reveals a lesion that has damaged his left angular and supramarginal gyrus. On examination, one would expect the following *except*:

a. Difficulty with left to right discrimination
b. Inappropriate affect
c. Finger agnosia
d. Inability to write

Answers

29. d	**30.** b	**31.** a	**32.** c	**33.** a	**34.** c	**35.** b

The angular gyrus is the part of the brain associated with complex language functions (i.e. reading, writing and interpretation of what is written). Lesion to this part of the brain shows symptoms of the Gerstmann syndrome: effects include finger agnosia, alexia (inability to read), acalculia (inability to use arithmetic operations), agraphia (inability to copy), and left-right confusion.

36. A 34-week pregnant nurse comes in contact with a patient with chickenpox at her workplace. She has never had chickenpox in the past and is unvaccinated. The best option for her is:

a. Varicella zoster immunoglobulin to be given within 7 days
b. Vaccinate for chicken pox
c. Start oral acyclovir
d. Wait and watch

Varicella (live attenuated vaccine) is not recommended in pregnancy. Varicella zoster immunoglobulin (VZIg) should be given to exposed non-immune patients as it reduces the morbidity.

37. A 24-years-old male presents with consumption of an unknown substance. His respiratory rate is 22/minute, pulse rate is 110/minute, BP is 150/94 mmHg and he has 2 episodes of seizures. There are tremors and hallucinations. The substance ingested most likely is:

a. Amphetamines b. Diazepam
c. Oxycodone d. Ethanol

Amphetamines increase the activity of the neurotransmitters dopamine and norepinephrine. Tachycardia and other arrhythmias are due to the sympathomimetic effects of amphetamines. Amphetamines cause tachycardia and hypertension and can cause significant cerebral blood flow which increases by 30%. Increased dopamine levels in the central nervous system (CNS) cause psychosis, euphoric effects, and other movement disorders. Amphetamine toxicity can also cause seizures due to neuronal death from the interaction between amphetamines and NMDA receptors.

38. An 18-years-old boy was brought to the emergency department after being bitten by a saw-scaled viper. The monitoring which is most crucial in this patient is:

a. Single breath count
b. Neck flop
c. Whole blood clotting time
d. Creatine phosphokinase

Most of saw-scaled viper species have venom that contains factors that can cause a consumption coagulopathy and defibrination, which may persist for days to weeks. This may result in bleeding anywhere in the body, including the possibility of an intracranial hemorrhage. The latter classically occurs a few days following the bite.

39. A 35-years-old man with history of alcoholism presents with ophthalmoplegia, ataxia and global confusion. The treatment of choice for this patient is:

a. IV glucose b. IV thiamine
c. IV mannitol d. IV immunoglobulin

Classically, Wernicke encephalopathy is characterized by the triad—ophthalmoplegia, ataxia, and confusion. In patients suspected of WE, thiamine treatment should be started immediately. Blood should be immediately taken to test for thiamine, other vitamins and minerals levels. Following this an immediate intravenous or intramuscular dose of thiamine should be administered two or three times daily.

40. Characteristic features of Horner's syndrome are:

a. Partial ptosis, enophthalmos, constricted pupil, decreased sweating
b. Partial ptosis, exophthalmos, constricted pupil, decreased sweating
c. Partial ptosis, enophthalmos, dilated pupil, decreased sweating
d. Partial ptosis, enophthalmos, constricted pupil, increased sweating

Horner's syndrome, also known as oculosympathetic paresis, is a combination of symptoms that arises when sympathetic trunk is damaged. The signs and symptoms occur on the same side (ipsilateral) as it is a lesion of the sympathetic trunk. It is characterized by miosis (a constricted pupil), partial ptosis (a weak, droopy eyelid), apparent anhydrosis (decreased sweating), with apparent enophthalmos (inset eyeball).

41. A 40-years-old woman presents with sudden onset palpitations. An ECG done reveals narrow-QRS complex tachycardia. The most likely diagnosis is:

a. Ventricular tachycardia
b. Pre-excited tachycardia
c. Paroxysmal supraventricular tachycardia with aberrancy
d. AV re-entry tachycardia

Findings on AV nodal re-entry tachycardia (AVNRT) on ECG include narrow complex tachycardia, a P wave that occurs after the QRS complex (a short RP interval) and tachycardia that quickly terminates with AV blocking manoeuvres (carotid massage or adenosine).

42. A 21-years-young man presents in emergency with high grade fever with inflammation of knee and ankle joints which is fleeting in nature. There is history of occasional palpitations. There is no history of antecedent sore throat. On examination, splenomegaly is present. The ECG shows prolongation of PR interval. What is the most likely diagnosis in India?

a. Still disease b. Enteric fever
c. Rheumatic fever d. Reiter's syndrome

Answers

36. a	37. a	38. c	39. b	40. a	41. d	42. c

Rheumatic arthritis is an asymmetric, migratory/fleeting polyarthritis with predominant involvement of large joints of lower limbs and migrates to the upper limb. Classically the joints are red, tender, swollen and the child cannot tolerate any movement about the joint.

43. A 50-years gentleman with Type-2 diabetes mellitus for 5 years presents in medical emergency with sudden onset of dyspnoea at rest, orthopnoea, and prostration. On examination, pulse is rapid and very weak in volume. His blood pressure is 100/70 mmHg. There are diffuse crepitations at lung bases. What is the most likely diagnosis of his conditions?

a. Mitral stenosis with bacterial endocarditis
b. Right heart failure
c. Left heart failure
d. Constrictive pericarditis

Common respiratory signs of left heart failure are increased rate of breathing (tachypnea) and increased *work* of breathing (nonspecific signs of respiratory distress). Rales or crackles, heard initially in the lung bases, and when severe, throughout the lung fields suggest the development of pulmonary edema (fluid in the). The person will have dyspnea (shortness of breath) on exertion and in severe cases, dyspnea at rest. Increasing breathlessness on lying flat, called orthopnea, occurs.

44. A 26-years-old HIV infected male presents with odynophagia. Upper GI endoscopy demonstrates serpiginous ulcers in a normal surrounding mucosa in distal esophagus. The most likely diagnosis is:

a. Gastroesophageal reflux disease
b. Cytomegalovirus esophagitis
c. Candida esophagitis
d. Herpetic esophagitis

CMV classically causes serpiginous ulcers in the distal esophagus that may coalesce to form giant ulcers. Brushings alone are insufficient for diagnosis, and biopsies must be performed. Biopsies reveal intranuclear and intracytoplasmic inclusions with enlarged nuclei in large fibroblasts and endothelial cells.

45. Which of the following is the most important complication in a patient with coeliac disease, who was previously doing well on a gluten-free diet and is now not responding to gluten restriction?

a. Intestinal infection
b. Intestinal lymphoma
c. Resistant coeliac disease
d. Type II diabetes mellitus

For a small number of people living with celiac disease, a gluten-free diet is not enough to stop the otherwise severe symptoms. These patients are classified as having refractory celiac disease (RCD), which usually affects between 2 and 5 percent of celiac disease patients. In one type of RCD called RCDII, the white blood cells found in the wall of the small intestine divide and multiply in excessive numbers. In approximately half of the RCDII patients, these cells, called lymphocytes, go on to develop into a particularly rare form of lymphoma. This rare and very aggressive form of white blood cell cancer is called enteropathy-associated T-cell lymphoma.

46. A middle-aged diabetic male who has recurrent chest pain undergoes coronary artery angiogram. The following day, he develops haematuria, proteinuria and renal impairment. What is the most likely diagnosis?

a. Renal artery stenosis
b. Acute renal infraction
c. Atheroembolism
d. Haemolytic uraemic syndrome

Cholesterol embolism occurs when cholesterol is released, usually from an atherosclerotic plaque, and travels as an embolus in the bloodstream to lodge (as an embolism) causing an obstruction in blood vessels further away. Most commonly this causes skin symptoms (usually livedo reticularis), gangrene of the extremities and sometimes kidney failure; problems with other organs may arise, depending on the site at which the cholesterol crystals enter the bloodstream. When the kidneys are involved, the disease is referred to as atheroembolic renal disease. it is a complication of medical procedures involving the blood vessels, such as vascular surgery or angiography.

47. Which one of the following is a cause of early (0–4 weeks) infection in recipients of haematopoietic stem cell transplantation?

a. Cytomegalovirus
b. Pneumocystis jirovecii
c. Varicella zoster
d. Herpes simplex

Herpes simplex virus (HSV) infection (especially of skin and mucous membranes) prior to the introduction of acyclovir was a major problem in the hematopoietic stem cell transplantation (HSCT) recipient. Occurring in the pre-engraftment period, HSV infection greatly exacerbated the severity of mucositis. Not only were ulcers observed in the oral cavity and anogenital areas, ulcerations of the esophagus, stomach and intestine were also observed. HSV pneumonia was also noted, with rare cases of cutaneous dissemination and encephalitis. The current standard of care is to test all candidates for HSCT for an antibody to HSV, with seropositive individuals then placed on antiviral prophylaxis, beginning prior to HSCT. Effective agents for HSV prophylaxis include acyclovir (intravenous or oral), valacyclovir or famciclovir.

Answers

43. c **44.** b **45.** b **46.** c **47.** d

48. A 24 years female presented with generalized weakness. Her thyroid function test is as follows. Serum T3 = Normal, T4 = Normal, TSH = 10 mU/L. What is the most likely diagnosis?

a. Primary hypothyroidism
b. Secondary hypothyroidism
c. Subclinical hypothyroidism
d. Non-thyroidal illness

Subclinical hypothyroidism (SCH), also called mild thyroid failure, is diagnosed when peripheral thyroid hormone levels are within normal reference laboratory range but serum thyroid-stimulating hormone (TSH) levels are mildly elevated. This condition occurs in 3% to 8% of the general population. It is more common in women than men, and its prevalence increases with age. Of patients with SCH, 80% have a serum TSH of less than 10 mIU/L.

49. A 32-years-old HIV infected male presents with shortness of breath and moderate fever of two-week duration. On examination, cyanosis is present, with respiratory rate of 22/minute and some basal crackles in chest. The CT chest shows bilateral ground-glass pattern. The most likely etiologic diagnosis is:

a. Streptococcus pneumoniae
b. Pneumocystis jirovecii
c. Mycobacterium tuberculosis
d. Staphylococcus sp.

The most common high-resolution CT finding of *Pneumocystis jiroveci pneumonia* is diffuse ground-glass opacity. The term ground-glass refers to parenchymal opacification, which does not obscure the underlying pulmonary architecture. This usually occurs in a bilateral, symmetrical, predominantly perihilar distribution and may be geographic or mosaic in appearance, with areas of normal lung adjacent to areas of affected lung.

50. A 22-years-old male is admitted with fever and altered consciousness for two days. Examination reveals nuchal rigidity and diffuse petechial rash on the trunk and lower extremities. The most likely etiologic agent is:

a. *Escherichia coli*
b. *Streptococcus pneumoniae*
c. *Neisseria meningitidis*
d. *Haemophilus infleunzae*

The average incubation period of meningococcal meningitis is four days, but can range between two and 10 days. The most common symptoms are a stiff neck, high fever, sensitivity to light, confusion, headaches and vomiting. In addition, in infants bulging fontanelle and ragdoll appearance are commonly found. A less common but even more severe (often fatal) form of meningococcal disease is meningococcal septicaemia, which is characterized by a haemorrhagic rash and rapid circulatory collapse.

51. A 36-years-old chronic alcoholic, malnourished male is hospitalized with pneumonia. His condition worsens after aggressive treatment with intravenous dextrose and antibiotics. This phenomenon of 'Refeeding Syndrome' is accompanied by which one of the following biochemical alterations?

a. Hypophosphatemia
b. Hyponatremia
c. Hyperkalemia
d. Hypermagnesemia

Hypophosphatemia is a potentially life-threatening complication of reinstating nutrition in a malnourished patient. Refeeding syndrome is a term that refers to various metabolic abnormalities that may complicate carbohydrate administration in subnourished patient populations.

52. A 31-years-young man presents with fever, weight loss, pain with swelling of knee joint and low backache with stiffness. Three weeks earlier, he was treated for symptoms of urinary tract infection by local practitioner. The joint aspirate is leucocyte rich and contains multinucleated macrophages. His urine culture is sterile. What is the most probable diagnosis?

a. Septic arthritis
b. Crystal arthritis
c. Reactive arthritis
d. Still disease

Reactive arthritis (ReA), formerly termed Reiter syndrome, is an autoimmune condition that develops in response to an infection. It has been associated with gastrointestinal (GI) infections with *Shigella, Salmonella, Campylobacter,* and other organisms, as well as with genitourinary (GU) infections (especially with *Chlamydia trachomatis*).

53. A 56-years-old man presented with acute onset aphasia. Speech output was markedly reduced with preserved comprehension of spoken language. The area of brain involved is:

a. Posterior part of temporal lobe
b. Cerebellum
c. Midbrain
d. Inferior frontal gyrus

Expressive aphasia, also known as Broca's aphasia, is a type of aphasia characterized by partial loss of the ability to produce language (spoken, manual, or written), although comprehension generally remains intact. Broca's area is located in inferior frontal gyrus.

54. A 30-years-old male was being evaluated for paraparesis. On examination, there was severe muscle atrophy, with absent deep tendon reflexes and absent Babinski sign. The most likely possibility is:

a. Upper motor neuron disease
b. Lower motor neuron disease
c. Psychogenic cause
d. Cerebellar disease

Answers

48. c **49.** b **50.** c **51.** a **52.** c **53.** d **54.** b

In LMN (lower motor neuron) disease, the extensor plantar reflex is usually absent. Muscle paresis/paralysis, hypotonia/atonia, and hyporeflexia/areflexia are usually seen immediately following an insult. Muscle wasting, fasciculations and fibrillations are typically signs of end-stage muscle denervation and are seen over a longer time period. Another feature is the segmentation of symptoms – only muscles innervated by the damaged nerves will be symptomatic.

55. A 16-years-old boy presented with fever and a diffuse maculopapular rash. Examination revealed generalized cervical lymphadenopathy and hepatosplenomegaly. After intake of Ampicillin (prescribed by a local practitioner), the rash worsened. The most likely diagnosis is:

a. Dengue fever
b. Measles
c. Drug-rash
d. Infectious mononucleosis

In adolescence and young adulthood, infectious mononucleosis presents with a characteristic triad: Fever – usually lasting 14 days; often mild; sore throat–usually severe for 3–5 days, before resolving in the next 7–10 days and swollen glands–mobile; usually located around the back of the neck (posterior cervical lymph nodes) and sometimes throughout the body. A small minority of people spontaneously present a rash, usually on the arms or trunk, which can be macular (morbiliform) or popular. Almost all people given amoxicillin or ampicillin eventually develop a generalized, itchy maculopapular rash, which however does not imply that the person will have adverse reactions to penicillins again in the future.

56. Following the bite of a snake, a patient develops generalized myalgias, rhabdomyolysis, and progressive flaccid paralysis. The most likely snake implicated is:

a. Cobra
b. Krait
c. Russel viper
d. Sea snake

The most important symptoms of sea snake bite are rhabdomyolysis (rapid breakdown of skeletal muscle tissue) and paralysis. Early symptoms include headache, a thick-feeling tongue, thirst, sweating, and vomiting. The venom is very slow acting and symptoms that happen from little as 30 minutes to several hours after the bite include generalized aching, stiffness, and tenderness of muscles all over the body. Passive stretching of the muscles is also painful, and trismus, which is similar to tetanus, is common. This is followed later on by symptoms typical of other elapid envenomations, a progressive flaccid paralysis, starting with ptosis and paralysis of voluntary muscles. Paralysis of muscles involved in swallowing and respiration can be fatal.

57. A 65-years-old man, on *Warfarin* treatment, is started on antitubercular treatment. The pharmacologic effect of *Warfarin* is likely to:

a. Increase
b. Decrease
c. Remain the same
d. Be unpredictable and variable

Rifampin has been reported to decrease the warfarin pharmacological effects in human subjects ingesting these agents simultaneously as rifampicin is an enzyme inducer (CYP2D6) enhancing the metabolism of warfarin. The concomitant administration of rifampin and warfarin resulted in the need for an unusually high maintenance dose of warfarin (20 mg per day) in order to produce a therapeutic effect.

58. A chronic alcoholic develops a paroxysm of palpitations after alcohol binge. Which of the following arrhythmia is most likely?

a. Ventricular fibrillation
b. Ventricular premature complex
c. Atrial flutter
d. Atrial fibrillation

In 1978, Philip Ettinger described "Holiday heart syndrome" (HHS) for the first time, as the occurrence, in healthy people without heart disease known to cause arrhythmia, of an acute cardiac rhythm disturbance, most frequently atrial fibrillation, after binge drinking.

59. An elderly man with history of diabetes mellitus and Coronary Artery Disease comes for follow-up, with complaints of muscle pains. Which one of the following drugs could be the most likely cause?

a. Aspirin
b. Glimepiride
c. Enalapril
d. Atorvastatin

Muscle aches are the commonest (10%) side effect of statins. Rise in CPK levels occur infrequently.

60. A 40-years-old lady comes to outdoor clinic with complaints of sudden onset chest pain. The chest X-ray shows bilateral pneumothorax. Examination reveals abnormalities of body habitus—including long arms, legs and finger (arachnodactyly), scoliosis, high arched palate, joint hypermobility, and a pansystolic murmur at cardiac apex. Which one of the following diseases is most likely?

a. Takayasu's arteritis
b. Raynaud's syndrome
c. Marfan's syndrome
d. Rheumatic heart disease—mitral regurgitation

Marfan syndrome (MFS) is a genetic disorder that affects the connective tissue. Those with the condition tend to be tall and thin, with long arms, legs, fingers and toes. They also typically have overly-flexible joints and scoliosis. The most serious complications involve the heart and aorta, with an increased risk of mitral valve prolapse and aortic aneurysm.

Answers

55. d **56.** d **57.** b **58.** d **59.** d **60.** c

61. An 18-years-old male has insulin dependent diabetes, with malabsorption syndrome and bilateral upper lobe bronchiectasis. A diagnostic work-up will include all *except*:

a. 24-hour fecal fat-estimation
b. CT-chest
c. Lung biopsy
d. DNA sequencing study

Clinical presentation suggests the diagnosis of cystic fibrosis (CF). Investigations done for CF include 24-hours fecal fat estimation (for malabsorption), CT scan chest (for bronchiectasis) and DNA sequencing study for CF.

62. A 26-years-old young lady attends medical emergency and is labelled as acute severe asthma by the emergency physician. Which one of the following is unlikely to be a part of the prescription?

a. Albuterol
b. Anti-leukotrienes
c. Aminophylline
d. Magnesium sulfate

Anti-leukotrienes (Montelukast) are used for maintenance therapy of asthma. They have no role in managing acute severe asthma.

63. Spontaneous oesophageal perforation after a bout of forceful vomiting or retching is characteristically seen in which one of the following conditions?

a. Menetrier's disease
b. Boerhaave's syndrome
c. Achalasia of the oesophagus
d. Barrett's oesophagus

Boerhaave syndrome is also known as spontaneous esophageal rupture or effort rupture of the esophagus. Although vomiting is thought to be the most common cause, other causes include those that can increase intra-esophageal pressure and cause a barogenic esophageal rupture.

64. A 13-years-old boy presents with hematuria, oliguria, edema and hypertension. He has history of sore throat two weeks prior to presentation. Laboratory investigations are remarkable for low C3 and increased titres of ASO and antiDNase. Which one of the following statements is NOT correct about management for this condition?

a. Renal biopsy is rarely required for making diagnosis
b. Antibiotic treatment is given for streptococcal infection
c. Treatment is largely supportive
d. Immunosuppressants are to be used for crescentic glomerulonephritis

Combination of glucocorticoids in pulsed doses, cytotoxic agents (azathioprine, cyclophosphamide), and intensive plasma exchange may be useful in crescentic GN.

65. A 60-years-old patient is admitted in emergency with seizure, aphasia and altered sensorium. He has history of fever and headache for the preceding 3 days. The CSF examination is unremarkable. What would be the probable diagnosis?

a. Multiple sclerosis
b. Tubercular meningitis
c. Pyogenic (bacterial) meningitis
d. Viral encephalitis

Sign and symptoms of encephalitis include headache, fever, fits, altered sensorium with or without neurological deficit, signs of increased intracranial tension, and meningeal signs. No organism is seen in CSF.

66. A 68-years-old male presented in OPD with complaints of progressive small handwriting. On examination, he had resting tremor, bradykinesia, rigidity and postural instability. This patient is suffering most likely from:

a. Parkinson's disease
b. Vascular dementia
c. Alzheimer's disease
d. Frontotemporal dementia

Features of Parkinson's disease include tremor (mainly at rest and described as pill rolling tremor in hands), bradykinesia, limb rigidity, gait and balance problems etc.

67. An elderly patient presents with abnormal gait. He has a wide base freezing gait with imbalance, comprising short strides, shuffling along the floor and difficulty with starts and turns. Heal-Shin test is normal. Which one of the following is most likely disorder?

a. Cerebellar ataxia
b. Sensory ataxia
c. Frontal gait disorder
d. Parkinson's disease

Frontal lobe gait apraxia: A broad-based (wide-based) gait with short stride, freezing, falls, and an inability to 'walk and talk', in the elderly, is most likely due to frontal lobe pathology. The commonest cause is cerebrovascular disease.

68. A 35-years-old man presents with history of low-grade fever and headache for last five weeks. Clinical examination is remarkable for signs of meningismus. He undergoes lumbar puncture (LP) and a day later reports worsening of headache. Which one of the following features is NOT consistent with diagnosis of "Post-LP" headache?

a. Post-LP headache usually begins within 48 hours
b. Post-LP headache worsens in sitting position
c. Post-LP headache is most severe upon waking up
d. Post-LP headache may improve with caffeine intake

Post-lumbar puncture headache is defined as "bilateral headaches that develop within 7 days after an lumbar puncture and disappears within 14 days. The headache worsens within 15 min of resuming the upright position, disappears or improves within 30 min of resuming the recumbent position". This definition helps to avoid

Answers

61. c 62. b 63. b 64. d 65. d 66. a 67. c
68. c

confusion with migraine or simple headache after lumbar puncture.

69. A young lady presents in outdoor clinic with complaints of menstrual irregularity, weight gain, hair loss, tiredness and weakness. What will be the investigation of choice?

a. FSH and LH level
b. Estrogen level
c. Free T3 and free T4 level
d. Free T4 and TSH level

Clinical findings suggest the diagnosis of hypothyroidism. Thyroid function tests include TSH, T3 and T4 levels estimation.

70. Every individual carries four alpha gene alleles. Deletion of three alleles leads to development of:

a. Haemoglobin X disease
b. Haemoglobin H disease
c. Haemoglobin F disease
d. Hydrops fetalis

Alpha-thalassemia (α-thalassemia) has two clinically significant forms: hemoglobin Bart hydrops fetalis (Hb Bart) syndrome (caused by deletion/inactivation of all four α-globin genes; –/–), and hemoglobin H (HbH) disease (most frequently caused by deletion/inactivation of three α-globin genes; –/–α).

Answers

69. d **70.** b

12 Surgery

1. **Mallory-Weiss tear causing haematemesis is seen over:**
   a. Oesophagus
   b. Gastroesophageal junction
   c. Anterior wall of stomach
   d. Fundus of stomach

   Mallory–Weiss syndrome or gastroesophageal laceration syndrome refers to bleeding from a laceration in the mucosa at the junction of the stomach and esophagus. This is usually caused by severe vomiting because of alcoholism or bulimia, but can be caused by any condition which causes violent vomiting and retching such as food poisoning. The syndrome presents with hematemesis. The laceration is sometimes referred to as a *Mallory-Weiss tear*.

2. **A 47-years-old post-menopausal lady was on adjuvant hormonal treatment with Tamoxifen for 3 years for Carcinoma Breast. She came to Outpatient Department with history of passing blood clots per vagina. She is probably suffering from:**
   a. Carcinoma vulva
   b. Carcinoma vagina
   c. Carcinoma endometrium
   d. Uterine fibroid

   Tamoxifen increases the incidence of uterine carcinoma.

3. **A 70-years-old male having comorbidities present with benign appearing parotid tumour. The best option is:**
   a. Tumour enucleation
   b. Superficial parotidectomy
   c. Aspiration biopsy confirmation
   d. Radio-therapy

   FNAC is very important and diagnostic in pleomorphic adenoma.

4. **A gentleman of 56 years underwent laparoscopic left hemicolectomy for diagnosed left colonic carcinoma. Histopathology revealed the tumour to be invading submucosa and muscularis propria. Among the 16 regional lymph nodes harvested, 2 were positive for malignant deposits. His staging as per AJCC will be:**
   a. T1, N1, M0
   b. T2, N1, M0
   c. T1, N0, M0
   d. T2, N1, M1

   The cancer has grown through the muscularis mucosa into the submucosa (T1), and it may also have grown into the muscularis propria (T2). It has not spread to nearby lymph nodes (N0) or to distant sites (M0). The cancer has grown into the outermost layers of the colon or rectum but has not gone through them (T3).

5. **A policeman of 45 years presented with lipodermatosclerosis over lower medial aspect of left leg, along with a healed venous ulcer. As per the CEAP (Clinical-etiology-anatomy-pathophysiology) classification his clinical classification will be:**
   a. C4a
   b. C4b
   c. C5
   d. C6

   The CEAP classification (Clinical-Etiological-Anatomical-Pathophysiological) was created in 1994 to standardize the diverse manifestations of chronic venous disease. It was modified in 2004 to refer more broadly to chronic venous disorders. Therefore, it covers the broad spectrum of morphological and functional alterations of the venous system. C5 denotes healed ulcer.

6. **A few days following viral fever, a 50-years-old female presented with pain in neck, fever, malaise and firm enlargement of both the lobes of thyroid. On investigation thyroid antibodies were normal and serum T4 was high normal. Probable diagnosis is:**
   a. Autoimmune thyroiditis
   b. Lymphoma of thyroid
   c. Granulomatous thyroiditis
   d. Riedel's thyroiditis

   Features of DeQuervain's subacute granulomatous thyroiditis include painful diffuse, swelling in thyroid which is tender; commonly seen in females and initially there is a transient hyperthyroidism with high T3 and T4 but poor radio-iodine uptake.

Answers

1. b	**2.** c	**3.** c	**4.** b	**5.** c	**6.** c

7. **A gentleman of 36 years presented with a long history of upper abdominal pain which was periodic and often occurred early morning. For last 3 months, he is having projectile vomiting, which is non-bilious, unpleasant in nature with undigested food materials. On examination he appears unwell, dehydrated and seemed to have lost weight. Probably he is suffering from:**
   a. Gastric outlet obstruction
   b. Carcinoma stomach
   c. Gastro-oesophageal reflux with oesophagitis
   d. Superior mesenteric artery syndrome

Gastric outlet obstruction (GOO) is a clinical syndrome that can manifest with a variety of symptoms, including abdominal pain, postprandial vomiting, early satiety, and weight loss. It is caused by either a benign or malignant mechanical obstruction or a motility disorder interfering with gastric emptying.

8. **A 40-years-old female patient presents with colicky abdominal pain associated with episodes of mild diarrhoea for last 6 months accompanied with intermittent fever and weight loss. There are multiple discharging sinuses on perineal examination. The most likely clinical diagnosis in this patient is:**
   a. Amoebic colitis
   b. Crohn disease
   c. Ulcerative colitis
   d. Ileocaecal tuberculosis

Symptoms of Crohn's disease often include abdominal pain, diarrhea (which may be bloody if inflammation is severe), fever, abdominal distension, and weight loss. In Crohn's disease, perianal region should be examined for evidence of induration and erythema, fistulous tract openings, multiple or eccentric anal fissures, ulcerations, and/or large, broad-based skin tags.

9. **A gentleman of 48 years was being worked up for hepatocellular function. He had no history or signs of encephalopathy. His serum bilirubin was 5 mg%, serum albumin was 3.9 gm%, International Normalized Ratio was 1.6. On ultrasound no free fluid was detected inside abdomen. As per Child-Turcotte-Pugh (CTP) classification, he was in:**
   a. CTP–A
   b. CTP–B
   c. CTP–C
   d. CTP–D

	1	*2*	*3*
Encephalopathy	None	Grade 1–2 (or precipitant-induced)	Grade 3–4 (or chronic)
Ascites	None	Mild/Moderate (diuretic-responsive)	Severe (diuretic-refractory)
Bilirubin (mg/dL)	< 2	2–3	> 3
Albumin (g/dL)	> 3.5	2.8–3.5	< 2.8
PT (sec prolonged) or INR	< 4 < 1.7	4–6 1.7–2.3	> 6 > 2.3

CTP score is obtained by adding the score for each parameter.

CTP class: *A = 5–6 points, B = 7–9 points, C = 10–15 points*

10. **A 48-years-old male with the history of chronic duodenal ulcer presented in surgical emergency with the complaints of sudden severe pain in the abdomen. At presentation:**
    Pulse = 120/m, BP = 90/60 mm of Hg
    Abdomen: Tenderness (+), Rigidity (+), Guarding (+)
    Respiratory Rate: 20/m
    X-ray: Gas under right dome of diaphragm
    The probable diagnosis is:
    a. Acute appendicitis
    b. Acute pancreatitis
    c. Acute myocardial infraction
    d. Perforation peritonitis

The majority of perforation peritonitis comprises of peptic ulcer perforations followed by typhoid ileal, appendicular and traumatic perforations. Peritonitis usually presents as an acute abdomen. Local findings include abdominal tenderness, guarding or rigidity, distension, diminished bowel sounds. Systemic findings include fever, chills or rigor, tachycardia, sweating, tachypnea, restlessness, dehydration, oliguria, disorientation and ultimately shock.

11. **A young sports person presented in surgical emergency with the complaints of severe pain in the groin area, extending into the scrotum and upper thigh. The pain is debilitating and he is not able to exercise. On examination there is tenderness in the region of inguinal canal and pubic tubercle. He is probably suffering from:**
    a. Varicocele
    b. Inguinal hernia
    c. Sportsman hernia
    d. Femoral hernia

A sports hernia is a painful, soft tissue injury that occurs in the groin area. It most often occurs during sports that require sudden changes of direction or intense twisting movements. Although a sports hernia may lead to a traditional, abdominal hernia, it is a different injury.

12. **Diaphragmatic injury is suspected in a 50 years gentleman with history of blunt abdominal trauma, having a normal chest X-ray. He is best managed by:**
    a. Diagnostic peritoneal lavage and proceed
    b. Upper GI contrast study
    c. CECT abdomen
    d. Diagnostic laparoscopy

Answers

7. a **8.** b **9.** b **10.** d **11.** c **12.** d

Laparoscopy is an excellent diagnostic and therapeutic procedure in the setting of suspected diagnostic rupture, with or without herniation of abdominal content. It is safe and effective in repairing the diaphragm following rupture due to blunt abdominal trauma.

13. A 20-years-old man had history of pain in the right side of abdomen. His X-ray abdomen AP view shows radio-opaque shadow, which on lateral film falls behind the vertebral column. The probable diagnosis is:

a. Gallstone disease
b. Renal calculus
c. Calcified mesenteric lymph node
d. Phlebolith

90% of the renal calculus are radio-opaque and only 10% of the gallstones are radio-opaque.

14. A 70-years-old man on anticoagulants due to some heart disease suffered a minor head injury. One month later he has severe headache with slowly developing neurological signs. The probable diagnosis is:

a. Extradural haematoma
b. Acute subdural haematoma
c. Chronic subdural haematoma
d. Subarachnoid haemorrhage

A chronic subdural hematoma (SDH) is a collection of blood on the brain's surface, under the outer covering of the brain (dura). It usually begins forming several days or weeks after bleeding initially starts. Bleeding is usually due to a head injury. A chronic SDH does not always produce symptoms.

15. A 50-years-old male presented with pain along the left arm and ptosis. His chest X-ray showed soft tissue opacity at the apex of the left lung along with the erosion of the adjacent rib. The probable diagnosis is:

a. Pancoast lung
b. Bronchial carcinoma
c. Lung abscess
d. Adenocarcinoma of lung

The combination of severe shoulder/arm pain along with the distribution of the C8, T1, T2 nerve trunks, Horner syndrome (ipsilateral ptosis, miosis, and anhidrosis; caused due to interruption of sympathetic nerve chain running to the head) and atrophy of the intrinsic hand muscles is termed "Pancoast-Tobias syndrome."

16. A young boy riding a motorcycle, met with a road traffic accident. On examination he had maxillofacial trauma with paraesthesia of the lower lip. Most likely underlying he has a:

a. Fracture involving infraorbital foramen
b. Fracture involving floor of orbit
c. Fracture of the mandibular body
d. Fracture of temporal bone

The mandible is reported to be the most commonly fractured bone of the facial skeleton. Mandibular fractures that occur between the mental and mandibular foramina frequently result in inferior alveolar nerve (IAN) injury. As a consequence of nerve injury, an altered neurosensory function of the skin and mucous membrane within the distribution of mental nerve on the side of fracture may be observed, though usually such condition gradually improves with time.

17. A 20-years-old patient underwent open hernia surgery four days back. He is running fever for the last one day and on local examination the operated site was wet with pus and surrounding redness and edema. The appropriate management would be:

a. Change of antibiotics
b. Daily dressing
c. Opening sutures and cleaning of wound
d. Sending pus for C/S

A surgical site infection (SSI) is an infection that occurs in the incision created by an invasive surgical procedure. Any sutures or clips present should be removed, allowing for the drainage of any pus and the opportunity for wound packing if required.

18. An eight-years-old male child complains of severe pain in right testes. The most probable diagnosis is:

a. Torsion of right testis
b. Strangulated inguinal hernia
c. Acute epididymo-orchitis
d. Undescended testis

Testicular torsion occurs when the spermatic cord (from which the testicle is suspended) twists, cutting off the testicle's blood supply. The most common symptom in children is rapid onset of severe testicular pain. The testicle may also be higher than usual and vomiting may occur. In newborns pain is often absent and instead the scrotum may become discolored or a testicle may disappear from its usual place.

19. A 32-years-old female underwent laparoscopic cholecystectomy which was difficult. On her second postoperative day, she develops jaundice. Her LFT parameters show serum bilirubin 6.8 mg/dL; direct bilirubin 5.6 and indirect bilirubin 1.2 mg/dL; and serum alkaline phosphatase 1226 IU/L. She is most likely suffering from obstructive jaundice due to:

a. Bile duct injury
b. Carcinoma gallbladder
c. Hepatocellular carcinoma
d. Carcinoma head of pancreas

Biliary injury (bile duct injury) is the traumatic damage of the bile ducts. It is most commonly an iatrogenic complication

Answers

13. b 14. c 15. a 16. c 17. c 18. a 19. a

of cholecystectomy—surgical removal of gallbladder, but can also be caused by other operations or by major trauma. The risk of biliary injury is more during laparoscopic cholecystectomy than during open cholecystectomy.

20. A 60-years-old man presents with painless progressive jaundice for two months. He has a history of weight loss. On examination, his gallbladder is palpable which is smooth, non-tender and globular. His serum bilirubin is 18.2 mg/dL. He is most likely suffering from:

a. Carcinoma head of pancreas
b. Carcinoma stomach
c. Choledocholithiasis
d. Klatskin tumour

Signs and symptoms of the most common form of pancreatic cancer may include jaundice, abdominal or back pain, unexplained weight loss, light-colored stools, dark urine and loss of appetite. There are usually no symptoms in the disease's early stages, and symptoms that are specific enough to suggest pancreatic cancer, typically do not develop until the disease has reached an advanced stage. By the time of diagnosis, pancreatic cancer has often spread to other parts of the body.

21. A young 23-years-old male riding his motorcycle meets with a road accident. He is tachypnoeic with HR 110/m and BP 112/74 mmHg. On examination, he has tenderness over left side of chest with decreased air entry. His trachea is pushed to opposite side. Abdominal examination is unremarkable. Most probably he is suffering from:

a. Haemothorax
b. Consolidation
c. Subcutaneous emphysema
d. Tracheal rupture

Hemothorax tends to occur following blunt or penetrating trauma to the thorax or thoracoabdominal area. It may also follow thoracic surgery, or may be spontaneous. Chest pain, dyspnea, and tachypnea are common presenting features. Other symptoms of hemothorax are dependent on the mechanism of injury, but may include cyanosis, decreased or absent breath sounds on affected side, tracheal deviation to unaffected side, dull resonance on percussion, unequal chest rise etc.

22. A 45-years-old underwent abdominal rectal prolapse surgery. At present, he complains of sexual dysfunction which is probably due to the injury of:

a. Pelvic autonomic nerves
b. Inferior mesenteric artery
c. Rectum
d. Urinary bladder

In pelvic surgery there is a risk of damage to the pelvic autonomic nerves with consequent urinary dysfunction, impotence and orgasmic failure.

23. A 40-years-old man, with a history of a reducible left groin swelling of two years, comes with severe pain over left groin. The swelling is now non-reducible and is very tender to touch. The most probable treatment plan for this patient would be:

a. Continue conservative management
b. Hot fomentation of groin area
c. Oral antibiotics
d. Prepare for emergency surgery

Irreducibility or incarceration is a complication, in which hernia cannot be reduced, or pushed back into place, at least not without very much external effort. In intestinal hernias, this also substantially increases the risk of bowel obstruction and strangulation.

24. A 35-years-old female had laparoscopic ventral hernia repair using polypropylene mesh in January 2021. In June 2021, she is again admitted with features of subacute intestinal obstruction and is managed conservatively. She continues to have recurrent colicky pain after that. Most probably she is suffering from:

a. Recurrence of hernia
b. New hernia
c. Acute appendicitis
d. Bowel adhesion to mesh

Ventral hernia mesh repair is a common surgical procedure and may be performed by open or laparoscopic technique. Most patients have favorable outcome after surgery, but some patients experience problems such as pain, discomfort, and hernia recurrences. Intra-abdominal adhesions may have deleterious effects, like intestinal obstruction followed by chronic pain and reduced quality of life. Adhesion seems to be associated with abdominal pain and discomfort.

25. A 35-years-old man presents to emergency with acute onset pain abdomen radiating to whole abdomen and abdominal distension for one day. On examination, he has tenderness and guarding all over abdomen with pulse rate of 100/m and BP 116/84 mmHg. Chest X-ray erect position shows gas under bilateral domes of diaphragm. Probably he is suffering from:

a. Acute pancreatitis
b. Ruptured liver abscess
c. Appendicular perforation
d. Colonic perforation

The most common cause of air under diaphragm (pneumoperitoneum) is a perforated abdominal viscus, generally a perforated peptic ulcer, although any part of the bowel may perforate from a benign ulcer, tumor or abdominal trauma. A perforated appendix seldom causes a pneumoperitoneum.

Answers

20. a	**21.** a	**22.** a	**23.** d	**24.** d	**25.** d

26. A 70-years-old man comes to emergency with pain lower abdomen and not passing urine for eight hours. He has a past history of urgency, hesitancy and frequency of urine. On examination, he has a lump up to the umbilicus which is slightly tender. What is the next step of management?

a. Get an urgent USG
b. Per rectal examination
c. Per urethral catheterize the patient
d. Start antibiotics

Urinary retention is characterized by poor urinary stream with intermittent flow, straining, a sense of incomplete voiding, and hesitancy (a delay between trying to urinate and the flow actually beginning). As the bladder remains full, it may lead to incontinence, nocturia (need to urinate at night), and high frequency. Acute retention, causing complete anuria, is a medical emergency, as the bladder can stretch to an enormous size, and possibly tear if not dealt with quickly. If the bladder distends enough, it becomes painful. In such a case, there may be suprapubic constant, dull, pain. In acute urinary retention, urinary catheterization, placement of a prostatic stent, or suprapubic cystostomy relieves the retention.

27. A 35-years-old male patient comes to casualty with acute pain abdomen; and on examination found to have cold, clammy extremities, sunken eyes, dry tongue, thready pulse, drawn and anxious face with abdominal guarding and rigidity. This clinical picture indicates:

a. Local peritonitis
b. Diffuse early peritonitis
c. Diffuse late peritonitis
d. Acute cholecystitis

Features of diffuse late peritonitis include rigid and distended abdomen, bowel sounds absent and shock (cold clammy extremities, sunken eyes, dry tongue, rapid thread pulse and anxious facies).

28. A young male is undergoing emergency surgery for a clinical diagnosis of acute appendicitis. Intraoperatively minimal pus was found but the appendix was normal. What is the next step of management?

a. Appendectomy
b. Right hemicolectomy
c. Close the abdomen without doing anything
d. Search for perforated Meckel's diverticulum

Meckel's diverticulum (MD) occurs when the omphalomesenteric duct fails to obliterate completely during fetal life. It is the most common congenital abnormality of the gastrointestinal tract, classically thought to represent about 2% of the population. Despite the fact that this condition is relatively common, only about 4–16% of cases will lead to complications, which include hemorrhage, intussusception, inflammation and, occasionally, perforation. Many of the other presenting symptoms, such as abdominal pain and nausea, are non-specific and may mimic appendicitis.

29. In a 65-years-old, double contrast barium enema shows cancer of colon with an apple core appearance. Colonoscopic biopsy shows adenocarcinoma. What will be the next step of management?

a. Surgery
b. Chemotherapy
c. CECT to stage disease
d. Radiotherapy

Colorectal cancer diagnosis is performed by sampling of areas of the colon suspicious for possible tumor development, typically during colonoscopy or sigmoidoscopy, depending on the location of the lesion. It is confirmed by microscopical examination of a tissue sample. Disease extent is usually determined by a CT scan of the chest, abdomen and pelvis. Other potential imaging tests such as PET and MRI may be used in certain cases.

30. A 35-years-old woman presented with a lump in her upper abdomen for two months which was slightly increasing. She also complained of early satiety. She gave a history of acute severe pain in upper abdomen for which she was admitted in hospital for 10 days, about three months ago. On examination, the mass was firm, smooth surfaced and not moving with respiration. She was most likely suffering from:

a. Cancer stomach
b. Cancer colon
c. Pseudocyst pancreas
d. Splenic cyst

A pancreatic pseudocyst is a circumscribed collection of fluid rich in pancreatic enzymes, blood, and necrotic tissue, typically located in the lesser sac of the abdomen. Pancreatic pseudocysts are usually complications of pancreatitis, although in children they frequently occur following abdominal trauma. Pancreatic pseudocysts account for approximately 75% of all pancreatic masses.

31. A patient has recurrent abdominal pain and jaundice. The blood investigations reveal reticulocytosis and hyperbilirubinemia. What is the clinical diagnosis?

a. Hereditary spherocytosis
b. Mirizzi's syndrome
c. Choledochal cyst
d. Sclerosing cholangitis

Symptoms of hereditary spherocytosis include anemia, jaundice, splenomegaly, and fatigue. Furthermore, the detritus of the broken-down blood cells—unconjugated or indirect bilirubin—accumulates in the gallbladder, and can cause pigmented gallstones to develop.

32. A 60-years-old male presents with bleeding p/r. Proctoscopy reveals 2nd degree haemorrhoids. The treatment of choice is:

a. Cryotherapy
b. Sclerotherapy
c. Banding
d. Surgery

Answers

26. c **27.** c **28.** d **29.** c **30.** c **31.** a **32.** c

Rubber band ligation is typically recommended as the first-line treatment in those with grade 1 to 3 disease. It is a procedure in which elastic bands are applied onto an internal hemorrhoid at least 1 cm above the dentate line to cut off its blood supply. Within 5–7 days, the withered hemorrhoid falls off.

33. A 30-years-old man met with an accident and presented with multiple fractures of ribs and paradoxical movement with severe respiratory distress. X-ray shows pulmonary contusion on right side without pneumothorax or haemothorax. Which one of the following is the initial choice of treatment?

a. Immediate internal fixation
b. Endotracheal intubation and mechanical ventilation
c. Thoracic epidural analgesia and O_2 therapy
d. Stabilization with towel clips

A person with flail chest (paradoxical respiration) may be intubated with a double lumen tracheal tube. In a double lumen endotracheal tube, each lumen may be connected to a different ventilator. Usually one side of the chest is affected more than the other, so each lung may require drastically different pressures and flows to adequately ventilate.

34. A 30-years-old lady sustained chest injury in an accident and presented with massive haemothorax on right side. Tube thoracostomy drained 1800 mL of blood. What is the most appropriate treatment?

a. Correction of hypovolemic shock
b. Put one more chest tube
c. Clamp the chest tube to cause the tamponade
d. Resuscitation and prepare for urgent thoracotomy

In some cases of hemothorax, bleeding continues and surgery is necessary to stop the source of bleeding. For example, if the hemothorax was caused by aortic rupture in high energy trauma, surgical intervention (thoracotomy) is mandatory.

35. A patient with burns died within 24 hours. What could be the most probable cause?

a. Circulatory shock
b. Physical burn injury to the airways above the larynx
c. Physical burn injury to the airways below the larynx
d. Circumferential burn

Inhaled burning gases can cause upper airway burns and laryngeal edema.

36. A third degree circumferential burn in the arm and forearm region, which of the following is the most important for monitoring?

a. Blood gases
b. Carboxy-oxygen levels
c. Macroglobinuria and cryoglobinuria
d. Peripheral pulse and circulation

Circumferential eschar in the upper limb, lower limb, neck, thorax can cause more oedema which initially causes venous compression and later arterial compression causing ischaemia, gangrene of the distal part. So distal area should be monitored for circulation.

37. Ideal management in an old and frail patient presenting with a mass situated 15 cm away from anal orifice:

a. Abdomino-perineal resection
b. Colonoscopic removal
c. Hartman's operation
d. Anterior resection

Hartmann's operation is an excellent palliative procedure —done in elderly people who are not fit for major surgery like AP resection and also in locally advanced tumours. Here rectal growth is resected and upper end of the rectum is closed completely. Proximal colon is brought out as end colostomy.

38. 3 cm breast carcinoma and involving 4 ipsilateral axillary lymph nodes is what stage as per TNM classification?

a. Stage IIA
b. Stage IIB
c. Stage IIIA
d. Stage IIIB

No tumor is found in the breast or the tumor may be any size; cancer is found in 4 to 9 axillary lymph nodes or in the lymph nodes near the breastbone (found during imaging tests or a physical exam) OR The tumor is larger than 5 centimeters; small groups of breast cancer cells (larger than 0.2 millimeter but not larger than 2 millimeters) are found in the lymph nodes OR The tumor is larger than 5 centimeters; cancer has spread to 1 to 3 axillary lymph nodes or to the lymph nodes near the breastbone (found during a sentinel lymph node biopsy) defines stage IIIA of breast carcinoma.

39. Congenital sensorineural deafness with abnormal iodine metabolism and goiter in children is:

a. Nome's syndrome
b. Gradenigo's syndrome
c. Pendred's syndrome
d. Cogan's syndrome

Pendred syndrome is characterized by defective organification of iodine, goiter and sensorineural deafness (typically associated with malformation of the inner ear bony labyrinth).

40. A patient after heavy drinking of alcohol presents with too much vomiting and haematemesis. Most likely diagnosis could be:

a. Mallory–Weiss syndrome
b. Oesophageal carcinoma
c. Achalasia cardia
d. Boerhaave syndrome

Answers

33. b **34.** d **35.** b **36.** d **37.** c **38.** c **39.** c
40. a

Mallory-Weiss syndrome is seen in adults with severe prolonged vomiting, causing longitudinal tear in the mucosa of stomach at and just below the cardia, leading to severe haematemesis. Violent vomiting often may be due to migraine or vertigo or following a bout of alcohol.

41. Cause of acute onset, large volume hematemesis in a patient with mild splenomegaly:

a. Gastric carcinoma b. Barret's esophagus
c. Esophageal varices d. Gastritis

Triad of portal hypertension include esophageal varices, splenomegaly and ascites.

42. A 60-years-old male has been operated for carcinoma of caecum and right hemicolectomy has been done. On the 4th postoperative day, the patient develops fever, swelling and pain in the legs. The most important clinical entity one should look for is:

a. Urinary tract infection
b. Intravenous line infection
c. Chest infection
d. Deep vein thrombosis

Postoperative thrombosis is the MC cause of DVT. It is common after the age of 40 years. Incidence following surgeries is 30%. In 30% of cases, both legs are affected.

43. Best management of a nodule of 2 cm in left thyroid, later found to be a papillary carcinoma:

a. Radiotherapy
b. Thyroidectomy with radical dissection
c. Total thyroidectomy
d. Hemi-thyroidectomy

For papillary carcinoma of thyroid, total or near total thyroidectomy, with central node compartment dissection (level VI) is done.

44. A lady presented with breast carcinoma. On investigation, it is noticed that other breast is also involved. Likely histological subtype is:

a. Inflammatory carcinoma b. Colloid carcinoma
c. Lobular carcinoma d. In situ carcinoma

Lobular carcinoma in situ (LCIS), multifocal breast cancer, family history are risk for development of bilateral breast cancer. There is 5 fold increases in 2nd breast cancer on opposite side in a female, who has had breast cancer on ipsilateral side.

45. A patient with head injury opens eyes on painful stimulus, uses inappropriate words and localizes pain. What is his GCS score?

a. 8 b. 10
c. 12 d. 14

Eye opening of painful stimuli is 2, inappropriate words in verbal response is 3 and localizing pain in motor response is 5.

46. A 60-years-old patient with a history of fall presents with headache and progressive neurological deterioration. The diagnosis is:

a. Acute subdural hemorrhage
b. Extradural hemorrhage
c. Chronic subdural hemorrhage
d. Fracture skull

Chronic subdural haematoma

- Common in old age, with history of minor trauma.
- Patient presents with confusion, disorientation, gradually with altered level of consciousness and drowsiness.
- Later convulsions, features of intracranial hypertension and features of coning develop.

47. Cystic, compressible, translucent swelling in the posterior triangle of neck:

a. Cystic hygroma b. Branchial cyst
c. Thyroglossal cyst d. Dermoid cyst

Important features of cystic hygroma include that swelling is present at birth in the posterior triangle of neck causing obstructed labor and the swelling is smooth, soft, fluctuant (cystic), partially compressible, brilliantly trans-illuminant. It is not reducible completely.

48. A young patient presented with dyspnea, bleeding and petechial hemorrhage in the chest after 2 days following fracture shaft femur of right side. Most likely cause is:

a. Air embolism b. Fat embolism
c. Pulmonary thromboembolism
d. Amniotic fluid embolism

Fat embolism is commonly seen after fracture femur, tibia, or multiple fractures and occasionally following electroconvulsive therapy, usually occurs in 72 hours. Clinical features include tachypneoa, petechial haemorrhages in the skin etc.

49. Normal anatomical narrowing of ureter are present in all *except*:

a. Ureteropelvic junction
b. Crossing the abdominal aorta
c. Entering bladder wall
d. Ureteric orifice

The ureter has a diameter of 3 mm but there are three constrictions, which are the most common sites of renal calculus obstruction: (i) At the pelviureteric junction (PUJ) of the renal pelvis and the ureter; (ii) As the ureter enters the pelvis (brim of pelvis) and crosses over the common iliac artery bifurcation and (iii) At the vesicoureteric junction (VUJ) as the ureter obliquely enters the bladder wall.

Answers

41. c	42. d	43. c	44. c	45. b	46. c	47. a
48. b	49. b					

50. Which of the following is NOT correct for breast abscess?

a. Drainage of abscess by a radial incision
b. Antibiotic is given if pus is already present
c. A counter-incision is made in the dependent part
d. Dressings are changed frequently

A breast abscess is a collection of pus that develops into the breast with different causes. During lactation, breast abscess develops only rarely, most sources cite about 0.4–0.5% of breastfeeding women. Known risk factors are age over 30, primiparous and late delivery. Antibiotics were not shown effective in prevention of lactation abscess but are useful to treat a secondary infection.

51. Which of these is a palliative shunt procedure created between the left subclavian artery and pulmonary artery to treat cyanotic congenital heart disease?

a. Gott's shunt
b. Lieno renal shunt
c. Blalock-Taussig shunt
d. Waterstons shunt

The Blalock–Thomas–Taussig shunt (commonly called the Blalock–Taussig shunt) is a surgical procedure used to increase pulmonary blood flow for palliation in duct dependent cyanotic heart defects like pulmonary atresia, which are common causes of blue baby syndrome. In modern surgery, this procedure is temporarily used to direct blood flow to the lungs and relieve cyanosis while the infant is waiting for corrective or definitive surgery. One branch of the subclavian artery or carotid artery is separated and connected with the pulmonary artery. The first area of application was tetralogy of Fallot.

52. During laparoscopic inguinal hernia repair, in the 'triangle of doom', the following are true *except*:

a. Vas deferens on medial side
b. Cord structures on lateral side
c. Base by iliac vessels
d. Dangerous area for dissection

The Triangle of Doom is an anatomical triangle defined by the vas deferens medially, spermatic vessels laterally and peritoneal fold inferiorly. This triangle contains external iliac artery and vein, the deep circumflex iliac vein, the genital branch of genitofemoral nerve and hidden by fascia, the femoral nerve. It bears significance in laparoscopic repair of groin hernia. Surgical staples are avoided here.

53. All of the following statements are true for keloids *except*:

a. It is rarely seen in white skinned persons and is more common over the sternum
b. True keloid continues to become worse even after one years
c. True keloid does not spread into surrounding tissue
d. The maturation and stabilization of the collagen fibrils is inhibited

Keloids should not be confused with hypertrophic scars, which are raised scars that do not grow beyond the boundaries of the original wound.

54. A patient has carcinoid tumour of appendix of size more than 2.5 cm. The management of choice is:

a. Appendicectomy
b. Appendicectomy and 24 hour urinary HIAA
c. Appendicectomy and abdominal CT scan
d. Right hemicolectomy

Open right hemicolectomy (open right colectomy) is a procedure that involves removing the cecum, the ascending colon, the hepatic flexure (where the ascending colon joins the transverse colon), the first third of the transverse colon, and part of the terminal ileum, along with fat and lymph nodes.

55. Regarding haemorrhagic shock, which one of the following statements is correct?

a. Clinically manifested when > 10% of loss of total blood volume occurs
b. Tachycardia presents in 100% of hypovolemic patients
c. Loss of 40% of circulating volume is life-threatening
d. In acute stage of shock, systemic vasodilation becomes evident

Hemorrhage classes			
Class	*Blood loss*	*Response*	*Treatment*
I	<15% (0.75 Litre)	Minimum fast heart rate, normal blood pressure	Minimal
II	15–30% (0.75–1.5 Litre)	Fast heart rate, min. low blood pressure	Intravenous fluids
III	30–40% (1.5–2 Litre)	Very fast heart rate, low blood pressure, confusion	Fluids and packed RBCs
IV	>40% (>2 Litre)	Critical blood pressure and heart rate	Aggressive interventions

56. The following conditions are associated with high incidence of pigment gallstones *except*:

a. Cirrhosis
b. Ileal disease
c. Thalassemia
d. Prosthetic heart valve

Risk factors for pigment stones include hemolytic anemias [such as from sickle-cell disease, hereditary spherocytosis, thalassemia, prosthetic heart valves (Low-grade hemolytic anemia occurs in 70% of prosthetic heart valve recipients, and severe hemolytic anemia occurs in 3%)], cirrhosis, and biliary tract infections. People with erythropoietic protoporphyria (EPP) are at increased risk to develop gallstones.

Answers

50. b **51.** c **52.** c **53.** c **54.** d **55.** c **56.** b

57. The capillary refill time is prolonged in all types of shock *except*:

a. Hypovolaemic shock b. Cardiogenic shock
c. Septic shock d. Obstructive shock

Among various complementary indices, the capillary refill time (CRT) is a parameter of shock. CRT tends to be prolonged in patients with sepsis; however, the CRT is determined subjectively, and its assessment lacks objectivity and reproducibility.

58. Ventral hernia includes all *except*:

a. Epigastric hernia b. Para-umbilical hernia
c. Lumbar hernia d. Inguinal hernia

Ventral hernias of the abdomen are defined as a non-inguinal, non-hiatal defect in the fascia of the abdominal wall.

59. Mainstay of an accurate diagnosis of pancreatic injury following blunt abdominal trauma is:

a. Computed Tomogram
b. Diagnostic peritoneal lavage
c. USG abdomen
d. MRI abdomen

High resolution CT scan is diagnostic for pancreatic injury.

60. Following are the factors for increased risk of wound infection *except*:

a. Malnutrition
b. Good blood supply
c. Metabolic diseases (diabetes, uraemia)
d. Immunosuppression

Poor blood supply results in delayed wound healing.

61. A 22-years-old young man came with history of occasional bleeding per rectum. On colonoscopy, numerous sessile polyps were seen in descending and sigmoid colon. On family history his elder brother was operated for thyroid malignancy. The young man should be advised:

a. Prophylactic panproctocolectomy
b. Prophylactic anterior resection
c. Surveillance colonoscopy every 6 months
d. Colonoscopic removal of all polyps

Cowden disease is an uncommon autosomal dominant disorder and is the family name of the original report patient, Rachel Cowden. This syndrome is a rare disorder that is inherited in autosomal dominant manner with intrafamilial and interfamilial differences in symptom expression. In Cowden disease, one sees facial trichilemmomas, acral keratosis and oral mucosal papillomas. This disorder is also associated with breast and thyroid cancer. There are numerous colic and small-intestinal polyps. They have been described as hamartomatous lesions consisting of mildly fibrotic, mildly disordered mucosa overlying a submucosa that display disorganization and splaying of smooth-muscle fibres. Conventional panproctocolectomy has the advantage of eliminating all colorectal polyps and virtually eliminating the risk of carcinoma of the large bowel.

62. NOT a presenting feature of burns:

a. Sepsis b. Shock
c. Acute kidney injury d. Hyperproteinemia

Hypoproteinemia is obvious in burns due to excessive loss of plasma proteins as a result of increase in the capillary permeability and infection.

63. Which of the following is NOT a complication of chronic lower limb edema?

a. Infection of soft tissue b. Thickening of skin
c. Ulceration d. Varicose vein

Varicose veins (due to incompetent valves of veins of lower limb) are more common in women than in men, and are linked with heredity. Other related factors are pregnancy, obesity, menopause, aging, prolonged standing, leg injury, and abdominal straining.

64. All of the following are true for thromboangiitis oblliterans/Berger disease *except*:

a. Phlebitis migrans
b. Nerves may be involved
c. Involvement of ulnar artery and peroneal arteries
d. Small acral vessels of limb are involved which result in hypohydrosis

Thromboangiitis obliterans (TAO), an inflammatory vasculopathy also known as Buerger disease, is characterized by an inflammatory endarteritis that causes a prothrombotic state and subsequent vaso-occlusive phenomena (NO hypohydrosis).

65. Which of the following parasite is associated with consumption of raw fish and may lead to the development of carcinoma of gallbladder?

a. H. nana b. Strongyloides
c. Schistosomiasis d. Clonorchis

Dwelling in the bile ducts, Clonorchis induces an inflammatory reaction, epithelial hyperplasia and sometimes even cholangiocarcinoma.

66. NOT a feature of achalasia cardia:

a. Bad smell from mouth
b. Regurgitation of food
c. Dysphagia more for liquids
d. Cork screw esophagus on barium meal

Diffuse esophageal spasm is sometimes referred to as corkscrew esophagus, due to a characteristic appearance of the esophagus as a corkscrew on barium swallow X-rays.

Answers

57. c	58. d	59. a	60. b	61. a	62. d	63. d
64. d	65. d	66. d				

67. Which of the following is FALSE for femoral hernia?

a. Most common to strangulate
b. Absent cough impulse
c. More common in females
d. Most common type of hernia in females

Femoral hernia is most common in females but most common hernia in females is indirect inguinal hernia (NOT femoral hernia).

68. A 60-years-old male alcoholic presents with acute upper GI bleeding following bouts of vigorous vomiting. Most likely diagnosis:

a. Acute gastritis
b. Boerhaave's syndrome
c. Mucosal and submucosal tear at cardiac orifice of stomach
d. Esophageal carcinoma

Mallory-Weiss syndrome is characterized by mucosal tear at the gastroesophageal junction following bout of forceful retching (or vomiting, coughing or straining).

69. A female patient is presenting with BP of 90/60 mm Hg and pulse rate of 150 beats/minute after blunt trauma abdomen. How would you assess this patient?

a. USG
b. CT scan
c. X-ray
d. MRI

If the patient is hemodynamically unstable (cannot be shifted to imaging centre), USG is the best investigation for evaluation of blunt trauma. If the patient is stable, CT scan is the best choice.

70. A newborn child is presenting with regurgitation of all feeds and develops coughing and cyanosis with feeding. Most likely diagnosis:

a. Congenital hypertrophic pyloric stenosis
b. Esophageal atresia
c. Zenker's diverticulum
d. Achalasia cardia

Clinical features of trachea-esophageal fistula include regurgitation of all the contents by the newborn, saliva pours almost continuously from the mouth and there are attacks of coughing and cyanosis on feeding.

Answers

67. d **68.** c **69.** a **70.** b

13 Obstetrics

1. **A 23-year-old presents with recurrent abortions at 16 weeks gestation. She should be investigated for:**
   a. TORCH infection
   b. Hepatitis B infection
   c. Incompetent cervix
   d. Balanced paternal translocation

   Cervical weakness/incompetent cervix may cause miscarriage or preterm birth during the second and third trimesters.

2. **A patient of ectopic pregnancy had beta-hCG less than 6000 IU/mL. Medical management was done by single dose methotrexate. Beta-hCG repeated after 48 hours was found 7000 IU/mL. What will you do further?**
   a. Repeat the injection of methotrexate
   b. Operate the patient
   c. Follow-up with Beta-hCG after one week
   d. Follow-up with Beta-hCG after 72 hours

   The drugs commonly used for salpingocentesis are: methotrexate (MTX), potassium chloride, prostaglandin ($PGF_{2\alpha}$), hyperosmolar glucose or actinomycin. For systemic therapy, a single dose of MTX 50 mg/M^2 is given intramuscularly. Monitoring is done by measuring serum beta-HCG on day 4 and day 7.

3. **Most probable cause of heavy bleeding in a P2L2 during tenth day post-partum is:**
   a. Retained bits of cotyledons and membranes
   b. Subinvolution of placental site
   c. Resumption of menstruation
   d. Infected episiotomy wound

Cause of PPH	Incidence
Uterine atony	70%
Trauma	20%
Retained tissue	10%
Coagulopathy	1%

4. **A 32-year-old woman is noted to have 1200 cc of blood loss following a spontaneous vaginal delivery and delivery of placenta. The uterine fundus is palpated and noted to be firm. Which of the following is the most likely treatment for this patient?**
   a. B′ lynch suture
   b. Surgical repair of cervical tear
   c. Intramuscular prostaglandin
   d. Replacement of inverted uterus

   Injury to the birth canal, which includes the uterus, cervix, vagina and the perineum, which can happen, even if the delivery is monitored properly. The bleeding is substantial as all these organs become more vascular during pregnancy.

5. **A 20-year-old Primigravida, comes at 35 weeks of gestation with complaints of swelling of feet. On examination her blood pressure is 170/110 mm Hg on 2 occasions; urine examination shows proteinuria. Which one of the following statements regarding her management is NOT true?**
   a. Can be labelled as preeclampsia
   b. Requires urgent admission
   c. Injection Dexamethasone is to be given for fetal lung maturity
   d. Both maternal and fetal monitoring are required

   Management of preeclampsia: (1) Admission in hospital and rest; (2) Adequate protein in diet (100 g); (3) Antihypertensives (methyldopa, labetalol); (4) Progress chart and (5) Fetal well-being assessment.

6. **A 25-year-old, $G_2P_1L_1$ came with amenorrhoea of two and half months followed by bleeding PV and pain abdomen. On examination cervical OS is open with slight bleeding. The uterus is 10 weeks size with no tenderness in the fornices. The probable clinical diagnosis is:**
   a. Ectopic pregnancy
   b. Incomplete abortion
   c. Missed abortion
   d. Inevitable abortion

   Inevitable miscarriage refers to the presence of an open internal os in the presence of bleeding in the first trimester of pregnancy. Most often the conception products are not expelled and intracervical contents are present at the time of examination.

Answers

1. c 2. d 3. a 4. b 5. c 6. d

7. A 15-year-old girl comes to the gynae casualty with a relative with complains of amenorrhoea 2 months. The urine pregnancy test is positive, ultrasound confirms 8 weeks pregnancy. The attendants are not willing to file a police case. What should the treating doctor do?

a. Take consent for abortion and proceed
b. Inform the police and make MLC
c. Take parents consent for MTP
d. None of these

Under POCSO Act, if any girl under 18 years of age is seeking abortion, the service provider is compelled to register a complaint of sexual assault with the police.

8. A 25-year-old $G_2P_1L_1$, Rh –ve woman presented at 30 weeks gestation to the antenatal clinic, the indirect Coomb's test (ICT) was found to be positive. What would be the next line of management?

a. Anti D to be given
b. ICT titers to be closely monitored at weekly intervals
c. Amniocentesis for estimation of bilirubin by Liley's chart is to be done
d. Baby is to be delivered as soon as possible

Once ICT for Rh-D antibodies becomes positive in critical titer, pregnancy is managed as iso-immunized pregnancy. The aim is to detect fetal anemia at the earliest and also to avoid events likely to increase the feto-maternal hemorrhage/FMH (like external cephalic version, external trauma over the abdomen or invasive testing). Weekly monitoring is performed with the antibody titer and ultrasonography. Antibody titers of 1:128 are considered to cause significant fetal anemia and once these titers are reached, the pregnancy is monitored closely by MCA-PSV (middle cerebral artery peak systolic velocity).

9. Given below are the obstetric maneuvers and their indications. Which one of the following is correctly matched?

a. McRobert's maneuver—after coming head of breech
b. Lovset's maneuver—delivery of foot in breech
c. Pinard's maneuver—delivery of extended arm
d. Ritgen's maneuver—controlled delivery of fetal head

The delivery of the fetal head should be managed by Ritgen's maneuver, i.e. lifting the fetal chin anteriorly, using the fingers of one hand placed between the anus and the coccyx, and thereby extending the fetal neck, whereas the other hand should be placed on the fetal occiput to control the pace of the expulsion of the fetal head.

10. A 29-year-old woman presents in emergency ward with amenorrhea of 6 weeks and pain. Urine pregnancy test shows positive. Examination shows diffuse significant lower abdomen tenderness. The pelvic examination is difficult to accomplish due to guarding. Her Beta-hCG level is 4000 mIU/mL. Transvaginal ultrasound shows no pregnancy in the uterus and no adnexal mass but moderate fluid in abdomen. Which of the following is the next best step?

a. Repeat Beta-hCG level in 48 hours
b. Institution of methotrexate
c. Emergency laparotomy
d. Wait and watch

Laparotomy is indicated if there is any evidence of rupture of ectopic pregnancy.

11. Rapid gain in weight, hypertension and proteinuria suggest the diagnosis of:

a. Eclampsia
b. Preeclampsia
c. Gestational hypertension
d. None of the above

Preeclampsia is a disorder of pregnancy characterized by high blood pressure and a large amount of protein in the urine. The disorder usually occurs in the third trimester of pregnancy and gets worse over time. In severe disease there may be red blood cell breakdown, a low blood platelet count, impaired liver function, kidney dysfunction, swelling (gain in weight), shortness of breath due to fluid in the lungs, or visual disturbances.

12. Investigation of choice in a pregnant lady at 16 weeks of pregnancy with past history of delivering a baby with Down syndrome:

a. Triple screen test
b. Amniocentesis
c. Chorionic villous sampling
d. USG

Genetic amniocentesis is an invasive procedure. It is performed after 15 weeks under ultrasonographic guidance. The fetal cells obtained in this procedure are subjected for cytogenetic analysis.

13. A 28-year-old female presented with history of 6 weeks amenorrhea and pain in abdomen. USG showed fluid in pouch of Douglas. Aspiration revealed a dark coloured blood that failed to clot. Most likely diagnosis is:

a. Ruptured ovarian cyst
b. Ruptured ectopic pregnancy
c. Red degeneration of fibroid
d. Pelvic abscess

Through an 18-gauze lumbar puncture needle fitted with a syringe, the posterior fornix is punctured to gain access to the pouch of Douglas (culdocentesis). Aspiration of nonclotting blood with hematocrit greater than 15% signifies ruptured ectopic pregnancy.

Answers

7. b **8.** b **9.** d **10.** c **11.** b **12.** b **13.** b

14. In second stage of labor, on per-vaginum examination, anterior fontanelle and supra-orbital ridge can be felt. The likely presentation is:

a. Face b. Flexed head
c. Deflexed head d. Brow

Brow is the rarest variety of cephalic presentation where the presenting part is the brow and the attitude of the head is short that of degree of extension necessary to produce face presentation, i.e. the head lies in between full extension and full flexion. The position is to be confirmed on vaginal examination by palpating supraorbital ridges and anterior fontanel.

15. Which of the following types of placenta complicate third stage of labor and is associated with a past history of caesarean section?

a. Placenta succenturita b. Placenta extracholis
c. Placenta membranecae d. Placenta accreta

Placenta accreta (morbid adherent placenta) is an extremely rare form in which the placenta is directly anchored to the myometrium partially or completely without any intervening deciduas. The probable cause is due to absence of deciduas basalis and poor development of fibrinoid layer. The most important risk factors are the placenta previa and previous cesarean section.

16. A 40-year-old lady with completed family has been diagnosed to have H. mole. The treatment would be:

a. Radiotherapy b. Chemotherapy
c. Total hysterectomy d. Radio + Chemotherapy

Hysterectomy is justified in H. mole in: (i) Women approaching 40 years. (ii) Patient completed her family irrespective of age. (iii) Uncontrolled hemorrhage or perforation during surgical evacuation. Hysterectomy reduces the risk of GTN (gestational trophoblastic neoplasia) by fivefold.

17. A 32 weeks pregnant lady presents in emergency room with continuous bleeding per vaginum. The uterus is painful and tender. Most likely diagnosis is:

a. Circumvallate placenta b. Rupture of membranes
c. Placenta previa d. Accidental hemorrhage

Abruptio placentae/accidental hemorrhage/premature separation of placenta is one form of antepartum hemorrhage where the bleeding occurs due to premature separation of normally situated placenta. Uterine tenderness may vary depending upon the grade of separation.

18. Painless, heavy and recurrent bleeding of sudden onset is seen in:

a. Cervical carcinoma b. Circumvallate placenta
c. Placenta previa d. Abruptio placentae

The only symptom of placenta previa is vaginal bleeding. The classical features of bleeding in placenta previa are sudden onset, painless, apparently causeless and recurrent.

19. A woman presents with amenorrhea of 2 months duration, lower abdominal pain, facial pallor, fainting and shock. The diagnosis is:

a. Ruptured ovarian cyst
b. Ruptured ectopic pregnancy
c. Threatened abortion
d. Septic abortion

The classic triad of symptom of disturbed tubal pregnancy is abdominal pain (100%), preceded by amenorrhea (75%) and lastly, appearance of vaginal bleeding (70%). Syncopal attack (10%) is due to reflex vasomotor disturbances following peritoneal irritation from hemoperitoneum.

20. A young woman with 6 weeks amenorrhea presents with mass in abdomen. USG shows an empty uterus. Likely diagnosis is:

a. Ovarian cyst b. Ectopic pregnancy
c. Complete abortion d. None of the above

Transvaginal sonography (TVS) is more informative for ectopic pregnancy. The diagnostic features are:

- Absence of intrauterine pregnancy with a positive pregnancy test
- Fluid (echogenic) in the pouch of Douglas
- Adnexal mass clearly separated from the ovary
- Rarely cardiac motion may be seen in an unruptured tubal ectopic pregnancy

21. A pregnant lady in her first trimester presents with vaginal bleeding. On examination the os is closed and uterine size corresponds to the period of amenorrhoea. The condition could be:

a. Septic abortion b. Complete abortion
c. Inevitable abortion d. Threatened abortion

Threatened abortion is a clinical entity where the process of miscarriage has started but has not progressed to a state from where recovery is impossible.

22. Which of the following is the earliest sign of magnesium toxicity in a patient with eclampsia on treatment with magnesium sulphate?

a. Loss of deep tendon reflexes
b. Respiratory depression
c. Cardiac arrest
d. Decreased urine output

Features of magnesium sulphate toxicity include: (1) Loss of deep tendon reflexes (magnesium levels >7 mEq/L); (2) Respiratory depression (more than 10 mEq/L) and (3) Cardiac arrest (more than 25 mEq/L).

Answers

14. d	15. d	16. c	17. d	18. c	19. b	20. b
21. d	22. a					

23. In the Manning scoring system of biophysical profile for foetal monitoring, which parameter is NOT included?

a. Fetal tone
b. Fetal gross body movements
c. Oxytocin challenge test
d. Non-stress test

Oxytocin challenge test/contraction stress test is an invasive method to assess the fetal well-being during pregnancy. Where there is alteration in FHR in response to uterine contractions, it suggests fetal hypoxia. The test is based on determination of the respiratory function of the fetoplacental unit during induced contractions when the blood flow through the unit is curtailed.

24. Parameter (biophysical profile) affected last in a state of fetal compromise:

a. Gross body movement b. Fetal tone
c. Breathing movement d. Liquor pocket

Earliest diagnosis of IUFD is possible with sonography. The evidences are: a. Lack of all fetal motions (including cardiac) during a 10-minute period of careful observation with a real-time sonar is a strong presumptive evidence of fetal death and b. oligohydramnios and collapsed cranial bones are evident.

25. Preferred management of occipito-posterior position during labor:

a. Artificial rupture of membranes
b. Cesarean section
c. Oxytocin drip
d. Wait and watch

In occipito-posterior position there is increased maternal morbidity, incidental to prolonged labor and increased incidence of operative delivery (1 in 5). There is also increased perinatal morbidity and mortality (10%) due to asphyxia or trauma during vaginal operative delivery. However, it is to be morbidity and remembered that in 4 out of 5 cases, there is usually no trouble and the fetus is delivered spontaneously.

26. External cephalic version (ECV) is CONTRAINDICATED in:

a. Primigravida b. Flexed breech
c. Anemia d. PIH

Contraindications of ECV include antepartum hemorrhage, fetal causes (hyperextension of the head, large fetus (>3.5 kg), major congenital abnormalities, dead fetus, IUGR), × pregnancy, rupture membranes—with drainage of liquor, abnormal cardiotocography, contracted pelvis, previous cesarean section, obstetrics complications (severe preeclampsia, obesity, elderly primigravida, bad obstetric history), oligohydramnios, rhesus isoimmunization etc.

27. Which of the following is true for Cephalohematoma?

a. Tension varies on crying b. May cause jaundice
c. Edematous fluid d. Cross suture line

Cephalohematoma is a hemorrhage of blood between the skull and the periosteum of a newborn baby secondary to rupture of blood vessels crossing the periosteum. Because the swelling is subperiosteal, its boundaries are limited by the individual bones (does not cross suture line), in contrast to a caput succedaneum. If severe the child may develop jaundice, anemia or hypotension.

28. In a patient with third degree perineal tear, presenting after 1 week, repair should be done:

a. Immediately b. 2 weeks
c. After 6 weeks d. After 12 weeks

Recent tear should be repaired immediately following the delivery of the placenta. This reduces the chances of infection and minimizes the blood loss. In case of delay beyond 24 hours, the repair is to be withheld. Antibiotics should be started to prevent infection. The complete tear should be repaired after 3 months if delay beyond 24 hours. In case if any doubt to grade of 3rd degree, it is advisable to classify to the higher degree rather than lower degree.

29. The essential investigation to be included in follow-up of hydatidiform mole is:

a. Ultrasound abdomen b. Chest X-ray
c. Serum levels of hCG d. Serum levels of TSH

Routine follow-up of H. mole is mandatory for all cases for at least 1 year. The occurrence of choriocarcinoma is mostly confined to this period. The prime objective is to diagnose persistent trophoblastic disease (20–30%) that is considered malignant. However, hCG levels following evacuation should regress to normal within 3 months time.

30. Which structure will remain intact in a lady with 3rd degree tear as a result of midline episiotomy and delivering a 9 lb baby:

a. Rectal mucosa b. Perineal muscles
c. Perineal body d. Anal sphincter

Risk factors for third degree perineal tears include big baby (weight > 3 kg), nulliparity, outlet contraction with narrow pubic arch, shoulder dystocia, forceps delivery, scar in the perineum (perineorrhaphy, episiotomy), face to pubis delivery, midline episiotomy, precipitate labor etc.

31. True about herpes simplex genitalis are all *except*:

a. Caused due to herpes simplex virus-2
b. Risk of fetal infection is high at term
c. May lead to malignancy
d. Treated by acyclovir

Genital tract infection is due to HSV-2. Infection may be primary, nonprimary, first episode and recurrent. It is

Answers

23. c	**24.** b	**25.** d	**26.** d	**27.** b	**28.** d	**29.** c
30. a	**31.** c					

transmitted by sexual contact. Primary infection may occur during pregnancy. If the primary infection is acquired in the last trimester there is chance of premature labor or IUGR.

32. Triple test for Down syndrome is by using all *except*:

a. Maternal hCG
b. Maternal estriol
c. Maternal α-fetoprotein
d. Maternal HPL

Triple test is a combined biochemical test which includes MSAFP, hCG and uE3 (unconjugated estriol). Maternal age in relation to confirmed gestation age is also taken into account. It is used for detection of Down's syndrome. In affected pregnancy, levels of MSAFP and uE3 tend to be low while that of hCG is high.

33. Ultrasound is done in 1st trimester for all *except*:

a. Multiple pregnancy
b. Fetal anomalies
c. To estimate gestational age
d. To know the position of the placenta

The relationship of placenta to the internal cervical os is important to define low lying placenta and placenta previa. This best evaluated in second trimester USG. Only 5% of placenta previa identified in the second trimester will persist to term.

34. True about abruptio placentae are all *except*:

a. Hypertension in the pregnancy is important predisposing factor
b. Placenta lying in the lower segment
c. Tender and hard uterus
d. Continuous bleeding per vaginum

When the placenta is implanted partially or completely over the lower uterine segment (over and adjacent to the internal os), it is called placenta previa.

35. Placenta pravia is characterized by all of the following *except*:

a. Painless bleeding
b. Causeless bleeding
c. Presents in first trimester
d. Recurrent bleeding

Painless and recurrent vaginal bleeding in the second half of pregnancy should be taken as placenta previa unless proved otherwise.

Answers

32. d **33.** d **34.** b **35.** c

14 Gynecology

1. **A 35-years-old nulliparous woman complains of menorrhagia and mass per abdomen. On examination, the positive findings are: she is anaemic, has a pelvic mass of 16–18 weeks size, firm in consistency which moves with the movement of cervix. What is the most likely clinical diagnosis?**
   a. Leiomyoma
   b. Adenomyosis
   c. Endometrial carcinoma
   d. Ovarian tumour

   Uterine fibroids are leiomyomata of the uterine smooth muscle. As other leiomyomata, they are benign, but may lead to excessive menstrual bleeding (menorrhagia), often cause anemia and may lead to infertility.

2. **A 58-years-old woman, post-menopausal for last 8 years comes with history of spotting per vaginum. What is the most likely cause?**
   a. Endometrial hyperplasia
   b. Endometrial carcinoma
   c. Atrophic endometritis
   d. Estrogen replacement therapy

   Atrophic endometritis is the most common cause of postmenopausal bleeding (66.67%), followed by endometrial carcinoma (13. 6%) and endometrial polyp (11.6%).

3. **A diabetic obese patient comes with history of post-menopausal bleeding. On examination, there is a supra-pubic mass and per vagina there is purulent discharge. The probable diagnosis is:**
   a. Carcinoma cervix
   b. Carcinoma endometrium
   c. Uterine myoma
   d. Ovarian carcinoma

   Approximately 40% of cases of endometrial carcinoma are related to obesity. Endometrial cancer is also associated with excessive estrogen exposure, high blood pressure and diabetes. Whereas taking estrogen alone increases the risk of endometrial cancer, taking both estrogen and a progestogen in combination, as in most birth control pills, decreases the risk.

4. **For a woman who has had unprotected intercourse two days ago, which one of the following emergency contraceptive methods *cannot* be suggested?**
   a. LNG IUD (LNg IUD)
   b. Ulipristal acetate
   c. Levonorgestrel 150 mg
   d. Yuzpe regimen

   Methods of emergency contraception/post-coital contraception include hormones (morning-after pills: levonorgestrel, 0.75 mg, two doses given at 12 hours interval; two tablets (150 mg) can be taken as a single dose also), copper IUCD, combined hormonal regimen (Yuzpe method), anti-progesterone (RU 486-Mifepristone) and ulipristal acetate.

5. **A 35-years-old married woman with no risk factors for cervical cancer is having Pap smear showing 'atypical squamous cells of undermined significance (ASCUS)' for the first time. What is the further step in the management?**
   a. Repeat Pap immediately
   b. Cryotherapy
   c. Large loop excision of the transformation zone
   d. To follow-up with Pap test at 6 months

   Atypical squamous cells of undetermined significance (ASCUS): Squamous cells are thin and flat and grow on the surface of a healthy cervix. In the case of ASCUS, the Pap smear reveals slightly abnormal squamous cells, but the changes do not clearly suggest that precancerous cells are present, so repeat Pap smear.

6. **For a primary amenorrhoea individual having an XY karyotype, normal infantile female external and internal genitalia fibrous bands in place of gonad, lack of development of secondary sexual characters, what is the most probable diagnosis?**
   a. Testicular feminization syndrome
   b. Mixed gonadal dysgenesis
   c. Swyer syndrome
   d. Defective antimullerian hormone

   Swyer syndrome, or XY gonadal dysgenesis, is a type of hypogonadism in a person whose karyotype is 46, XY. The

Answers

1. a	**2.** c	**3.** b	**4.** a	**5.** d	**6.** c

person is externally female with streak gonads, and if left untreated, will not experience puberty. Such gonads are typically surgically removed (as they have a significant risk of developing tumors) and a typical medical treatment would include hormone replacement therapy.

7. A lady who is using oral contraceptive pills comes with a complaint of vaginal discharge and pruritus vulvae. On local examination, there is curdy white discharge from the vagina. What is the most likely clinical diagnosis?

a. Trichomonal vaginitis
b. Monilial vaginitis
c. Gardnerella vaginalis
d. Atrophic vaginitis

Candida infection of the vagina or vulva may cause severe itching, burning, soreness, irritation, and a whitish or whitish-gray cottage cheese-like discharge.

8. A 30-years-old female has severe dysmenorrhoea and dyspareunia. On examination, uterus is 8 weeks size, uniformly enlarged and there is tenderness in posterior fornix. What is the most probable diagnosis?

a. Fibroid uterus
b. Dysfunctional uterine bleeding
c. Adenomyosis
d. Endometrial carcinoma

Patients with adenomyosis often present with painful menses (dysmenorrhea), profuse menses (menorrhagia, or both). Other possible symptoms are pain during sexual intercourse (dyspareunia), chronic pelvic pain and irritation of the urinary bladder.

9. An infertile woman presents with yellow or green vaginal discharge, Bartholin cyst and proctitis. What is the most probable diagnosis?

a. Syphilis
b. Trichomoniasis
c. Gonorrhoea
d. Candidiasis

Symptoms of gonorrhea in women include vaginal discharge, dysuria, intermenstrual bleeding, dyspareunia and abdominal pain. In men, gonorrhea causes anterior urethritis. Many people with gonococcal proctitis do not have any symptoms. In a small fraction of men, ascending urethritis progresses to epididymitis. Discharge is usually described as thin, purulent, and mildly odorous; however, many patients have minimal or no symptoms from gonococcal cervicitis.

10. A 28-years-old P1L1 presents with severe pain in her abdomen and is taken for laparotomy. On opening the abdomen pseudomyxoma of the peritoneum is present. What should be the probable reason?

a. Mucinous cystadenoma of ovary
b. Serous cystadenoma of ovary
c. Rupture of dermoid tumor
d. Endometriosis

Pseudomyxoma peritonei (PMP) is a clinical condition caused by cancerous cells (mucinous adenocarcinoma) that produce abundant mucin or gelatinous ascites. This disease is most commonly caused by an appendiceal primary cancer (cancer of the appendix); mucinous tumors of the ovary have also been implicated, although in most cases ovarian involvement is favoured to be a metastasis from an appendiceal or other gastrointestinal source.

11. In a 40-years-old woman, Pap smear shows atypical glandular cells. The next step of management should be:

a. Repeat Pap smear after three months
b. Colposcopic directed cervical biopsy
c. Colposcopy, cervical biopsy, endocervical curettage and endometrial biopsy
d. Hysteroscopy and directed endometrial biopsy

The Papanicolaou test (abbreviated as Pap test, also known as Pap smear, cervical smear, or smear test) is a method of cervical screening used to detect potentially pre-cancerous and cancerous processes in the cervix. Abnormal findings are often followed up by more sensitive diagnostic procedures, and, if warranted, interventions that aim to prevent progression to cervical cancer. Thorough evaluation of endocervix, ectocervix and endometrium is required.

12. A 50-years-old P4L4 has a simple left ovarian cyst of 10 cm. CA-125 is 30 u/mL. Treatment of choice would be:

a. TAH + BSO (Total abdominal hysterectomy + Bilateral salpingo-oophorectomy)
b. Laparoscopic cystectomy
c. Laparoscopic oophorectomy
d. Medical management with oral contraceptives

CA-125 is useful in differential diagnosis and in follow-up of the disease of ovarian tumours. CA-125 levels in premenopausal people over 200 U/ mL may indicate ovarian cancer, as may any elevation in CA-125 above 35 U/mL in post-menopausal people. If a tumor in a premenopausal woman is determined to be a low malignant potential tumor during surgery, and it is clearly stage I cancer, only the affected ovary is removed. For postmenopausal women with low malignant potential tumors, hysterectomy with bilateral salpingo-oophorectomy is still the preferred option.

13. A seven-years-old girl with precocious puberty is found to be having a 10 cm ovarian cyst on USG. The most likely etiology is:

a. Benign cystic teratoma
b. Brenner tumour
c. Choriocarcinoma
d. Granulosa cell tumour

Granulosa cell tumours (or granulosa-theca cell tumours or folliculoma) are a ovarian stomal tumour which produces estrogen. So, in a pre-pubertal girl, it might lead to precocious puberty.

Answers

7. b **8.** c **9.** c **10.** a **11.** c **12.** a **13.** d

14. A 17-years-old girl presents with an ovarian cyst of 5 cm. The cyst is echo free, unilocular and CA 125 of 8 U/mL. What is most appropriate management?

a. Laparoscopy for cyst removal
b. Laparotomy for cyst removal
c. Conservative with follow-up ultrasound
d. Medical treatment

Follow-up imaging in women of reproductive age for incidentally discovered simple cysts on ultrasound is not needed until 5 cm, as these are usually normal ovarian follicles. Simple cysts 5 to 7 cm in premenopausal females should be followed yearly. Simple cysts larger than 7 cm require further imaging with MRI or surgical assessment. Because they are large, they cannot be reliably assessed by ultrasound alone because it may be difficult to see the soft tissue nodularity or thickened septation at their posterior wall due to limited penetrance of the ultrasound beam.

15. The contraceptive choice for a 38-years-old P1L1 woman having chronic hypertension, dysmenorrhoea and menorrhagia is:

a. Copper intrauterine device
b. Sterilization
c. Levonorgestrel intrauterine device
d. Combined oral contraceptive pills

Intrauterine device (IUD) with progestogen, sold under the brand name Mirena among others, is a intrauterine device that releases the hormone levonorgestrel. It is used for birth control, heavy menstrual periods (menorrhagia), and to prevent excessive build of the lining of the uterus in those on estrogen replacement therapy. It is one of the most effective forms of birth control with a one-year failure rate around 0.2%. The device is placed in the uterus and lasts three to five years. Following removal fertility returns quickly.

16. A woman presents with heavy foul smelling discharge with sharply demarcated ulcers without induration on the perineum and the labia majora. Inguinal lymphadenopathy is also present. What is the most probable diagnosis?

a. Gonorrhoea
b. Tuberculosis
c. Chancroid
d. Trichomoniasis

The ulcer of chancroid characteristically: (1) ranges in size dramatically from 3 to 50 mm (1/8 inch to two inches) across; (2) is painful; (3) has sharply defined, undermined borders; (4) has irregular or ragged borders; (5) has a base that is covered with a gray or yellowish-gray material; (6) has a base that bleeds easily if traumatized or scraped; (7) painful swollen lymph nodes occurs in 30 to 60% of patients and (8) dysuria (pain with urination) and dyspareunia (pain with intercourse) in females.

17. A 28-years-old woman develops amenorrhoea after having dilatation and curettage. The most likely diagnosis is:

a. Kallmann syndrome
b. Asherman syndrome
c. Anorexia nervosa
d. Turner syndrome

Asherman syndrome (AS) which is also referred to as intrauterine adhesions (IUA) or intrauterine synechiae, is an acquired uterine condition that occurs when scar tissue (adhesions) form inside the uterus and/or the cervix. It is characterized by variable scarring inside the uterine cavity, where in many cases the front and back walls of the uterus stick to one another. AS can be the cause of menstrual disturbances (amenorrhoea), infertility, and placental abnormalities etc.

18. A 26-years-old woman $P_1 L_1$ reports with High Grade Squamous Intraepithelial Lesion (HGSIL) on Pap smear (Papanicolaou smear). Further management for her is:

a. VIA, VILI
b. Colposcopy and directed biopsy
c. LEEP
d. Conization

Colposcopy is a medical diagnostic procedure to examine an illuminated, magnified view of the cervix and the tissues of the vagina and vulva. It is done using a colposcope, which provides an enlarged view of the areas, allowing the colposcopist to visually distinguish normal from abnormal appearing tissue and take directed biopsies for further pathological examination.

19. A 16-years-old girl presents with primary amenorrhea with absent vagina, cervix and uterus in the presence of normal secondary sexual characteristics. Ovaries are present on USG. The most probable diagnosis is:

a. Klinefelter's syndrome
b. Androgen insensitivity syndrome
c. Mayer–Rokitansky–Kuster–Hauser syndrome
d. Prader–Willi syndrome

Müllerian agenesis, also known as Mayer–Rokitansky–Küster–Hauser syndrome (MRKH) or vaginal agenesis, is a congenital malformation characterized by a failure of the Müllerian duct to develop, resulting in a missing uterus and variable degrees of vaginal hypoplasia of its upper portion. Müllerian agenesis (including absence of the uterus, cervix and/or vagina) is the cause in 15% of cases of primary amenorrhoea. Because ovaries do not develop from the Müllerian ducts, affected women might have normal secondary sexual characteristics but are infertile due to the lack of a functional uterus.

20. A 50-years-old post-menopausal woman comes with complaints of bleeding per vaginum. Which one of the following investigations is NOT required?

a. Endometrial biopsy
b. Diagnostic laparoscopy
c. Hysteroscopy
d. Pap smear

Evaluation of post-menopausal bleeding: (1) Abnormal endometrium may have to be investigated by a hysteroscopy

Answers

14. c	15. c	16. c	17. b	18. b	19. c	20. b

with a biopsy or a dilation and curettage; (2) Pap smear is done to rule out carcinoma cervix.

21. In the process of MTP (Medical Termination of Pregnancy) done by suction and evacuation, it was realized that perforation of uterus occurred with cannula. The next step should be:

a. Laparotomy with exploration of bowel
b. Manual vacuum aspiration
c. Wait and watch
d. Complete the evacuation with curette

If perforation is caused by suction cannula, diagnostic laparoscopy is helpful to assess the size and site of perforation and the amount of hemorrhage. Operative laparoscopy or laparotomy may be needed to tackle the situation. One should not forget to inspect the intestine or omentum for evidence of injury.

22. An 18-years-old unmarried girl comes with complaints of heavy, prolonged bleeding during menses. Which among the following investigations is NOT usually advised?

a. Urine pregnancy test
b. Ultrasound uterus and adnexa
c. Coagulation profile
d. Dilatation and curettage

In adolescent dysfunctional uterine bleeding, d and c is rarely needed only if bleeding fails to stop or is severe in nature.

23. A 58-years-old woman with suspected ovarian cancer was operated for surgical staging. On laparotomy and subsequent histopathological examination of the specimen it was found that both ovaries were involved, capsule was ruptured, ascites was present containing malignant cells. Uterus and tubes were normal and there were no peritoneal implants. The FIGO stage for this patient would be:

a. Stage I b. Stage II
c. Stage III d. Stage IV

In stage 1, the cancer has not spread beyond the ovaries. Stage 1A means the cancer is only in one ovary. In stage 1B, the cancer is in both ovaries. Stage 1C means that one or both ovaries contain cancer cells and one of the following are also found: the outer capsule broke during surgery, the capsule burst before surgery, there are cancer cells on the outside of an ovary, or cancer cells are found in fluid washings from the abdomen.

24. A 22-years-old woman comes with complaints of pain and discomfort in vaginal region. On examination there is unilateral tender swelling in the posterior half of labium minus, overlying skin is red and edematous. What is the most probable diagnosis?

a. Utero vaginal prolapse b. Inversion of uterus
c. Bartholin's abscess d. Trichomoniasis

On examination of Bartholin's abscess, there is a unilateral tender swelling beneath the posterior half of the labium majus expanding medially to the posterior part of the labium minus. The overlying skin appears red and oedematous.

25. A 29-years-old woman is noted to have three consecutive first trimester spontaneous abortion. Examination reveals fibroid uterus. Which of the following types of uterine fibroids would most likely lead to recurrent abortions?

a. Submucosal b. Intramural
c. Subserosal d. Cervical

Uterine fibroids, especially the submucosal type, are associated with increased risks of spontaneous abortion, preterm delivery, abnormal presentation in labor, pelvic outlet obstruction, postpartum hemorrhage, and puerperal sepsis.

26. A 25-years-old infertile woman is noted to have blocked fallopian tube on Hysterosalpingography (HSG). Which of the following is the best next step for this woman?

a. Clomiphene citrate therapy
b. Gonadotropin therapy
c. Laparoscopy
d. Intrauterine insemination

The results of HSG and those of laparoscopy are complementary in tubal infertility evaluation. While HSG seems to be reliable when the tubes are patent, laparoscopy helps to reveal false tubal obstructions observed with HSG, and also helps in the diagnosis of pelvic adhesive bands and endometriosis.

27. The contraceptive choice for a 38-years-old woman with chronic hypertension and history of dysmenorrhea and menorrhagia (malignancy ruled out) is:

a. Copper intrauterine device
b. Levonorgestrel intrauterine device
c. Combined oral contraceptive pills
d. Sterilization

The levonorgestrel (LNg) intrauterine device releases small amounts of levonorgestrel, a form of progesterone, into the uterus each day. This type of IUD reduces cramping and heavy menstrual bleeding. And it is a highly effective method of birth control.

28. A 60-years-old woman presents with postmenopausal bleeding. On endometrial curettage she is diagnosed as endometrial carcinoma (EC). Which one of the following is a risk factor for endometrial cancer?

a. Multiparity b. Oral contraceptive use
c. Smoking d. Diabetes mellitus

Major risk factors for EC are obesity, diabetes, and hypertension.

Answers

21. a 22. d 23. a 24. c 25. a 26. c 27. b
28. d

29. A 40-years-old woman presented to the gynaecologist with complaints of profuse vaginal discharge. There was no discharge from the cervix on the speculum examination. The diagnosis of bacterial vaginosis was made based upon all of the following findings on microscopy *except*:

a. Abundance of gram variable coccobacilli
b. Absence of lactobacilli
c. Abundance of polymorphs
d. Presence of clue cells

Bacterial vaginosis is characterized by malodorous vaginal discharge. The term vaginosis is preferred as there is no vaginal inflammation.

30. A 36-years-old woman has absence of menses for the last 4 months. Pregnancy test is negative. Serum levels of LH and FSH are raised. Serum estradiol level is low. These findings suggest:

a. Bilateral tubal obstruction
b. PCOD
c. Premature menopause
d. Exogenous estrogen administration

Diagnosis of premature ovarian insufficiency include a history of amenorrhea in less than 35 years of age, serum gonadotropin level (FSH >40 mIU/mL) is high and serum E_2 level is low (<20 pg/mL).

31. In a woman presenting with amenorrhea, headache, blurred vision and galactorrhea, the appropriate investigation is:

a. Prolactin level
b. LH
c. FSH
d. hCG

Hyperprolactinemia inhibits ovarian steroidogenesis. Hyperprolactinemia causes secondary amenorrhea in about 30% of women. Hyperprolactinemia is commonly due to pituitary adenomas (microadenoma or macroadenoma). Visual field examination is essential to detect any compression effect on the optic nerves.

32. A patient presented with primary amenorrhoea with developed secondary characters and a bulging at hymen. Most probable diagnosis is:

a. PCOS
b. Rokitansky-Kuster-Hauser syndrome
c. Imperforate hymen
d. Kallman's syndrome

The chief complains of imperforate hymen are periodic lower abdominal pain, which may be continuous, primary amenorrhoea and urinary symptoms, such as frequency, dysuria or even retention of urine. Vulval inspection reveals a tense bulging membrane of bluish coloration.

33. A 46-years-old lady has abnormal uterine bleeding with simple hyperplasia of endometrium. The treatment of choice would be:

a. Total hysterectomy
b. Progesteron
c. Estrogen + progestogen
d. Estrogen

In perimenopausal and postmenopausal women with hyperplasia without atypia, continuous progestin therapy may be considered. However, hysterectomy with bilateral salpingo-oophorectomy is done as an alternative as the risk of carcinoma increases with age.

34. A female with primary amenorrhoea has normal breast and normal pubic hairs. USG showed absent uterus, absent cervix and short vaginal pouch but normal ovaries. Most likely diagnosis:

a. Klinefelter's syndrome
b. Mullerian agenesis
c. Gonadal dysgenesis
d. Turner's syndrome

An individual with Mullerian agenesis/MRKH syndrome is hormonally normal; that is, they will enter puberty with development of secondary sexual characteristics including thelarche and adrenarche (pubic hair). Their chromosome constellation will be 46, XX. Ovaries are intact and ovulation usually occurs. Typically, the vagina is shortened and intercourse may, in some cases, be difficult and painful. Medical examination supported by gynecologic ultrasonography demonstrates a complete or partial absence of the cervix, uterus, and vagina.

35. A 10-years-old girl presented with primary amenorrhea, absent breasts, malformed uterus. The most likely diagnosis is:

a. Mayer–Rokitansky–Kuster–Hauser syndrome
b. Turner's syndrome
c. Swyer's syndrome
d. Mixed gonadal dysgenesis

Turner's syndrome cases usually present as primary amenorrhea with delayed secondary sex characters. Vagina, uterus and fallopian tubes are present. The uterus is small but is responsive to exogenous estrogen.

Answers

29. c **30.** c **31.** a **32.** c **33.** a **34.** b **35.** b

15 Dermatology

1. **A 50-years-old patient presented with erythematous scaly plaques over trunk and extremities for last 10 years. Lesions are occasionally itchy. There is history of remission and relapse with exacerbation during winters. Most likely diagnosis:**
   a. Pityriasis rosea b. Lichen planus
   c. Contact dermatitis d. Psoriasis vulgaris

   Psoriasis is characterized by a course of remission and relapse and presence of silvery white scaly papules on erythematous base. Lesions are mildly pruritic or non-pruritic. The condition is aggravated in winters.

2. **A 30-years-old sexually active male presented with painful, grouped vesicular eruption on penile shaft for 4 days. He gave past history of similar lesions four times in the past one year. Such lesions are associated with:**
   a. Herpes simplex virus-2
   b. Treponema pallidum
   c. Chlamydia trachomatis serotype L2
   d. Hemophilus ducreyi

   In males, the lesions of HSV-2 occur on the glans penis or shaft of penis. Classically, it consists of macular or popular skin and mucous membrane lesions occurring about 5–7 days after a sexual contact. These lesions then progress to multiple vesicles, which are often very painful. The characteristic feature of herpes genitalis is that it tends to recur.

3. **A 24-years-old male complains of mild urethral discharge after sexual contact with a sex-worker. Drug used to treat such a patient:**
   a. Azithromycin 1 mg single dose
   b. Azithromycin 1 mg for 3 weeks
   c. Azithromycin 500 mg single dose
   d. Azithromycin 1 gram single dose

   Chlamydia trachomatis non-gonococcal urethritis is managed by Azithromycin 1 g single stat dose, which also take care of mycoplasma.

4. **A 30-year-old male presented with pruritic, flat topped, polygonal, shiny violaceous papules with flexural distribution. The most likely diagnosis is:**
   a. Psoriasis b. Pityriasis rosea
   c. Lichen planus d. Lichenoid dermatitis

   Cutaneous lesions of lichen planus present as purplish, plain topped, pruritic, polygonal, papules on peripheral parts of body with mild scaling in a bilateral symmetrical manner.

5. **A 50-years-old man has a 2-year-old history of facial bullae and oral ulcers. Microscopic smear from skin lesions is most likely to disclose:**
   a. Tzanck cells b. Acantholytic cells
   c. Necrosis d. Koilocytes

   Tzanck smear is prepared in pemphigus vulgaris. The scrapings from floor of blister are smeared on a microscopic slide and examine under light microscope after staining with Leishman's stain. Acantholytic cells are seen as large round cells lying free with no attachment with other epidermal cells.

6. **A 23-year-old lady presents with vesicular lesions in the buccal mucosa and flaccid blisters on the skin. The possible diagnosis is:**
   a. Pemphigus vulgaris b. Pemphigus foliaceous
   c. Pemphigoid d. Dermatitis herpetiformis

   Oral lesions are present in 50–70% of patients of pemphigus vulgaris. Cutaneous lesions erupt in crops and consists of flaccid blisters filled with fluid.

7. **A six-year-old boy presents with generalized seizure disorder and hypopigmented skin lesions. On examination he has tiny red nodules over the nose and cheeks. The most likely diagnosis is:**
   a. Tuberous sclerosis b. Sturge–Weber disease
   c. PHACE syndrome d. Neurofibromatosis

   Tuberous sclerosis complex (TSC) is a rare multisystem genetic disease that causes benign tumours to grow in the brain and on other vital organs such as the kidneys, heart, liver, eyes, lungs, and skin. A combination of symptoms may include seizures, intellectual disability, developmental delay, behavioural problems, skin abnormalities, and lung and kidney disease. TSC is caused by a mutation of either of two genes, TSC1 and TSC2, which code for the proteins hamartin and tuberin, respectively. These proteins act as tumour growth suppressors, agents that regulate cell proliferation and differentiation.

Answers

1. d **2.** a **3.** d **4.** c **5.** b **6.** a **7.** a

8. A 7-years-old child with history of asthma has developed itching and rashes in the axilla, groin and popliteal region. Most likely diagnosis:

a. Seborrheic dermatitis
b. Contact dermatitis
c. Atopic dermatitis
d. Irritant dermatitis

Childhood and adolescent form pattern of atopic dermatitis presents with intensively pruritic lesions on flexural areas (popliteal fossa, antecubital fossa, axilla and groin). There is a personal or family history of other atopic conditions like asthma, hay fever, allergic rhinitis or conjunctivitis.

9. A lady has family history of asthma. She presented with itching in cubital fossa and popliteal fossa. Most likely diagnosis:

a. Xeroderma pigmentosum
b. Psoriasis vulgaris
c. Contact dermatitis
d. Atopic dermatitis

Adult phase of atopic dermatitis is characterized by itchy lesions which are lichenified. These lesions are present in flexural (cubital and popliteal fossa). One of the very important feature of atopic dermatitis is the presence of personal or family history of other atopic conditions like asthma.

10. A patient presented with recurrent oral aphthous ulcers with genital ulcers. Ophthalmologic examination show uveitis. History of fever is present. Most likely diagnosis:

a. Measles
b. Henoch-Schonlein purpura
c. Behcet's disease
d. Ankylosing spondylitis

Behcet's syndrome is characterized by genital ulcers, aphthous (oral) ulcers and uveitis.

Answers

8. c **9.** d **10.** c

16 Anesthesia

1. **Which of the following inhalational anaesthetic agents has rapid onset of action and rapid recovery actions and is most desirous for day care (OPD/outpatient) surgical procedures?**
   a. Ether b. Halothane
   c. Trichloroethylene d. Desflurane

   Desflurane is the fastest acting induction agent (B/G coefficient 0.42) and its potency is medium (MAC is 6%). It undergoes minimal metabolism (<1%) and does not produce any fluoride. Therefore, desflurane is the agent of choice for prolonged duration surgeries, old age patients and hepatic and renal disease patients.

2. **A 20-year-old patient presented with early pregnancy for medical termination of pregnancy (MTP) in day care facility. What will be the induction agent of choice?**
   a. Thiopentone b. Ketamine
   c. Propofol d. Diazepam

   Because of propofol's (i) early induction (ii) early and smooth recovery (iii) inactive metabolites and (iv) antiemetic effects it is, the IV agent of choice for day care surgery.

3. **Administration of succinylcholine to a paraplegic patient led to the development of dysrhythmia, conduction abnormalities and finally cardiac arrest. The most likely cause is:**
   a. Hypercalcemia
   b. Hyperkalemia
   c. Anaphlaxia
   d. Hypermagnesemia

   Succinylcholine is contraindicated for up to 2–3 months after trauma, up to 6 months after hemiplegia/paraplegia and up to 1 year after burns (the greatest risk is between 1 week to 2 months). In these conditions denervated/regenerating nerve develops extrajunctional receptors which can produce hyperkalemia.

4. **Proper technique of endotracheal intubation involves:**
   a. Flexion of neck
   b. Flexion of the neck and extension of the atlanto-occipital joint
   c. Extension of the neck
   d. Extension of the neck and flexion of the atlanto-occipital joint

   Technique of intubation: (1) The patient should lie supine; (2) There should be extension at atlanto-occipital joint and flexion at cervical spine and (3) This position is achieved by putting a 6 to 8 cm thick pillow under the occiput.

5. **Ratio of chest compression to breathing while CPR in adults, without advanced airway in place:**
   a. 15:2 b. 30:2
   c. 45:2 d. 60:2

   Before advanced airway (i.e. by mouth to mouth, bag and mask ventilation), the ratio should be 30:2 (30 compressions followed by 2 breaths) irrespective of duration of resuscitation (previously this ratio was 15:2). The reason for change in ratio is to minimize interruption in chest compression (this is the most important goal of latest recommendation).

6. **A patient was undergoing surgical procedure under general anesthesia. Suddenly he developed tachycardia, sweating, hypertension and tachypnea. Best step to manage such a condition would be:**
   a. Intravenous beta-blockers
   b. End the surgical procedure
   c. Wait and watch
   d. Deepen the plane of anesthesia

   Signs of light anesthesia/intra-operative awareness include tachycardia, sweating (perspiration), hypertension, tachypnea, lacrimation, coughing (preserved reflexes) etc. In such cases, anesthesia should be deepened immediately.

7. **A 10-years-old child was undergoing surgery for squint. During surgery, there was a sudden fall in heart rate from 140 bpm to 40 bpm (beats per minute). As an anesthetist, how will you manage this situation?**
   a. Wait and watch
   b. Ask the surgeon to stop surgery for some time
   c. Deepen the plane of anesthesia
   d. Give I/V beta blockers

Answers

1. d	**2.** c	**3.** b	**4.** b	**5.** b	**6.** d	**7.** b

Sudden and sudden bradycardia during an ophthalmic surgical procedure suggest the possibility of oculo-cardiac reflex. As soon as the oculo-cardiac reflex is noticed, the ophthalmic surgeon should relieve the traction on the rectus muscles till the episodes ends and there is an increase in heart rate. Otherwise, intravenous atropine needs to be given.

8. **While assessing the adequacy of mouth opening preoperatively in a patient, only soft palate was visible. This is which grade as per Mallampati grading:**
   a. I
   b. II
   c. III
   d. IV

In class III of Mallampati grading, only soft palate is visible.

9. **A 55-years-old hypertensive male is on ACE inhibitors. There is a past history of CABG (coronary artery bypass grafting) done 3 years back. Now he is planned for hernia surgery. He has good effort tolerance. What should be the initial plan of preoperative evaluation of this patient?**
   a. Routine preoperative examination plus stress testing
   b. Routine preoperative examination plus clinical examination
   c. Routine preoperative examination plus clinical examination plus angiography
   d. Routine preoperative examination plus clinical examination plus ventilation-perfusion scan

Initial step in investigating such a patient would be general preoperative examination and clinical examination. If everything is good, he can be planned for non-cardiac surgery. If there are some abnormal findings on clinical examination, then only he needs to be evaluated further with 2D-echocardiography or angiography.

10. **During abdominal surgery under local anaesthetic, patient suddenly felt sharp pain. Injury to which structure is likely?**
    a. Liver parenchyma
    b. Large gut
    c. Small gut
    d. Parietal peritoneum

The parietal peritoneum is supplied by nerves (e.g., phrenic and thoraco-abdominal) to the adjacent body wall, and most of it is very sensitive to pain. Painful stimuli to the central part of the diaphragmatic peritoneum are referred to the shoulder. The visceral peritoneum is insensitive to pain.

Answers

8. c **9.** b **10.** d

17 Radiology

1. **There is consolidation in middle lobe of right lung. Which of the heart border will be obliterated on chest X-ray?**
   a. Right heart border　b. Left heart border
   c. Anterior heart border　d. Posterior heart border

   As the right middle lobe of lung lies adjacent to the right cardiac border, diseases like consolidation of the right middle lobe will obliterate the right cardiac border.

2. **Which of the following combination of heart configuration and its cause is NOT correct?**
   a. Flask-shaped heart: Pericardial effusion
   b. Egg on side heart: Transposition of great arteries
   c. Snowman's sign: Ebstein's anomaly
   d. Pentagon-shaped heart: Mitral incompetence

   Snowman's sign/Figure of 8/Cottage loaf sign is seen in transposition of great arteries.

3. **In mitral stenosis, barium swallow will show indentation/compression on esophagus due to the enlargement of:**
   a. Left atrium　b. Left ventricle
   c. Right atrium　d. Right ventricle

   Left atrium enlargement can cause compression of the esophagus from anterior side as it lies just anterior to the thoracic part of the esophagus.

4. **Which sign is seen on USG when common femoral vein meets with great saphenous vein and femoral artery at great saphenous opening?**
   a. String sign
   b. Tillaux sign
   c. Stemmer's sign
   d. Mickey mouse sign

   The normal anatomy of the common femoral artery, common femoral vein and great saphenous vein at the level just below the inguinal crease is shown as Mickey mouse sign on USG.

5. **Radiation dose monitoring in occupational personnel (like X-ray technician) is done by:**
   a. TLD badge　b. Grid
   c. Tungsten　d. Lead apron

   For monitoring radiation dose in occupational personnel in imaging centers, TLD (thermos-luminescent dosimeter) body badges and rings are used.

6. **A 7-weeks pregnant lady is accidentally exposed to chest X-ray in a hospital. What needs to be done next?**
   a. Continue pregnancy　b. Terminate pregnancy
   c. Chromosomal checking　d. Amniocentesis

   In first trimester of pregnancy, any radiation exposure of more than 5 rads needs consideration for continuing pregnancy. Single exposure rarely causes such a large exposure so pregnancy can be continued.

7. **FALSE for MRI:**
   a. Imaging perfusion of brain
   b. Presence of hydrogen ions
   c. Blood vessels visualized without contrast
   d. Superior to CT for bone scanning

   CT scan is best to detect cortical bony lesions and fine osseous details.

8. **Investigation of choice for detection and characterization of interstitial lung disease is:**
   a. MRI
   b. Chest X-ray
   c. High resolution CT scan
   d. Ventilation perfusion scan

   HRCT is of proven value in the diagnosis of diffuse lung disease (like interstitial lung diseases), particularly in the early stages when the chest radiograph is normal and for follow-up.

9. **MIBG scan is done for:**
   a. Gastrointestinal stromal tumours
   b. Acute pancreatitis
   c. Phaeochromocytoma
   d. Meckel's diverticulum

   MIBG is accumulated by pheochromocytoma and neuroblastoma.

10. **What dose of radiation would affect hematological system?**
    a. 0–250 cGY　b. 250–500 cGY
    c. 500–750 cGY　d. 750–1000 cGY

    250–500 cGY of radiation affects hemopoietic system and death can occur in weeks post-exposure. Hemopoietic and gastrointestinal syndromes are reversible with good symptomatic and supportive care.

Answers

1. a	2. c	3. a	4. d	5. a	6. a	7. d
8. c	9. c	10. b				

18 Psychiatry

1. Sallu, an occasional alcoholic has got a change in his behavior. He has become suspicious that people are trying to conspire against him though his father says that there is no reason for his fears. He is having hallucinations of voices commenting on his actions. Most likely diagnosis is:

a. Delirium tremens
b. Alcohol induced psychosis
c. Schizophrenia
d. Delusional disorder

Schizophrenia is characterized by disturbances in thought and verbal behavior, perception, affect, motor behavior and relationship to the external world. The diagnosis is entirely clinical.

2. A 40-year-old female had headache for last 6 months. She had several consultations. All her investigations were normal. She still insists that there is something wrong and seeks another consultant. Most likely diagnosis is:

a. Phobia
b. Psychogenic headache
c. Hypochondriasis
d. Depression

Hypochondriasis is defined as a persistent preoccupation with a fear (or belief) of having one (or more) serious diseases (s), based on person's own interpretation of normal body function or a minor physical abnormality.

3. A patient is depressed for last 3 years, do not go out of his house much and is isolated from the society. He is having normal weight and normal sleep. Most probably he is having:

a. No psychiatric illness
b. Chronic fatigue syndrome
c. Dysthymia
d. Major depression

If the symptoms consist of persistent mild depression, the disorder is called as Dysthymia; and if symptoms consist of persistent instability of mood between mild depression and mild elation, the disorder is called as cyclothymia.

4. A young patient with self-mutilating behaviour and impulsivity is having:

a. Paranoid personality disorder
b. Adjustment disorder
c. Borderline personality disorder
d. Dependent personality disorder

The borderline type of personality is also known as borderline personality disorder (DSM-IV-TR), the characteristic features of which include impulsivity, deliberate self harm (in the form of self-mutilation, suicidal gestures, or accident proneness) etc.

5. A 16-year-old male is found to have a mental age of 9 years on IQ testing. He has:

a. Mild mental retardation
b. Moderate mental retardation
c. Severe mental retardation
d. Profound mental retardation

IQ of 50–70 is categorized as mild MR.

6. A 30-year-old lady complained of sudden onset of breathlessness, anxiety, palpitation and feeling of impending doom. Physical examination is normal. What is the diagnosis?

a. Panic attack
b. Schizophrenia
c. Conversion disorder
d. Acute psychosis

Panic disorder is characterized by discrete episodes of acute anxiety. The onset is usually in early third decade with often a chronic course. The episode is usually sudden, lasts for a few minutes and is characterized by very severe anxiety.

7. Female patient presented with acute restlessness and fear of impending doom. Most probable diagnosis is:

a. Schizophrenia
b. Delirium
c. Anxiety neurosis
d. MDP

Anxiety is a 'normal' phenomenon, which is characterized by a state of apprehension or unease arising out of anticipation of danger.

Answers

1. c **2.** c **3.** c **4.** c **5.** a **6.** a **7.** c

8. A 30-year-old male presented with symptoms of palpitations and sweating on meeting seniors and on making public presentations. This makes him avoid such situations. The diagnosis is:

a. Panic reaction
b. Social phobia
c. Avoidance personality
d. Adjustment disorder

Social phobia is an example of irrational fear of activities of social interaction, characterized by an irrational fear of performing activities in the presence of other people or interacting with others. The patient is afraid of his own actions being viewed by others critically, resulting in embarrassment or humiliation.

9. A girl with normal milestones spends her time seeing her own hand and do not interact with others. Likely diagnosis is:

a. ADHD
b. Autism
c. Asperger's syndrome
d. Rett's syndrome

Autism is characterized by stereotyped behaviours such as head banging, body-spinning, hand-flicking, lining-up objects, rocking, clapping, twirling etc. and marked impairment in making friends.

10. A 10-year-old child is very restless and hyperactive. His activities and running in school are very disturbing to his friends. Likely diagnosis is:

a. Schizophrenia
b. Attention deficit hyperactivity disorder
c. Autistic disorder
d. Conduct disorder

ADHD is commonest type of attention deficit disorder (ADD) which is characterized by poor attention span with distractibility (does not seem to listen), hyperactivity (moving about here and there and difficulty in sitting still at one place for long) and impulsivity (acts before thinking, on the spur of the moment).

Answers

8. b **9.** b **10.** b

19 Orthopedics

1. **A 1-year-old child presents with multiple fractures seen in various stages of healing. The most probable diagnosis in this case is:**
   a. Scurvy
   b. Rickets
   c. Battered baby syndrome
   d. Sickle cell disease

   Physical examination of a child with battered child syndrome (BCS) with detect injuries such as bruises, burns, swelling, retinal hemorrhages, internal damage such as bleeding or rupture of an organ, fractures of long bones or spiral fractures that result from twisting, and fractured ribs or skull. The presence of injuries at different stages of healing (i.e., having occurred at different times) is nearly indicative of BCS.

2. **An army recruit, smoker and 6 months into training started complaining of pain at posterior medial aspect of both legs. There was acute point tenderness and the pain was aggravated on physical activity. The most likely diagnosis is:**
   a. Burger's disease
   b. Gout
   c. Lumbar canal stenosis
   d. Stress fracture

   Stress fracture is a special type of fracture sustained due to the chronic repetitive injury (stress) causing a break in bony trabeculae. These often present as only pain and may not be visible on X-rays.

3. **A young lady presented to the OPD with tingling sensation in thumb, index and middle finger. This sensation can be aggravated by palmar flexing the wrist for 1 minute. Findings are suggestive of:**
   a. Carpal Tunnel syndrome
   b. Cubital Tunnel syndrome
   c. Tarsal Tunnel syndrome
   d. Impingement syndrome

   Phalen's maneuver (palmar flexing wrist) can moderately increase the pressure in the Carpal Tunnel via this mass effect, pinching the median nerve between the proximal edge of the transverse Carpal ligament and the anterior border of the distal end of the radius. By compressing the median nerve within the Carpal Tunnel, characteristic symptoms (such as burning, tingling or numb sensation over the thumb, index, middle and ring fingers) conveys a positive test result and suggests Carpal Tunnel syndrome.

4. **Pain and tenderness over the lateral condyle of humerus with painful dorsiflexion of the wrist is indicative of:**
   a. Golfer's elbow
   b. Tennis elbow
   c. Pitcher's elbow
   d. Cricket elbow

   Tennis elbow (lateral epicondylitis) is a condition characterized by pain and tenderness at the lateral epicondyle of the humerus due to nonspecific inflammation at the origin of the extensor muscles of the forearm.

5. **A 15-year-old boy presented with mass in the distal femur. X-ray from the lesion showed features of Codman's triangle and sun-ray appearance. The diagnosis is:**
   a. Osteosarcoma
   b. Ewing's sarcoma
   c. Osteoclastoma
   d. Chondroblastoma

   Radiological examination in osteosarcoma include an area of irregular destruction in the metaphysis, sometimes overshadowed by the new bone formation, periosteal reaction, Codman's triangle and sun-ray appearance.

6. **A 24-year-old male, known epileptic, presented following a seizure with pain in the right shoulder region. Examination revealed that the right upper limb was adducted and internally rotated and the movements could not be performed. Likely diagnosis is:**
   a. Posterior dislocation of shoulder
   b. Luxation erecta
   c. Intrathoracic dislocation of shoulder
   d. Subglenoid dislocation of shoulder

   A posterior dislocation of the shoulder may result from a direct blow on the front of the shoulder, driving the head backwards. More often, however, posterior dislocation is the consequence of an electric shock or an epileptiform convulsion.

Answers

1. c **2.** d **3.** a **4.** b **5.** a **6.** a

7. A 3-year-old child falls from 2 metres height. On X-ray, no abnormality was detected. After 2 years, the child presents with calcaneal valgus. Probable cause is:

a. Undiagnosed
b. Tibial epiphyseal plate injury
c. Avascular necrosis of talus
d. Rocker bottom foot

Epiphyseal injuries is a group of injuries seen in a growing skeleton. An injury involving the growth plate result in deformities due to irregular growth. Shortening may occur because of premature epiphyseal closure.

8. Position of lower limb in synovitis stage of TB hip joint:

a. Flexion, adduction and internal rotation
b. Flexion, abduction and internal rotation
c. Flexion, adduction and external rotation
d. Flexion, abduction and external rotation

TB Hip stages: (1) Stage of synovitis (FABER–AL): Flexion, abduction and external rotation with apparent lengthening; (2) Stage of arthritis (FADIR–AS): Flexion, adduction and internal rotation with apparent shortening and (3) Stage of erosion (FADIR–TS): Flexion, adduction and internal rotation with true shortening.

9. A patient with recurrent dislocation of the shoulder presents to the hospital. The doctor tries to abduct his arm and to extend the elbow and external rotation, but the patient does not allow to do so. This test is called:

a. Duga's test
b. Hamilton test
c. Callaway's test
d. Apprehension test

Apprehension test is a test to detect an unstable shoulder. The shoulder is abducted and externally rotated. As the examiner loads the shoulder along the long axis of the arm, the patient becomes apprehensive, and tries to resist any further movement by using his hand or by making the shoulder stiff by muscle spasm.

10. A 5-years-old child presented with knee pain irritability and gum bleeding. Radiograph showed significantly thin cortex and a white line at the metaphysis. Most likely diagnosis:

a. Fluorosis
b. Rickets
c. Scurvy
d. Caffey's disease

Patients of scurvy may present with lethargy and malaise, bone pain, bleeding tendencies (e.g., bleeding gums) and impaired wound healing. Radiological changes include generalized osteopaenia, cortical thinning: "pencil-point" cortex, scorbutic rosary (expansion of the costochondral junctions), Wimberger's ring sign (circular, opaque radiologic shadow surrounding epiphyseal centers of ossification, which may result from bleeding), Frankel's line (dense zone of provisional calcification), Pelken spur (metaphyseal spurs which result in cupping of the metaphysis) etc.

Answers

7. b **8.** d **9.** d **10.** c

20 Pediatrics

1. **A 6-years-old child presents with oliguria, haematuria, puffiness of face, convulsions, BP of 200/100 mm Hg and blood urea 80 mg%. What is the most likely diagnosis?**
   a. Haemolytic uraemic syndrome
   b. Nephrotic syndrome
   c. Acute glomerulonephritis with hypertensive encephalopathy
   d. Obstructive uropathy

Hypertensive encephalopathy (HE) is general brain dysfunction due to significantly high blood pressure. Symptoms may include headache, vomiting, trouble with balance, and confusion. In hypertensive encephalopathy, generally the blood pressure is greater than 200/130 mmHg. Hypertensive encephalopathy is caused by an increase in blood pressure. Several conditions may evoke blood pressure elevation: acute nephritis, eclampsia, crises in chronic essential hypertension, sudden withdrawal of antihypertensive treatment.

2. **A 3-years-old child is brought for sudden inability to walk following fever of two days duration. On clinical examination, sensorium is normal, both the lower limbs are hypotonic with the right limb more affected than the left. Plantar reflex is equivocal and deep tendon reflexes are not elicitable in the lower limbs on both sides. The most probable diagnosis is:**
   a. Acute poliomyelitis
   b. Acute rheumatic fever
   c. Acute transverse myelitis
   d. Acute infective polyneuritis

Poliomyelitis, often called polio or infantile paralysis, is an infectious disease caused by the poliovirus. In about 0.5 percent of cases there is muscle weakness resulting in an inability to move. This can occur over a few hours to a few days. The weakness most often involves the legs but may less commonly involve the muscles of the head, neck and diaphragm. Many people fully recover. In those with muscle weakness about 2 to 5% of children and 15 to 30% of adults die. Another 25% of people have minor symptoms such as fever and a sore throat and up to 5% have headache, neck stiffness and pains in the arms and legs. These people are usually back to normal within one or two weeks. In up to 70% of infections there are no symptoms. Years after recovery post-polio syndrome may occur, with a slow development of muscle weakness similar to that which the person had during the initial infection.

3. **A 4-years-old boy diagnosed as a case of sickle cell disease presents with pain and swelling of bones, marked in small bones of hand and feet along with severe pain in abdomen. Investigation reveals necrosis of femoral head and upper third of tibia. The symptoms have resolved after one week. The possible explanation is:**
   a. Aplastic crisis
   b. Sequestration crisis
   c. Vaso-occlusive crisis
   d. Hemolytic crisis

Sickle cell disease (SCD) usually manifests early in childhood. For the first 6 months of life, infants are protected largely by elevated levels of HbF; soon thereafter, the condition becomes evident. The most common clinical manifestation of SCD is vaso-occlusive crisis. A vaso-occlusive crisis occurs when the microcirculation is obstructed by sickled RBCs, causing ischemic injury to the organ supplied and resultant pain.

4. **A three-years-old male child has a poor stream of urine and strains at micturition. After voiding, the bladder is still palpable. The patient should be advised:**
   a. Abdomen X-ray
   b. Urine examination
   c. Circumcision
   d. Excretory urogram

Presentation of a boy with posterior urethral valve will depend on the severity of obstruction. The boy may present at birth or as late as 3–4 years. The symptoms are the same—difficulty in passing urine, straining to pass urine, dribbling of urine, poor stream of urine. There may be distension of the lower abdomen caused by a stretched out filled-up bladder. The common mistake that can be made is to diagnose this condition as phimosis and then get a circumcision done. Investigations are done to look for the complications associated with this entity—like electrolyte imbalances and infection of urine and also in the blood stream by sending both blood and urine for culture studies and treating the infection first before specific therapy for the PUV.

Answers

1. c 2. a 3. c 4. b

5. A two-years-old child has weight less than 3 SD (less than 3 Z score) as per WHO growth chart and mid-upper arm circumference (MUAC) less than 11 cm. What is the correct diagnosis for this child?

a. Acute malnutrition
b. Chronic malnutrition
c. Severe acute malnutrition
d. Moderate acute malnutrition

Severe acute malnutrition (SAM) is defined as a weight to height ratio less than-3 Standard Deviations on the Z-score for the reference population and MUAC (mid-upper arm circumference) < 110 mm with or without oedema corresponds to SAM.

6. For a three-years-old male child, the height for age is 82% of the expected for that age and weight for height is 65% of the expected value. The child is labelled as:

a. Normal
b. Wasted
c. Stunted
d. Wasted and stunted

Low weight-for-height: Wasting or thinness indicates in most cases a recent and severe process of weight loss, which is often associated with acute starvation and/or severe disease. The definition of stunting according to the WHO is for the "height for age" value to be less than two standard deviations of the WHO Child Growth Standards median.

7. A 7-years-old child presents with intermittent claudication, pain and weakness of legs and dyspnea on running. Examination shows delayed and weak femorals compared to brachial arteries. The heart size is normal with a left ventricular forcible apex. The most probable diagnosis is:

a. Ventricular septal defect
b. Patent ductus arteriosus
c. Atrial septal defect
d. Coarctation of aorta

Patients with COA have cold legs and feet or have pain in their legs with exercise (intermittent claudication). Patients may experience dizziness or shortness of breath, fainting or near-fainting episodes, chest pain, abnormal tiredness or fatigue, headaches, or nose-bleeds. Arterial hypertension in the arms with low blood pressure in the lower extremities is classic. In the lower extremities, weak pulses in the femoral arteries and arteries of the feet are found.

8. A seven days old baby presents with complaints of vomiting and diarrhoea. Examination reveals cataract in both the eyes and jaundice. What is the most probable diagnosis?

a. Rh incompatibility
b. Galactosemia
c. Congenital rubella syndrome
d. Congenital syphilis

Infants affected by galactosemia typically present with symptoms of lethargy, vomiting, diarrhea, failure to thrive, and jaundice. The presence of presenile cataract, noticeable in galactosemic infants as young as a few days old, is highly associated with two distinct types of galactosemia: GALT deficiency and to a greater extent, GALK deficiency.

9. A two-years-old child is admitted with history of fever for two weeks and convulsions for the last one day. CSF examination shows CSF pressure elevated to 30–40 cm H_2O, clear CSF, lymphocytic pleocytosis (250 cells/mm^3), elevated protein and low chloride levels. What is the most probable diagnosis?

a. Pyogenic meningitis
b. Tubercular meningitis
c. Acute encephalitis
d. Subacute sclerosing panencephalitis (SSPE)

Fever and headache are the cardinal features of tubercular meningitis; confusion is a late feature and coma bears a poor prognosis. Meningism is absent in a fifth of patients with TB meningitis. Patients may also have focal neurological deficits. The CSF in TBM usually has a high protein, low glucose and a raised number of lymphocytes. Acid-fast bacilli are sometimes seen on a CSF smear, but more commonly, *M. tuberculosis* is grown in culture. A spiderweb clot in the collected CSF is characteristic of TB meningitis, but is a rare finding.

10. A five-years-old child was diagnosed with nephrotic syndrome, 18 months back. He was treated and successfully went into remission at that time. Following, the initial episode, the child has had 3 relapses, each of which was successfully treated with oral prednisolone (60 mg/m^2/24 h) until remission, followed by 40 mg/m^2 single dose, alternate days for four weeks. What is the diagnosis?

a. Nephrotic syndrome, infrequent relapses
b. Nephrotic syndrome, frequent relapses
c. Nephrotic syndrome, steroid dependent
d. Nephrotic syndrome, steroid resistant

Infrequent relapser nephrotic syndrome are defined as patients having less than two relapses within 6 months or less than four relapses within 12 months of response.

11. A 7-years-old girl presents to you with non-specific abdominal pain, mild abdominal distension, and not growing well. The child weighs 14 kg and height is 95 cm. Systemic examination is normal. The haemoglobin was 7.5 g/dL (microcytic hypochromic RBCs) and has not responded to iron therapy. Which of the following will be the first investigation you will like to do for diagnosing the condition?

a. Bone marrow aspiration
b. Tissue transglutaminase antibodies
c. Lower GI contrast examination
d. Colonoscopy/sigmoidoscopy

Answers

5. c	6. d	7. d	8. b	9. b	10. a	11. b

Coeliac disease is a long-term autoimmune disorder that primarily affects the small intestine. Classic symptoms include gastrointestinal problems such as chronic diarrhoea, abdominal distension, malabsorption, loss of appetite and among children failure to grow normally. This often begins between six months and two years of age. Non-classic symptoms are more common, especially in people older than two years. For most children and adults, the best way to screen for celiac disease is with the Tissue Transglutaminase IgA antibody, plus an IgA antibody in order to ensure that the patient generates enough of this antibody to render the celiac disease test accurate.

12. A seven-years-old boy weighing 20 kg presented with bleeding from upper GI tract (hematemesis) for last 18 hours. On examination, PR-86/m, RR-16/m and BP-100/70 mmHg; and spleen is palpable 5 cm below costal margin. There is no other abnormality. Liver function tests are normal. What is the next best step in management?

a. Fluid resuscitation with crystalloids
b. Intravenous vasopressin
c. Intravenous propranolol
d. Transdermal nitroglycerine

Esophageal varices result can from portal hypertension, regardless of the age group. The increased resistance to blood flow through the portal system is due to prehepatic, intrahepatic, and suprahepatic obstruction, but the most common causes of portal hypertension in children include portal vein thrombosis (prehepatic) and biliary atresia (intrahepatic).

13. A seven-years-old girl presents in emergency room with hypertension, lethargy, headache, seizures, and visual disturbances. Fundus examination reveals haemorrhages and exudates. Which of the following treatment regimen will be the most appropriate for this child?

a. Sublingual nifedipine
b. Intravenous labetalol infusion
c. Intravenous minoxidil
d. Furosemide

Labetalol is effective in the management of hypertensive emergencies, postoperative hypertension, pheochromocytoma-associated hypertension, and rebound hypertension from beta blocker withdrawal.

14. On routine newborn screening at day 3 of life, the baby was found to have TSH level 40 mU/L. What should be the next step?

a. Repeat thyroid profile within one week
b. Start child on thyroxine immediately
c. Repeat thyroid profile after four weeks
d. Repeat thyroid profile/start thyroxine, if the child has clinical features of congenital hypothyroidism, otherwise wait and watch

TSH concentrations in children are normally higher than in adults. In 2002, the NACB recommended age-related reference limits starting from about 1.3 to 19 μIU/mL for normal-term infants at birth, dropping to 0.6–10 μIU/mL at 10 weeks old, 0.4–7.0 μIU/mL at 14 months and gradually dropping during childhood and puberty to adult levels, 0.3–3.0 μIU/mL.

15. A five-years-old girl is brought to you with history of fever for seven days associated with rash, anorexia, myalgia and petechial haemorrhages. Which of the following investigations will be most appropriate for making a diagnosis of dengue fever?

a. Detection of NS1 antigen
b. Platelet count
c. IgG capture ELISA
d. Detection of IgM antibodies for dengue

Detection of NS1 (non-structural protein-1) during the febrile phase of a primary infection may be greater than 90% sensitive, However is only 60–80% in subsequent infections. Tests for dengue virus-specific antibodies, types IgG and IgM, can be useful in confirming a diagnosis in the later stages of the infection. Both IgG and IgM are produced after 5–7 days. The highest levels (titres) of IgM are detected following a primary infection, but IgM is also produced in reinfection. IgM becomes undetectable 30–90 days after a primary infection, but earlier following re-infections.

16. An eight-years-old boy was diagnosed to have *P. vivax* malaria and was treated with appropriate dosages of chloroquine. The fever subsided but recurred after 3 weeks. Peripheral smear was again positive for *P. vivax*. This child should now be treated as a case with:

a. Relapse
b. Recrudescence
c. Either relapse/recrudescence
d. Fresh infection

The plasmodium parasites, which are responsible for malaria, can persist in the blood without causing apparent symptoms for a few months (recrudescence). Relapse in this context occurs due to activation of hypnozoites in the liver.

17. A two-days-old neonate is brought with cyanosis, single second heart sound, and pansystolic murmur on the left sternal border. ECG reveals left axis deviation, right atrial overload and left ventricular hypertrophy. What is the most likely diagnosis?

a. Tetralogy of Fallot
b. Tricuspid atresia
c. Transposition of great arteries
d. Total anomalous pulmonary venous connection

Tricuspid atresia presents with progressive cyanosis, tachipnea over the first 2 weeks of life, holosystolic murmur

Answers

12. b **13.** b **14.** a **15.** d **16.** c **17.** b

due to the VSD, left axis deviation on electrocardiography and left ventricular hypertrophy (since it must pump blood to both the pulmonary and systemic systems) and normal heart size.

18. A three-years-old girl is brought with complaint of not being able to ever stand or walk. She achieved head control at one year of age. Examination reveals generalized hypotonia, brisk knee jerk, and ankle clonus. What is the likely diagnosis?

a. Cerebral palsy
b. Spinal muscular atrophy
c. Congenital hypothyroidism
d. Congenital myotonic dystrophy

Abnormal muscle tone, delayed motor development and persistence of primitive reflexes are the main early symptoms of CP. Symptoms and diagnosis typically occur by the age of 2, although persons with milder forms of cerebral palsy may be over the age of 5, if not in adulthood, when finally diagnosed. It is a developmental disability.

19. A 5-years-old boy is brought to the Emergency Room following a crushing injury. The ECG reveals peaked T waves, prolonged PR interval and widened QRS complexes. Which of the following treatments should be administered immediately?

a. Sodium bicarbonate infusion
b. Intravenous bolus procainamide
c. Insulin infusion
d. Intravenous magnesium sulphate

With mild to moderate hyperkalemia, there is prolongation of the PR interval and development of peaked T waves. Severe hyperkalemia results in a widening of the QRS complex, and the ECG complex can evolve to a sinusoidal shape. Insulin (e.g. intravenous injection of 10–15 units of regular insulin along with 50 mL of 50% dextrose to prevent the blood sugar from dropping too low) leads to a shift of potassium ions into cells, secondary to increased activity of the sodium-potassium ATPase. Its effects last a few hours, so it sometimes must be repeated while other measures are taken to suppress potassium levels more permanently. The insulin is usually given with an appropriate amount of glucose to prevent hypoglycemia following the insulin administration.

20. A seven-years-old boy presents with acute onset of mild intermittent pain in the right groin and a limp. Abduction and internal rotation of the hip were restricted on the affected side. There was no fever. Radiographs of the pelvis were normal. The most likely diagnosis is:

a. Transient monoarticular synovitis
b. Legg–Calve–Perthes disease
c. Slipped capital femoral epiphyses
d. Osteochondritis dissecans

Transient synovitis causes pain in the hip, thigh, groin or knee on the affected side. There may be a limp (or abnormal crawling in infants) with or without pain. On clinical examination, the child typically holds the hip slightly bent, turned outwards and away from the middle line (flexion, external rotation and abduction). Active and passive movements may be limited because of pain, especially abduction and internal rotation. The hip can be tender to palpation.

21. A child is brought with history of ingestion of an unknown substance. On examination child has excess salivation, lacrimation, miosis, gastrointestinal cramps and emesis. What was the most likely substance ingested?

a. Carbamates
b. Phenothiazines
c. Opioids
d. Tricyclic antidepressants

Carbamate insecticides target human melatonin receptors, along with inhibiting acetylcholinesterase.

22. A term newborn presents with respiratory failure which is refractory to mechanical ventilation, surfactant replacement therapy, glucocorticoid administration and extra corporeal membrane oxygenation. The most likely diagnosis is:

a. Surfactant protein B deficiency
b. Primary ciliary dyskinesia
c. Persistent tachypnea of infancy
d. Lymphocytic interstitial pneumonitis

Surfactant protein B is an essential lipid-associated protein found in pulmonary surfactant. Without it, the lung would not be able to inflate after a deep breath out. It rearranges lipid molecules in the fluid lining the lung so that tiny air sacs in the lung, called alveoli, can more easily inflate.

23. A child after snake bite develops petechiae and ecchymosis on the skin. In addition, child develops bleeding from venipuncture site and oliguria. The most likely snake species is:

a. Pit viper
b. Cobra
c. Mamba
d. Python

Hemotoxic snake includes viperids, Vipers and Russell's vipers. Clinical presentation include local swelling and pain, ecchymosis, hemorrhagic bullae, renal dysfunction etc.

24. A six-years-old boy presents with short neck, low hairline and restriction of neck movements. The child also has Sprengel anomaly, scoliosis, and fused cervical vertebrae. The most likely diagnosis is:

a. Atlantoaxial instability
b. Klippel–Feil syndrome
c. Noonan syndrome
d. Sandifer syndrome

Answers

18. a	19. c	20. a	21. a	22. a	23. a	24. b

The most common sign of Klipper–Feil syndrome is restricted mobility of the neck and upper spine. A short neck and low hairline at the back of the head may occur in some patients. Associated abnormalities may include scoliosis (side-to-side curvature of the spine), which is abnormal curving of the spine. The spine sometimes appears as a "C" or an "S". Approximately 35% of patients with Klippel–Feil syndrome will also have a congenital elevation of the scapula known as Sprengel's deformity.

25. A 10-years-old boy presents with recurrent bouts of nasal congestion, itching, sneezing, clear rhinorrhoea and conjunctival irritation. On examination he has conjunctival hyperaemia, allergic gape and a transverse nasal crease. Which of the following drugs is preferred for management of this child?

a. Diphenhydramine
b. Fluticasone
c. Cetirizine
d. Ipratropium bromide

Allergic rhinitis is characterized by nasal congestion, frequent sneezing, nasal obstruction and clear or mucoid rhinorrhoea. It is managed by topical nasal steroid spray for prevention and oral antihistamines for symptomatic relief.

26. A two-years-old child presents with partial albinism and susceptibility to infection. Peripheral smear examination reveals giant peroxidase positive lysosomal granules in granulocytes. Which of the following is most likely diagnosis?

a. Angelman syndrome
b. Hermansky–Pudlak syndrome
c. Waardenburg syndrome
d. Chediak–Higashi syndrome

Chédiak–Higashi syndrome is a rare autosomal recessive disorder that arises from a mutation of a lysosomal trafficking regulator protein, which leads to a decrease in phagocytosis. The decrease in phagocytosis results in recurrent pyogenic infections, albinism and peripheral neuropathy.

27. A one-year-old child on exclusive milk feeds presents with constipation. On examination there is no fecal impaction. What is the next step in management?

a. Oral lactulose
b. Increasing intake of vegetables and cereals
c. Colonic enemas using polyethylene glycol
d. Milk of magnesia

This is a case of functional constipation. Measures that may help include drinking enough fluids, eating more fibers.

28. A 10-years old girl is brought to the emergency following a road traffic accident. The child is comatose with GCS score of 4. She is hypertensive, has bradycardia and extensor posturing. CT imaging reveals comminuted skull fractures and intraparenchymal hemorrhage. The initial management should include all of the following measures *except*:

a. Head of bed elevation
b. Mechanical ventilation
c. Intravenous dexamethasone
d. Hypertonic saline administration

In a patient with intra-parenchymal hemorrhage, the head should be elevated to 30°C, 1.0–1.5 g/kg of 20% mannitol should be given by a rapid infusion, and the patient should be hyperventilated to a pCO_2 of 30–35 mmHg. These measures are designed to lower ICP as quickly as possible prior to a definitive neurosurgical procedure (craniotomy, ventriculostomy, or placement of an ICP monitor) can be done. Corticosteroids are not recommended in the management of IPH because they have been proven to offer no benefit in randomized trials.

29. A 3-years old boy is brought with complaints of staying aloof. He also has delayed speech. Rest of the developmental milestones were attained normally. The most likely diagnosis is:

a. Selective mutism
b. Attention deficit hyperactivity disorder
c. Autism
d. Phonological disorder

Autism is a developmental disorder characterized by troubles with social interaction and communication, and by restricted and repetitive behavior. Parents usually notice signs during the first two or three years of their child's life.

30. A 6-years-old boy comes to the immunization clinic having received all vaccines as per schedule till 18 months of age. Which vaccine should be administered now?

a. DTPw booster
b. TdaP booster
c. DT booster
d. TT booster

The primary series of three doses of DTP (DTwP or DTaP) should be given in infancy, with a booster dose of a tetanus toxoid containing vaccine ideally at age 4–7 years (DTPw) and another booster in adolescence, e.g., at age 12–15 years (TdaP).

Answers

25. b **26.** d **27.** b **28.** c **29.** c **30.** a

All Subject MCQs

MCQs with Answers

1. Protein content of cow milk differs from human milk:

a. 2 times b. 3 times
c. 4 times d. 5 times

Ans. b. 3 times

2. Time of administration of antibiotics in a patient planned for surgery:

a. 30 minutes before surgical procedure
b. In the morning of day of surgery
c. A night before the day of surgery
d. 30 minutes after surgical procedure

Ans. a. 30 minutes before surgical procedure

3. Which of the following is a long-acting insulin, but does NOT attain peak concentration in plasma?

a. Apidra b. Humulin R
c. Novolin R d. Glargine

Ans. d. Glargine

4. Which of the following type of hepatitis, most commonly results in chronicity?

a. Hepatitis A b. Hepatitis B
c. Hepatitis C d. Hepatitis D

Ans. c. Hepatitis C

5. Which of the following is a first line of defence against viruses and tumour?

a. Granzymes b. Apoptotic bodies
c. Immunoglobulins d. NK cells

Ans. d. NK cells

6. Which of the following types of emphysema is most commonly associated with smoking?

a. Centriacinar b. Panacinar
c. Mixed d. Irregular

Ans. a. Centriacinar

7. Evisceration means removal of:

a. Scleral shell b. Extraocular muscles of eye
c. Content of eye d. Whole eye

Ans. c. Content of eye

8. All of the following causes nephrotic syndrome *except*:

a. Minimal change disease
b. Focal segmental glomerulosclerosis
c. Membranous glomerulonephritis
d. Post-streptococcal glomerulonephritis

Ans. d. Post-streptococcal glomerulonephritis

9. Paralysis of which of the following results in winging of scapula?

a. Serratus anterior muscle b. Latissimus dorsi muscle
c. Pectoralis major muscle d. Pectoralis minor muscle

Ans. a. Serratus anterior muscle

10. Barrett's esophagus can lead to:

a. Squamous cell carcinoma
b. Transitional cell carcinoma
c. Adenocarcinoma
d. Clear cell carcinoma

Ans. c. Adenocarcinoma

11. Which of the following condition occurs because of loss of migration of neural crest cells?

a. Pyloric stenosis b. Intussusception
c. Achalasia cardia d. Hirschsprung's disease

Ans. d. Hirschsprung's disease

12. Acute graft rejection occurs within:

a. 1 day b. 1 week
c. 1 month d. 1 year

Ans. c. 1 month

13. A young female presented to the Psychiatry OPD with elevated mood, hyperactivity, spending excessive money and reduced sleep. Most appropriate drug to be used for long-term treatment of such a patient:

a. Barbiturates b. Carbamazepine
c. Phenytoin d. Lithium

Ans. d. Lithium

14. Which of the following gland is supplied by glossopharyngeal nerve?

a. Sublingual gland b. Submandibular gland
c. Parotid gland d. Thyroid gland

Ans. c. Parotid gland

15. Which of the following in NOT true for anemia of chronic diseases?

a. High ferritin
b. Low reticulocyte count
c. Low to normal iron levels
d. Raised TIBC

Ans. d. Raised TIBC

16. Diluent used to reconstitute BCG vaccine is:

a. Distilled water b. Normal saline
c. Dextrose 5% d. Ringer lactate

Ans. d. Ringer lactate

17. Which of the following increases in a case of chronic disease?

a. IgM b. IgG
c. IgA d. IgE

Ans. b. IgG

18. Glycogen storage disease presenting with exercise intolerance and muscle cramps:

a. Von Gierke's disease b. Her's disease
c. McArdle's disease d. Pompe's disease

Ans. c. McArdle's disease

19. A 52-years-old male presented with a painful, red eye and seeing coloured halos. Pupil is mid-dilated, vertically oval and nonreacting to light. Most likely diagnosis:

a. Acute congestive glaucoma
b. Open angle glaucoma
c. Mucopurulent conjunctivitis
d. Cataract

Ans. a. Acute congestive glaucoma

20. A young female patient had a clinical history of tuberculosis. She had now developed pleural effusion. Pleural tapping was done. Which of the following parameter is NOT routinely analysed in pleural fluid to confirm tubercular nature of pleural effusion?

a. Pleural fluid smear b. Gamma interferon
c. Adenosine deaminase d. Polymerase chain reaction

Ans. a. Pleural fluid smear

21. Which of the following enzyme is deficient in Maple syrup urine disease?

a. Alpha ketoacid decarboxylase
b. Sphingomyelinase
c. Glucose-6-phosphatase
d. Branched chain amino acid transaminase

Ans. d. Branched chain amino acid transaminase

22. Which of the following is the most common cause of blindness in India?

a. Refractive errors b. Cataract
c. Glaucoma d Anterior uveitis

Ans. b. Cataract

23. KOH mount is helpful in diagnosing infections caused by:

a. Candida albicans
b. Treponema pallidum
c. Mycobacterium tuberculosis
d. Mycobacterium leprae

Ans. a. Candida albicans

24. Example of uncoupler of oxidative phosphorylation:

a. 2, 4-Dinitrophenol
b. Antimycin-A
c. Carbon monoxide
d. Hydrogen sulphide

Ans. a. 2, 4-Dinitrophenol

25. Abductor of vocal cord:

a. Transverse arytenoid muscle
b. Posterior crico-arytenoid muscle
c. Cricothyroid muscle
d. Oblique arytenoid muscle

Ans. b. Posterior crico-arytenoid muscle

26. Titres of which of the following antibodies are increased in Rheumatic fever?

a. Anti-streptolysin O b. Anti-centromere
c. Anti-mitochondrial d. Anti-endomysial

Ans. a. Anti-streptolysin O

27. What is the ratio of WHR (waist-hip ratio) of female to male?

a. 1:2 b. 2:1
c. 0.85:0.9 d. 0.9:0.85

Ans. c. 0.85:0.9

28. Amongst the following, which is the best indicator of community health status?

a. Maternal mortality rate
b. Infant mortality rate
c. Proportional mortality rate
d. Kuppuswamy's index

Ans. b. Infant mortality rate

29. An example of blood stain test:

a. Hemin crystal
b. Acid phosphatase reaction
c. Florence test
d. Barberio's test

Ans. a. Hemin crystal

30. Which of the following is characterised by subperiosteal hemorrhages in the long bones?

a. Hemophilia b. Scurvy
c. Rickets d. Hypothyroidism

Ans. b. Scurvy

31. Which of the following glucose transporters, transport glucose in intestine?

a. SGLT1 b. SGLT2
c. SGLT3 d. SGLT4

Ans. a. SGLT1

32. Which of the following is considered as a marker for pheochromocytoma?

a. PSA b. CEA
c. CA-125 d. Vanillyl-Mandelic acid

Ans. d. Vanillyl-mandelic acid

33. Which type of malignancy may develop in a long-standing case of Barrett's esophagus?

a. Squamous cell carcinoma
b. Adenocarcinoma
c. Transitional cell carcinoma
d. Papillary carcinoma

Ans. b. Adenocarcinoma

34. **Pappenheimer bodies are composed of:**
 a. Iron b. Copper
 c. Zinc d. Arsenic

Ans. a. Iron

35. **Couvelaire uterus is associated with:**
 a. Post-dated pregnancy b. Placenta accreta
 c. Placenta previa d. Abruptio placentae

Ans. d. Abruptio placentae

36. **Site of lumbar puncture in an adult:**
 a. C6-C7 vertebral level b. T11-T12 vertebral level
 c. L1-L2 vertebral level d. L3-L4 vertebral level

Ans. d. L3-L4 vertebral level

37. **Deficiency of which of the vitamin result in night blindness?**
 a. Vitamin A b. Vitamin B
 c. Vitamin C d. Vitamin D

Ans. a. Vitamin A

38. **Which of the following is also known as surgery for 'Bag of worms'?**
 a. Herniotomy b. Varicocelectomy
 c. Non-scalpel vasectomy d. Varicose vein stripping

Ans. b. Varicocelectomy

39. **Dinner fork deformity is associated with:**
 a. Fracture scaphoid
 b. Colle's fracture
 c. Smith's fracture
 d. Barton's fracture

Ans. b. Colle's fracture

40. **When a fracture is taking more time for union, it is known as:**
 a. Non-union b. Malunion
 c. Delayed union d. Exuberant union

Ans. c. Delayed union

41. **Inhibitor of type IV complex of electron transport chain:**
 a. Cyanide b. Carbon dioxide
 c. Oligomycin d. Antimycin

Ans. a. Cyanide

42. **Type of GLUT transporter present in skeletal muscle:**
 a. GLUT1 b. GLUT2
 c. GLUT3 d. GLUT4

Ans. d. GLUT4

43. **Which of the following is present in synovial fluid?**
 a. Dermatan sulphate b. Keratan sulphate
 c. Hyaluronic acid d. Chondroitin sulphate

Ans. c. Hyaluronic acid

44. **Source of melanin:**
 a. Tryptophan b. Tyrosine
 c. Threonine d. Thiamine

Ans. b. Tyrosine

45. **Bases present in human DNA:**
 a. Adenine, guanine, cytosine and thymine
 b. Adenine, guanine, cytosine and thiamine
 c. Adenosine, guanine, cytosine and thymine
 d. Adenosine, guanine, cytosine and thiamine

Ans. a. Adenine, guanine, cytosine and thymine

46. **Keshan's disease is due to deficiency of:**
 a. Copper b. Mercury
 c. Magnesium d. Selenium

Ans. d. Selenium

47. **Validity of Yellow fever vaccine:**
 a. 10 weeks b. 10 months
 c. 10 years d. Lifelong

Ans. d. Lifelong

48. **In an endemic area, vaccination was planned for a particular disease to immunize the people against that disease. Which level of prevention is this?**
 a. Primordial level b. Primary level
 c. Secondary level d. Tertiary level

Ans. b. Primary level

49. **In a case of natural disaster, patients are categorized on the basis of their chances of survival. This is known as:**
 a. Tagging b. Triad
 c. Triage d. Treatment

Ans. c. Triage

50. **Which of the following condition has been added recently in VISION-2020 in India?**
 a. Cataract b. Refractive errors
 c. Childhood blindness d. Glaucoma

Ans. d. Glaucoma

51. **Condition caused by Leishmania donovani:**
 a. Dengue
 b. Visceral leishmaniasis
 c. Cutaneous leishmaniasis
 d. Kala-azar

Ans. d. Kala-azar

52. **A condition is very fatal and there is 100% mortality. Relationship between incidence (I) and prevalence (P) would be:**
 a. Prevalence < incidence
 b. Prevalence = incidence
 c. Prevalence > incidence
 d. No relationship between P and I

Ans. a. Prevalence < incidence

53. **SARS is caused by a novel variant of:**
 a. Coxsackie virus
 b. Coronavirus
 c. Respiratory synctial virus
 d. Poxvirus

Ans. b. Coronavirus

54. N95 masks provide barrier protection against:
a. Respiratory droplets b. All micro-organism
c. Air pollutants d. Aerosols

Ans. a. Respiratory droplets

55. All of the following are measure of dispersion *except*:
a. Range
b. Coefficient of dispersion
c. Standard deviation
d. Mean

Ans. d. Mean

56. Anthracosis is caused by inhalation of:
a. Cotton dust b. Coal dust
c. Sugar cane dust d. Asbestos

Ans. b. Coal dust

57. Which of the following enzyme need zinc as a cofactor?
a. Phosphofructokinase b. Carboxylase
c. Lysyl oxidase d. Carbonic anhydrase

Ans. d. Carbonic anhydrase

58. Ammonia formed in the brain is finally converted into:
a. Glycine b. Glutamic acid
c. Glutamine d. Glycogen

Ans. c. Glutamine

59. Which of the following enzyme is inhibited by Allopurinol?
a. Phosphofructokinase
b. Xanthine oxidase
c. Aldehyde dehydrogenase
d. HMG CoA reductase

Ans. b. Xanthine oxidase

60. How much energy is obtained from 1 gram of protein?
a. 1 Cal b. 4 Cal
c. 1 KCal d. 4 Kcal

Ans. d. 4 Kcal

61. A patient had anemia. Laboratory values were MCV of <80 and MCH of <23. Most likely type of anemia:
a. Macrocytic anemia
b. Microcytic, hypochromic anemia
c. Normocytic anemia
d. Megaloblastic anemia

Ans. b. Microcytic, hypochromic anemia

62. Ion, playing a major role in cell injury:
a. Sodium b. Potassium
c. Calcium d. Chloride

Ans. c. Calcium

63. Vitamin B_{12} deficiency is characterised by:
a. Macrocytic, hyperchromic anemia
b. Microcytic, hypochromic anemia
c. Normocytic, normochromic anemia
d. Microcytoic, hyperchromic anemia

Ans. a. Macrocytic, hyperchromic anemia

64. Which one of the following is a property of fertilized egg?
a. Multipotent b. Unipotent
c. Oligopotent d. Totipotent

Ans. d. Totipotent

65. A short statured girl, with primary amenorrhoea had webbing of neck and widely spaced nipple. Most likely karyotype:
a. 47XXY b. 45XO
c. 47XXX d. 46XX

Ans. b. 45XO

66. Type of necrosis seen in brain infarction:
a. Coagulative necrosis b. Fat necrosis
c. Liquefactive necrosis d. Caseous necrosis

Ans. c. Liquefactive necrosis

67. In pregnancy, which of the following is always pathological?
a. Diastolic murmur b. Systolic murmur
c. Loud first heart sound d. Loud second heart sound

Ans. a. Diastolic murmur

68. Koplik spot is a pathognomonic feature of:
a. Measles b. Rubella
c. Herpes zoster d. Herpes simplex

Ans. a. Measles

69. Full form of 'NITI' in NITI aayog:
a. National Institute of Tracking India
b. National Institute of Telecommunication in India
c. National Institute of Technology in India
d. National Institute for Transforming India

Ans. d. National Institute for Transforming India

70. A camp was organized for people above 40 years of age. Their BP and blood sugar levels were checked to rule out hypertension and diabetes mellitus. Which level of prevention is this?
a. Primordial level b. Primary level
c. Secondary level d. Tertiary level

Ans. c. Secondary level

71. Inability of a person to count fingers from a distance of 6 metres/20 feet should be classified as:
a. Social blindness b. Economic blindness
c. Manifest blindness d. Complete blindness

Ans. b. Economic blindness

72. As per Biomedical Waste Management Rule, plastic tubings, urobags and catheters should be disposed off in which colour bags?
a. Blue b. Red
c. White d. Yellow

Ans. b. Red

73. UNICEF focusses mainly on:
a. Monetary affairs b. Agriculture
c. Epidemic control d. Child health

Ans. d. Child health

74. **SSPE (subacute sclerosing panencephalitis) is a dangerous, though luckily rare, complication of:**
   a. Rubella b. Measles
   c. Mumps d. Tuberculosis

Ans. b. Measles

75. **Which of the following is used as a spermicidal gel for contraception?**
   a. Clomiphene b. Misoprostol
   c. Nonoxynol-9 d. Levonorgestrel

Ans. c. Nonoxynol-9

76. **Kyoto Protocol aims at:**
   a. Reducing greenhouse gas emission
   b. Water sanitization
   c. Reducing water pollution
   d. Reducing population of world

Ans. a. Reducing greenhouse gas emission

77. **Which of the following international body designed Sustainable Development Goals?**
   a. FAO b. UNICEF
   c. United Nations d. WHO

Ans. c. United Nations

78. **A person is planning to travel to malaria endemic area. He should be started on chemoprophylaxis with:**
   a. Quinine b. Primaquine
   c. Chloroquine d. Artesunate

Ans. c. Chloroquine

79. **Ticks or bugs are present on the surface of the host or are attached to the clothing of the host. This is defined as:**
   a. Infection b. Infestation
   c. Inflammation d. Contagion

Ans. b. Infestation

80. **Which of the following defines target couple?**
   a. Unmarried couple
   b. Couple with no children even after 15 years of marriage
   c. Married couple that is eligible for practising family planning
   d. Married couple in which the female is more than 45 years of age

Ans. c. Married couple that is eligible for practising family planning

81. **Exclusive breastfeeding should be continued till:**
   a. 3 months b. 6 months
   c. 9 months d. 12 months

Ans. b. 6 months

82. **Which is true for Kuppuswamy's scale?**
   a. Education, housing and income
   b. Education, occupation and housing
   c. Education, housing and occupation
   d. Education, occupation and income

Ans. d. Education, occupation and income

83. **Transfer of DNA from one bacterium to another through bacteriophage:**
   a. Transcription b. Transformation
   c. Transduction d. Translation

Ans. c. Transduction

84. **Which of the following is associated with carcinoma of urinary bladder?**
   a. Clonorchis sinensis
   b. Fasciola hepatica
   c. Echinococcus granulosus
   d. Schistosoma

Ans. d. Schistosoma

85. **A child developed high-grade fever and sore throat. Oral cavity examination shows a membrane. Which of the following media is used to make a final diagnosis?**
   a. LJ media b. Thayer martin
   c. Loeffler's serum slope d. Bordet Gengou media

Ans. c. Loeffler's serum slope

86. **Parasite which resides in lymphatics:**
   a. Tinea saginata b. Ancylostoma duodenale
   c. Ascaris lumbricoides d. Wuchereria bancrofti

Ans. d. Wuchereria bancrofti

87. **Which of the following is the most sensitive test for microfilariae?**
   a. Thick films
   b. Membrane filter concentration technique
   c. ELISA
   d. Immunofluorescence test

Ans. b. Membrane filter concentration technique

88. **Causative agent for malignant otitis externa:**
   a. Pseudomonas
   b. Streptococcus pneumoniae
   c. Staphylococcus aureus
   d. Hemophilus influenzae

Ans. a. Pseudomonas

89. **Which of the following is the smallest cestode?**
   a. Taenia saginata b. Taenia solium
   c. Hymenolepis nana d. Schistosoma japonicum

Ans. c. Hymenolepis nana

90. **Which of the following Ig is raised in recent infection?**
   a. IgM b. IgG
   c. IgA d. IgE

Ans. a. IgM

91. **Oral examination of a patient with HIV shows oral thrush, which bleeds on scrapping. Causative organism for this condition:**
   a. Candida
   b. Cryptococcus
   c. Corynebacterium diphtheriae
   d. Mycobacterium tuberculosis

Ans. a. Candida

92. Which of the following is NOT a causative agent of Bacterial vaginosis?
a. Mobiluncus b. Gardnerella
c. Pseudomonas d. Coccobacillus

Ans. c. Pseudomonas

93. Chances of Kala-azar occurrence are LESS at an altitude of:
a. 700 meters b. 500 meters
c. 300 meters d. 100 meters

Ans. a. 700 meters

94. Bacterium which can tolerate a temperature of more than 100 degrees C is defined as:
a. Halophilic b. Halophobic
c. Thermophobic d. Thermophilic

Ans. d. Thermophilic

95. Nerve supply of teres minor:
a. Radial nerve b. Axillary nerve
c. Ulnar nerve d. Median nerve

Ans. b. Axillary nerve

96. Which of the following bacterium is associated with duodenal ulcer?
a. E. coli
b. Hemophilus ducreyi
c. Hemophilus influenzae
d. Helicobacter pylori

Ans. d. Helicobacter pylori

97. p24 antigen is useful in diagnosis of:
a. HIV b. Influenza virus
c. Hepatitis B virus d. Rabies virus

Ans. a. HIV

98. Which of the following is cardioprotective?
a. Chylomicron b. VLDL
c. LDL d. HDL

Ans. d. HDL

99. Which of the following inhibits gluconeogenesis?
a. Glucagon b. Cortisol
c. Growth hormone d. Insulin

Ans. d. Insulin

100. A protein specimen was heated at a temperature of 100 degrees C. Which of the following protein structure would NOT be denatured?
a. Primary structure b. Secondary structure
c. Tertiary structure d. Quaternary structure

Ans. a. Primary structure

101. Safety muscle of tongue is:
a. Palatoglossus b. Styloglossus
c. Genioglossus d. Hyoglossus

Ans. c. Genioglossus

102. Sartorius muscle originates from:
a. Iliac crest
b. Anterior superior iliac spine
c. Obturator foramen
d. Pubis symphysis

Ans. b. Anterior superior iliac spine

103. Origin of celiac artery from abdominal aorta occurs at the level of:
a. Thoracic 9 vertebra b. Thoracic 10 vertebra
c. Thoracic 12 vertebra d. Lumbar 2 vertebra

Ans. c. Thoracic 12 vertebra

104. Trigone of bladder develops from:
a. Urogenital sinus
b. Distal part of mesonephric duct
c. Paramesonephric duct
d. Mullerian duct

Ans. d. Mullerian duct

105. While eliciting patellar tendon reflex, which of the following tendon is stretched?
a. Quadriceps femoris b. Biceps femoris
c. Quadratus femoris d. Adductor longus

Ans. c. Quadratus femoris

106. Vertebral level of highest point of iliac crest lies at the level of:
a. L2 vertebrae b. L3 vertebrae
c. L4 vertebrae d. L5 vertebrae

Ans. c. L4 vertebrae

107. Nerve supply of coracobrachialis muscle:
a. Musculocutaneous nerve
b. Radial nerve
c. Median nerve
d. Ulnar nerve

Ans. c. Median nerve

108. A 50-years-old male complained of pain in left thigh and calf region. On examination, left femoral and popliteal arteries were not palpable. Opposite side was normal. Most probable site of arterial blockage:
a. Aorto-iliac level b. Iliac artery level
c. Femoral artery level d. Popliteal artery level

Ans. b. Iliac artery level

109. Parasympathetic system supplies lacrimal gland through which ganglion?
a. Submandibular ganglion b. Pterygopalatine ganglion
c. Otic ganglion d. Trigeminal ganglion

Ans. b. Pterygopalatine ganglion

110. All of the following structures passes through the substance of parotid gland *except*:
a. Internal carotid artery b. Facial nerve
c. Retromandibular vein d. None of the above

Ans. a. Internal carotid artery

111. One of the weaker area of skull:
a. Nasion b. Pterion
c. Glabella d. Asterion

Ans. b. Pterion

112. Protraction of the mandible is done by:
a. Posterior fibres of temporalis
b. Lateral pterygoid
c. Serratus anterior
d. Buccinator

Ans. b. Lateral pterygoid

113. Middle meningeal artery arises from:
a. Facial artery b. Mandibular artery
c. Ophthalmic artery d. Maxillary artery

Ans. d. Maxillary artery

114. Which of the following muscle is mainly responsible for opening of eustachian tube?
a. Tensor tympani b. Tensor veli palatini
c. Salpingopharyngeus d. Stapedius

Ans. b. Tensor veli palatini

115. Which artery is palpated behind medial malleolus?
a. Dorsalis pedis artery b. Posterior tibial artery
c. Medial plantar artery d. Lateral plantar artery

Ans. b. Posterior tibial artery

116. Which of the following is the most common tumour of mediastinum?
a. Neurogenic tumour b. Thymoma
c. Lymphoma d. Heart tumours

Ans. a. Neurogenic tumour

117. Which of the following is an embryonic neural tumour:
a. Ependymoma b. Medulloblastoma
c. Neuroglioma d. Fibrous astrocytoma

Ans. b. Medulloblastoma

118. All of the following are components of SIRS (Systemic Inflammatory Response System) *except*:
a. Temperature more than 38 degree C
b. Temperature less than 36 degree C
c. Leucocytosis <12,000/microlitre
d. Heart rate >90 betas/minute

Ans. c. Leucocytosis <12,000/microlitre

119. An autosomal recessive condition:
a. Achondroplasia b. Hereditary spherocytosis
c. Hemophilia d. Sickle cell anemia

Ans. d. Sickle cell anemia

120. An autosomal dominant condition:
a. Sickle cell anemia b. Wilson disease
c. von Willebrand disease d. Hemophilia

Ans. c. von Willebrand disease

121. Use of keratometer:
a. Assessing diameter of cornea
b. Assessing curvature of cornea
c. Assessing the thickness of cornea
d. Assessing the corneal cell count

Ans. b. Assessing curvature of cornea

122. Internal hordeolum is defined as:
a. Inflammation of Meibomian gland
b. Inflammation of Zeis gland
c. Inflammation of lacrimal gland
d. Inflammation of nasolacrimal duct

Ans. a. Inflammation of Meibomian gland

123. Dendritic ulcers are seen in:
a. Vernal keratoconjunctivitis
b. Mycotic keratitis
c. Herpes simplex keratitis
d. Bacterial keratitis

Ans. c. Herpes simplex keratitis

124. In which of the following condition, Fleischer's ring are seen?
a. Wilson disease b. Keratoconus
c. Keratomalacia d. Trachoma

Ans. b. Keratoconus

125. True regarding phlyctenular conjunctivitis:
a. Post-fungal b. Post-protozoal
c. Post-tubercular d. Post-viral

Ans. c. Post-tubercular

126. Chronic, granulomatous inflammation in upper lid presenting as a painless swelling is:
a. Chalazion b. Internal hordeolum
c. Stye d. Trachoma

Ans. a. Chalazion

127. Formation of image in myopia occurs:
a. In front of lens
b. On retina
c. In front of retina
d. Behind retina

Ans. c. In front of retina

128. A 20-years-old male is complaining of defective vision and irregular astigmatism, which does not improve fully despite full correction with glasses, might be suffering from:
a. Cataract b. Wilson disease
c. Keratoconus d. Keratomalacia

Ans. c. Keratoconus

129. Fleischer's ring is found in:
a. Iridodialysis b. Keratoconus
c. Corneal dystrophy d. Herpetic keratitis

Ans. b. Keratoconus

130. Visual loss may occur because of involvement of:
a. Anterior cerebral artery b. Middle cerebral artery
c. Posterior cerebral artery d. Internal carotid artery

Ans. c. Posterior cerebral artery

131. Which of the following is the appropriate management for mild congenital ptosis?
a. Levator lengthening
b. Antibiotics and hot compression
c. Levator palpebrae superioris resection
d. Wedge resection of palpebral conjunctiva

Ans. c. Levator palpebrae superioris resection

132. A male patient presented with convergent squint in right eye. The vision in right eye is 6/60. There is no squint in left eye and the vision in left eye is 6/60. Next step in managing such a case:
a. Spectacles
b. Injection of botulinum toxin
c. MRI
d. Squint surgery

Ans. d. Squint surgery

133. In India, which of the following disease has been added recently in Vision-2020?
a. Glaucoma
b. Cataract
c. Errors of refraction
d. Childhood blindness

Ans. a. Glaucoma

134. A known case of diabetes mellitus presented with sudden loss of vision. Fundus picture is shown below. Most likely diagnosis:
a. Hypertensive retinopathy
b. Vitreous detachment
c. Central retinal arterial occlusion
d. Central retinal venous occlusion

Ans. d. Central retinal venous occlusion

135. In the management of aphakia, advantage of contact lens over normal glasses is that:
a. Cheap
b. No corneal complications
c. Ease of use in childhood
d. Prismatic effect would be less

Ans. d. Prismatic effect would be less

136. Drug which can cause postural hypotension:
a. Alpha blockers
b. Beta blockers
c. ACE inhibitors
d. Angiotensin receptor blockers

Ans. a. Alpha blockers

137. Which of the following is the mechanism of action of allopurinol?
a. Inhibition of HMG CoA reductase
b. Inhibition of HMG CoA synthase
c. Inhibition of xanthine oxidase
d. Inhibition of tyrosinase

Ans. c Inhibition of xanthine oxidase

138. Which of the following drug follows zero order kinetics?
a. Penicillin b. Phenytoin
c. Penicillamine d. Propranolol

Ans. b. Phenytoin

139. An example of oral direct thrombin inhibitor:
a. Aspirin b. Heparin
c. Protamine sulphate d. Dabigatran etexilate

Ans. d. Dabigatran etexilate

140. Which of the following drug requires therapeutic drug monitoring?
a. Penicillin b. Ciprofloxacin
c. Phenytoin d. Isoniazid

Ans. c. Phenytoin

141. A pregnant lady was found to be hepatitis B positive at 37 weeks of gestation. What is the ideal management to prevent transmission of HBV infection to neonate?
a. Hepatitis B immunoglobulin to mother
b. HBV vaccination of mother
c. Hepatitis B immunoglobulin to baby at birth
d. Hepatitis B vaccination + Hepatitis B immunoglobulin to baby at birth

Ans. a. Hepatitis B immunoglobulin to mother

142. A 25-years-old short statured pregnant lady was subjected to normal vaginal delivery. In puerperal period, she complained of passing urine per vaginum. What is the most likely diagnosis?
a. Urinary bladder rupture b. Stress incontinence
c. Vesicovaginal fistula d. Urge incontinence

Ans. c. Vesicovaginal fistula

143. A 32-years-old hypertensive lady, with 36 weeks pregnancy presented with convulsions. A provisional diagnosis of eclampsia was made. Management of such a case:
a. Methyldopa b. Labetalol
c. Magnesium sulphate
d. Magnesium sulphate + Labetalol

Ans. d. Magnesium sulphate + Labetalol

144. A 35-years-old lady, who had 4 living children, underwent normal vaginal delivery for her 5th pregnancy. After delivery of the placenta, she had excessive bleeding. Most likely cause:
a. Cephalopelvic disproportion
b. Postpartum hemorrhage
c. Retained placental bits
d. Pelvic injury

Ans. b. Postpartum hemorrhage

145. What is the most appropriate management of a 32-years-old lady with dichorionic diamniotic twin pregnancy, in which one baby is in cephalic presentation and other in breech presentation?
a. Normal vaginal delivery b. Vacuum extraction
c. Forceps application d. Cesarean section

Ans. d. Cesarean section

146. A 36-weeks-old pregnant lady presented to the casualty with hypotension and tachycardia. She had a history of Cesarean section. USG was done and it showed fluid in pouch of Douglas. Most likely diagnosis and appropriate management:

a. Rupture of ectopic pregnancy; Laparotomy
b. Rupture of ectopic pregnancy; Laparoscopic repair
c. Rupture of uterine scar; Laparotomy
d. Rupture of uterine scar; Laparoscopic repair

Ans. c. Rupture of uterine scar; Laparotomy

147. Most likely diagnosis of a 30-years-old pregnant lady presenting with mild bleeding, pain, tender uterus with absent fetal heart sounds:

a. Placenta previa b. Abruptio placentae
c. Intrauterine fetal death d. Ectopic pregnancy

Ans. b. Abruptio placentae

148. Likely diagnosis of a lady with 12 weeks pregnancy presenting with bleeding per vaginum and examination showed normal vagina, closed internal os, fundal height of 13 weeks and a live fetus on ultrasonographic examination:

a. Missed abortion b. Complete abortion
c. Incomplete abortion d. Threatened abortion

Ans. d. Threatened abortion

149. Most likely diagnosis and appropriate management of a lady with 36-weeks gestation, G2P1 presenting with hematuria and absent fetal heart rate on examination:

a. Obstructed labor; Normal vaginal delivery
b. Obstructed labor; Cesarean section
c. Placenta previa; Cesarean section
d. Abruptio placenta; Cesarean section

Ans. b. Obstructed labor; Cesarean section

150. What is the value for angle of cut in episiotomy?

a. 15 degree b. 30 degree
c. 45 degree d. 60 degree

Ans. d. 60 degree

151. What could be the most common cause of bleeding in a multigravida woman in labor having uncontrolled bleeding after delivery and removal of placenta?

a. Retained bits of placenta
b. Post-term pregnancy
c. Uterine atony
d. Perineal injuries

Ans. c. Uterine atony

152. In which of the following conditions, double decidual sac sign is related to?

a. Ectopic pregnancy
b. Hydatidiform mole
c. Uterine gestational sac
d. Threatened abortion

Ans. c. Uterine gestational sac

153. In case of tubal ectopic pregnancy, rupture occurs lately in case of:

a. Isthmic pregnancy b. Interstitial pregnancy
c. Ampullary pregnancy d. Infundibular pregnancy

Ans. b. Interstitial pregnancy

154. Which of the following defines delusion?

a. Disorder of perception b. Disorder of memory
c. Disorder of thought d. Disorder of mood

Ans. c. Disorder of thought

155. A 30-years-old male had a very severe road-traffic accident 6 weeks back, while going to office. Now he is very fearful of driving. He had flashbacks of that accident and is not going to even his office as he has to pass through that route. Most likely diagnosis:

a. Mania
b. Depression
c. Post-traumatic stress disorder
d. Delirium tremens

Ans. c. Post-traumatic stress disorder

156. A 25-years-old lady is having fear of taking elevator. She prefers to go by stairs to her flat on 7th floor. Most likely diagnosis:

a. Agoraphobia b. Claustrophobia
c. Zoophobia d. Social phobia

Ans. b. Claustrophobia

157. A 25-years-old lady, who had a normal vaginal delivery 5 weeks back, is now having fearfulness, irritability and suicidal thoughts. Most likely diagnosis:

a. Schizophrenia
b. Bipolar disorder
c. Post-partum psychosis
d. Post-partum depression

Ans. d. Post-partum depression

158. A person previously used to enjoy driving, but now he does not find any pleasure in it. This is known as:

a. Delusion of perception b. Anhedonia
c. Depression d. Autism

Ans. b. Anhedonia

159. A psychiatrist asked a patient that how is his mood. The patient replied that his mood is up and down. But ups and downs are part of life. One should live life to the fullest. This is:

a. Echolalia b. Tangential speech
c. Neologism d. Circumstantial speech

Ans. b. Tangential speech

160. Ocular condition associated with HLA-B27:

a. Glaucoma b. Cataract
c. Anterior uveitis d. Keratomalacia

Ans. c. Anterior uveitis

161. Which of the following test is specific for gout?

a. Serum uric acid levels b. Urinary uric acid levels
c. Synovial uric acid levels d. CSF uric acid levels

Ans. c. Synovial uric acid levels

162. Which of the following is the most abundant amino acid found in collagen?

a. Hydroxyproline
b. Glycine
c. Proline
d. Alanine

Ans. b. Glycine

163. Which enzyme is associated with deficiency of the vitamin thiamine?

a. Pyruvate kinase
b. RBC transketolase
c. Pyruvate dehydrogenase
d. FIGLU

Ans. b. RBC transketolase

164. Which of the following is a screening test for deficiency of vitamin A?

a. Nyctalopia
b. Bitot spots on conjunctiva
c. Retinol levels <10 mcg/dL
d. Beta carotene levels <10 mcg/dL

Ans. c. Retinol levels <10 mcg/dL

165. True for dietary fibers:

a. May result in constipation
b. Unrelated to metabolism
c. Reduces intestinal transit time
d. Causes hyperglycemia

Ans. c. Reduces intestinal transit time

166. Contraception of choice in a lady presenting after 96 hours of unprotected coitus:

a. Oral contraceptive pills
b. Mifepristone
c. Minipill
d. Intrauterine uterine contraceptive device

Ans. d. Intrauterine uterine contraceptive device

167. A lady presented to the Gynecology department with complaint of infertility. Hysterosalpingography showed bilateral cornual block. Next best step in management:

a. Tuboplasty
b. Hysterectomy
c. Salpingectomy
d. Laparoscopy

Ans. d. Laparoscopy

168. Amsel's criteria is used for diagnosing:

a. Trichomoniasis
b. Moniliasis
c. Gardnerella vaginosis
d. TB fallopian tube

Ans. c. Gardnerella vaginosis

169. A 16-years-old girl presented to the Gynecology department with bleeding per vaginum of acute onset. Immediate management of such a case:

a. Progesterone
b. Uterine artery embolization
c. Uterine artery ligation
d. Hysteroscopic examination

Ans. a. Progesterone

170. A lady presented to the gynecology clinic with the complaints of galactorrhoea and amenorrhoea. What could be the most likely diagnosis?

a. Cushing syndrome
b. Adrenal hyperplasia
c. Pituitary adenoma
d. Addison's disease

Ans. c. Pituitary adenoma

171. Management of choice in a 65-years-old, hypertensive and diabetic lady with heavy bleeding per vaginum:

a. Oral contraceptive pills
b. Hysterectomy
c. Laparoscopic evaluation
d. Uterine artery embolization

Ans. a. Oral contraceptive pills

172. Ideal contraceptive in a newly married couple when the woman is having irregular menstruation:

a. IUCD
b. Barrier contraceptive
c. Billing's method
d. Oral contraceptive pills

Ans. d. Oral contraceptive pills

173. Which of the following method of contraception should NEVER be used in deep venous thrombosis?

a. IUCD
b. Barrier contraceptive
c. Oral contraceptive pills
d. Coitus interruptus

Ans. c. Oral contraceptive pills

174. Which of the following is an absolute CONTRAINDICATION for use of Intrauterine Contraceptive Device?

a. Breast carcinoma
b. Deep venous thrombosis
c. Polycystic ovarian disease
d. Acute pelvic inflammatory disease

Ans. d. Acute pelvic inflammatory disease

175. Which of the following is the investigation of choice in evaluating a case of endometriosis?

a. Laparoscopy
b. Hysteroscopy
c. USG pelvis
d. CT scan pelvis

Ans. a. Laparoscopy

176. For emergency contraception, dose of mifepristone used is:

a. 100 mg
b. 200 mg
c. 300 mg
d. 600 mg

Ans. d. 600 mg

177. Which of the following is the most common cause of pelvic inflammatory disease?

a. Chlamydia
b. Neisseria gonorrhoeae
c. Mycobacterium tuberculosis
d. Trichomonas vaginalis

Ans. a. Chlamydia

178. **Which of the following is the best method of emergency contraception in a lady presenting after 96 hours of unprotected sex?**
  a. Minipill b. Mifepristone
  c. Oral contraceptive pills d. IUCD

Ans. b. Mifepristone

179. **Source of HCG:**
  a. Cytotrophoblast b. Syncytiotrophoblast
  c. Amnion d. Chorion

Ans. b. Syncytiotrophoblast

180. **In a 25-years-old female lady, delivery of the baby was conducted normally but the placenta remained attached to uterus. What complication is likely to occur if one tries forceful cord traction?**
  a. Post-partum hemorrhage
  b. Rupture of uterus
  c. Puerperal pyrexia
  d. Uterine inversion

Ans. d. Uterine inversion

181. **Which of the following is a surgical emergency?**
  a. Hydrocoele b. Testicular cancer
  c. Testicular torsion d. Varicocoele

Ans. c. Testicular torsion

182. **Alvarado Score 2 denotes:**
  a. Leukocytosis
  b. Migratory pain
  c. Temperature
  d. Tenderness in left iliac fossa

Ans. a. Leukocytosis

183. **Which of the following condition presents with almost odourless stools?**
  a. Cholera b. Arsenic poisoning
  c. Typhoid d. Amoebiasis

Ans. d. Amoebiasis

184. **Which of the following can result in hypoxic hypoxia?**
  a. Cyanide poisoning
  b. Arterio-venous shunt
  c. Carbon monoxide poisoning
  d. Anemia

Ans. b. Arterio-venous shunt

185. **Which of the following is a metaphyseal tumour?**
  a. Ewing sarcoma b. Giant cell tumour
  c. Osteosarcoma d. All of the above

Ans. c. Osteosarcoma

186. **A 34-years-old male had a road traffic accident, after which he became dyspneic. His BP was low and on auscultation, breath sounds were absent on one side. Most likely diagnosis:**
  a. Pleural effusion b. Pneumothorax
  c. Pulmonary embolism d. Pulmonary infarction

Ans. b. Pneumothorax

187. **Which of the following is a monoclonal antibody used in cancer chemotherapy?**
  a. Cisplatin b. Methotrexate
  c. 5-FluoroUracil d. Ritumixab

Ans. d. Ritumixab

188. **While performing autopsy, multiple cut injuries were found on scrotum. This is suggestive of:**
  a. Accident b. Suicide
  c. Homicide d. Artefacts

Ans. c. Homicide

189. **Which of the following condition is present at birth and persists throughout life?**
  a. Strawberry nevus b. Port-wine stain
  c. Allergic reaction d. Acanthosis nigricans

Ans. b. Port-wine stain

190. **Carcinoma of prostate commonly arises from which lobe?**
  a. Median lobe b. Lateral lobe
  c. Anterior lobe d. Posterior lobe

Ans. d. Posterior lobe

191. **All of the following are risk factors for development of carcinoma esophagus *except*:**
  a. Spicy food b. Barrett's esophagus
  c. Betel nut chewing d. Achalasia cardia

Ans. a. Spicy food

192. **In hyperkalemia, serum potassium value is more than:**
  a. 3.5 meq/L b. 4.5 meq/L
  c. 5.5. med/L d. 6.5 meq/L

Ans. c. 5.5. med/L

193. **What is the most common cause of respiratory obstruction in an unconscious patient?**
  a. Respiratory centre inhibition
  b. Traumatic asphyxia
  c. Injury to hyoid bone
  d. Tongue falling backward

Ans. d. Tongue falling backward

194. **Rupture of middle meningeal artery will result in:**
  a. Subdural hemorrhage
  b. Epidural hemorrhage
  c. Intracerebral hemorrhage
  d. Subarachnoid hemorrhage

Ans. b. Epidural hemorrhage

195. **A 65-years-old post-menopausal woman had a history of fall in bathroom over outstretched hand and sustained a bony fracture. Most likely fracture type is:**
  a. Colle's fracture
  b. Smith's fracture
  c. Dorsal Barton fracture
  d. Volar Barton fracture

Ans. a. Colle's fracture

196. Fracture of tibia-fibula in later stages of healing can be managed by:

a. Patellar tendon bearing brace
b. SOMI brace
c. Milwaukee brace
d. Boston brace

Ans. a. Patellar tendon bearing brace

197. A patient developed amoebiasis and was started on some drug. Later on she attended a party and took alcohol. After that she developed nausea, vomiting and dizziness. Which of the following drug is the likely agent which could have produced such an interaction with alcohol?

a. Clindamycin
b. Diloxamide
c. Azithromycin
d. Metronidazole

Ans. d. Metronidazole

198. Which of the following is the most potent opioid?

a. Morphine
b. Bupropion
c. Fentanyl
d. Naproxen

Ans. c. Fentanyl

199. Which of the following is the most cardiotoxic anticancer drugs?

a. Methotrexate
b. Anthracycline
c. 5-Fluorouracil
d. Cyclophosphamide

Ans. b. Anthracycline

200. Which of the following drug inhibits carbonic anhydrase enzyme?

a. Mannitol
b. Thiazide
c. Furosemide
d. Acetazolamide

Ans. d. Acetazolamide

201. A young lady presented to Medicine OPD with the complaints of palpitations. Her mother had died recently due to renal cancer. On examination, her pulse rate was 110/minute and respiratory rate was 12 breaths/minute. Which investigation is most relevant in such a case?

a. Serum Hydroxyindole Acetic Acid (HIAA) estimation
b. Measurement of plasma free metanephrines
c. 24 hours urinary Vanillylmandelic acid (VMA)
d. Urinary catecholamines

Ans. b. Measurement of plasma free metanephrines

202. Angiosarcoma of liver can be caused by exposure to:

a. Arsenic
b. Copper
c. Iron
d. Cadmium

Ans. a. Arsenic

203. A young patient had angina and recurrent syncopal attacks. He was referred to a physician, who provisionally diagnosed him as a case of Aortic stenosis. He was advised chest X-ray (PA and lateral view). Which of the following X-ray feature would suggest the diagnosis of aortic stenosis?

a. Straightening of the left border of heart
b. Dilatation of aortic valve
c. Post-stenotic dilatation of the aorta
d. Widening of the aortic knob

Ans. c. Post-stenotic dilatation of the aorta

204. A chronic alcoholic patient developed tremors, confusion, amnesia and gait abnormalities. All these symptoms can occur because of deficiency of:

a. Thiamine
b. Riboflavin
c. Niacin
d. Pyridoxine

Ans. a. Thiamine

205. A known case of hiatus hernia was operated and laparoscopic fundoplication was done. Intraoperatively patient develops mild pneumothorax but the vitals were stable. Next best step in the management of such a case would be:

a. Emergency needle compression
b. Thoracotomy
c. Wait and watch
d. Intercostal drainage

Ans. c. Wait and watch

206. Which of the following is a specific tumour marker for pancreatic carcinoma?

a. Alpha Fetoprotein
b. Lactate Dehydrogenase
c. CA 19-9
d. CA 125

Ans. c. CA 19-9

207. A patient is HBsAg positive, IgG anti-HBcAg positive and anti-HBs negative. This suggest:

a. Acute hepatitis B infection
b. Chronic hepatitis B infection
c. Carrier state of hepatitis B virus infection
d. Complete recovery from hepatitis B infection

Ans. b. Chronic hepatitis B infection

208. Nerve supply of flexor digitorum profundus muscle:

a. Ulnar nerve
b. Median nerve
c. Both
d. None

Ans. c. Both

209. A patient attended Surgery OPD with the complaints of swelling in thyroid region and weight loss. On examination, cervical lymphadenopathy was present. Histopathology of thyroid swelling showed the presence of cells with Orphan Annie eyed nuclei. Findings are consistent with the diagnosis of:

a. Medullary carcinoma of thyroid
b. Follicular carcinoma of thyroid
c. Papillary carcinoma of thyroid
d. Anaplastic carcinoma of thyroid

Ans. c. Papillary carcinoma of thyroid

210. A 30-years-old male has divorced his wife recently. Now he is having palpitations, headache and episodes of excessive sweating. This use to happen on recurrent basis. He visited psychiatrist multiple times but found no relief. Next best step in managing such a case:
   a. Check for catecholamine levels to exclude phaeochromocytoma
   b. He needs psychological counselling
   c. He should be investigated for hyperthyroidism
   d. Needs to switch on to some other anti-anxiety drug

Ans. a. Check for catecholamine levels to exclude phaeochromocytoma

211. PAIR technique is employed in managing:
   a. Simple liver cyst b. Amoebic liver abscess
   c. Pyogenic liver abscess d. Hepatic hydatid cyst

Ans. d. Hepatic hydatid cyst

212. KDIGO staging of a child with urine output less than 0.4 mL/kg/hour for the last 14 hours:
   a. Stage 1 b. Stage 2
   c. Stage 3 d. Stage 4

Ans. b. Stage 2

213. A lactating female presented to the Surgery OPD with complain of throbbing pain in right breast and high-grade fever. On examination, it was found that the breast was engorged and tender. What is the best line of management of such condition?
   a. Incision and drainage + Antibiotics
   b. Antibiotics only
   c. Pain killers
   d. Warm compressions

Ans. a. Incision and drainage + Antibiotics

214. Curschman's spiral is a sputum finding of:
   a. Normal person
   b. Chronic obstructive pulmonary disease
   c. Restrictive lung disease
   d. Interstitial lung disease

Ans. b. Chronic obstructive pulmonary disease

215. A known case of HIV presented to the Medicine OPD with the complaints of fever and cough of 2 weeks duration. Examining physician made a presumptive diagnosis of tuberculosis. What is the next best investigation?
   a. Sputum culture b. CB-NAAT
   c. X-ray chest d. CT scan chest

Ans. b. CB-NAAT

216. A patient had many episodes of vomiting and diarrhoea for past 48 hours. His urine frequency has also reduced. What would be the finding in such a case?
   a. Acute glomerulonephritis
   b. Urinary sodium >40
   c. Hyperosmolar urine
   d. None of the above

Ans. c. Hyperosmolar urine

217. In which of the following conditions, artificial pacemaker is required?
   a. Supraventricular tachycardia
   b. Severe atrioventricular nodal delay
   c. Atrial fibrillation
   d. After myocardial infarction

Ans. b. Severe atrioventricular nodal delay

218. Adenomyoma of gallbladder can progress to:
   a. Polyp of gallbladder
   b. Cholesterol stone in gallbladder
   c. Strawberry gallbladder
   d. Gallbladder carcinoma

Ans. d. Gallbladder carcinoma

219. A young lean female presented with complains of palpitations and weight loss. She also has intolerance to heat. On examination, sinus tachycardia was present. Most likely diagnosis:
   a. Hyperthyroidism b. Hypothyroidism
   c. Filariasis d. Cushing's syndrome

Ans. a. Hyperthyroidism

220. A patient presented with thyroid surgery. Before doing any operative procedure, what you would advise?
   a. FNAC
   b. TFT/Thyroid Function Tests
   c. USG
   d. Biopsy

Ans. b. TFT/Thyroid Function Tests

221. A patient of rheumatoid arthritis is treated with DMARD. Which of the following agent requires fundus examination and regular monitoring of visual acuity?
   a. Sulfasalazine b. Leflunomide
   c. Hydroxychloroquine d. Methotrexate

Ans. c. Hydroxychloroquine

222. For future management purposes in a hospital, a systemic observation and recording were made with regard to doctors spending time in patient care and those doctors spending time in hospital without patient care. This type of management technique is an example of:
   a. Work sampling b. Network analysis
   c. System analysis d. Surveillance

Ans. a. Work sampling

223. A 50-years-old heavy smoker developed severe chest pain. He was given sublingual nitroglycerine which relieved the pain within 10 minutes. Nitroglycerine terminated severe chest pain by:
   a. Release of nitrous oxide b. Release of nitric oxide
   c. Release of endothelins d. Release of free radicals

Ans. b. Release of nitric oxide

224. Mid-year population is counted on:
   a. 01 January b. 01 March
   c. 01 June d. 01 July

Ans. d. 01 July

225. A non-vegetarian adult male developed pain and redness over 1st metatarsophalangeal joint of right foot. There is a past history of similar episodes, which were relieved after taking analgesics. Physician ordered for serum uric acid, which was found to be more than 10 mg/dL. To manage such a case, physician would order a drug, which acts by inhibiting:

a. Dihydrofolate reductase b. HMG CoA reductase
c. Cyclo-oxygenase d. Xanthine oxidase

Ans. d. Xanthine oxidase

226. A 28-years-old lady with 3 months pregnancy developed burning sensation while micturition. Which of the following antibiotic is safer to use?

a. Doxycycline b. Cotrimoxazole
c. Amoxycillin d. Ofloxacin

Ans. c. Amoxycillin

227. A hypertensive elderly male had a cerebrovascular accident and he developed left sided hemipareisis. He was brought to Medicine department for treatment. This is which level of prevention?

a. Primordial prevention b. Primary prevention
c. Secondary prevention d. Tertiary prevention

Ans. c. Secondary prevention

228. Which of the following drug is LEAST effective in a male patient presenting with burning micturition and clinical features suggestive of urinary tract infection?

a. Moxifloxacin b. Nitrofurantoin
c. Ciprofloxacin d. Nalidixic acid

Ans. a. Moxifloxacin

229. A known case of carcinoma pancreas developed severe pain. To relieve pain, morphine was started. Patient responded nicely and pain was relieved. But after some time, relief in pain was not achieved. What could be the reason?

a. Desensitization of opioid receptors
b. Change in pharmacokinetics of morphine over a period of time
c. Upregulation of opioid receptors
d. Increase in intensity of pain

Ans. a. Desensitization of opioid receptors

230. A patient was on anticancer therapy and later on he developed fever and features suggestive of severe infection. Blood examination showed a Total Leucocyte Count of 2000/cmm. In such a case, which drug might prove effective?

a. Erythropoietin b. Cilastatin + Imipenem
c. Filgrastim d. Penicillin-G

Ans. c. Filgrastim

231. Delphi technique is related to:

a. Individual b. Group
c. Community d. Country

Ans. b. Group

232. Best agent used to disinfect blood spills on floor in hospital wards:

a. Cidex
b. Formalin
c. 1% Sodium hypochlorite
d. 90% ethyl alcohol

Ans. c. 1% Sodium hypochlorite

233. Which of the following foodstuff contains LEAST iron?

a. Apple b. Milk
c. Liver d. Spinach

Ans. b. Milk

234. All of the following are constrained by existing resources or time *except*:

a. Goal b. Mission
c. Vision d. Target

Ans. a. Goal

235. Trethowan's sign is related to:

a. Perthe's disease
b. Slipped capital femoral epiphysis
c. Developmental dysplasia of hip
d. Clubfoot

Ans. b. Slipped capital femoral epiphysis

236. A 65-years-old male presented to Surgery OPD with difficulty in urination and backache. His Prostate Specific Antigen level was found to be 100 ng/mL. Such a case is best treated with:

a. Goserelin b. Tamsulosin
c. Steroid d. Testosterone

Ans. a. Goserelin

237. An elderly male presented with festinating gait and resting tremors. Which of the following drug is NOT indicated in such a case?

a. Levo-dopa plus Carbi-dopa combination
b. Pramipexole
c. Selegiline
d. Rivastigmine

Ans. d. Rivastigmine

238. Which of the following is NOT a principle of Primary Health Care?

a. Appropriate facility
b. Community participation
c. Equitable distribution
d. Inter-sectoral coordination

Ans. a. Appropriate facility

239. Maltotriose, a oligosaccharide is made up of:

a. Glucose + Glucose + Glucose
b. Glucose + Fructose + Galactose
c. Glucose + Glucose + Fructose
d. Glucose + Glucose + Galactose

Ans. a. Glucose + Glucose + Glucose

240. Mechanism of action of furosemide:
a. Inhibition of Na-K-2Cl symporter in loop of Henle
b. Inhibition of Angiotensin Converting Enzyme
c. Antagonizing aldosterone in distal convoluted tubule
d. Inhibition of Na-Cl symporter in distal convoluted tubule

Ans. a. Inhibition of Na-K-2Cl symporter in loop of Henle

241. A known case of bronchial asthma was on theophylline. Physician started him on one more drug which leads to onset of theophylline toxicity. Most likely drug responsible for such a presentation:
a. Rifampicin
b. Sodium valproate
c. Phenobarbitone
d. Erythromycin

Ans. d. Erythromycin

242. A patient presenting with diarrhoea is found to be allergic to wheat. He was found to be positive for anti-endomysial antibodies. Most likely diagnosis:
a. Tropical sprue
b. Coeliac sprue
c. Pseudomembranous colitis
d. Ulcerative colitis

Ans. b. Coeliac sprue

243. A 15-years-old girl presented to Gynecology OPD with the complaints of heavy bleeding per vaginum since last 2 weeks. Which of the following should be checked?
a. Kidney function test
b. Liver function test
c. D-dimer ELISA
d. Coagulation profile

Ans. d. Coagulation profile

244. Caspases are involved in:
a. Apoptosis
b. Inflammation
c. Vasodilation
d. Increase in vascular permeability

Ans. a. Apoptosis

245. Which of the following enzyme is deficient in Von-Gierke's disease?
a. Glucose-6-phosphatase
b. Glucose-6-phosphate dehydrogenase
c. Muscle phosphorylase
d. Branching enzyme

Ans. a. Glucose-6-phosphatase

246. A surgeon operated on a patient and following surgery, the patient died. Now patient's relative wants to file a police case against the surgeon. Police would register the case under which of the following IPC?
a. IPC 84 b. IPC-302
c. IPC-304A d. IPC-304B

Ans. c. IPC-304A

247. Which of the following condition can lead to pulsation of the ipsilateral tonsil?
a. External carotid artery aneurysm
b. Internal carotid artery aneurysm
c. Common carotid artery aneurysm
d. Facial artery aneurysm

Ans. b. Internal carotid artery aneurysm

248. A 26-years-old lady presented with secondary amenorrhoea. There is a past history of dilatation and curettage. Blood test revealed FSH level of 7 IU/L. Findings are consistent with the diagnosis of:
a. Uterine synechiae b. Ovarian failure
c. Pituitary failure d. Pregnancy

Ans. a. Uterine synechiae

249. Anatomic/True conjugate is measured from:
a. Mid-point of sacral promontory to the upper border of pubis symphysis
b. Mid-point of sacral promontory to mid-point on posterior surface of pubis symphysis
c. Mid-point of sacral promontory to the lower border of pubis symphysis
d. Mid-point of sacral promontory to the iliac spine

Ans. a. Mid-point of sacral promontory to the upper border of pubis symphysis

250. A child presented to the Pediatric OPD with the complaint of fatigue. On per-abdominal examination, he was having hepatosplenomegaly. Blood test revealed anemia. Peripheral blood smear of this patient shows target cells. Most likely diagnosis:
a. Sickle cell anemia b. Iron deficiency anemia
c. Thalassemia d. Anemia of chronic diseases

Ans. c. Thalassemia

251. In India, Rabies free state/Union Territory is:
a. Puducherry b. Andaman and Nicobar
c. Jammu and Kashmir d. Kerala

Ans. b. Andaman and Nicobar

252. A patient postoperatively developed hallucinations and confusion. His family member said that he used to drink alcohol occasionally. Most likely diagnosis:
a. Alcoholic hallucinosis
b. Schizophrenia
c. Delirium
d. Wernicke's Korsakoff psychosis

Ans. c. Delirium

253. A patient presented to the Medical OPD with the complaints of headache and fever. On examination, neck stiffness was noticed and lumbar puncture was done. CSF analysis report showed CSF pressure: Increased; Proteins: Mildly increased; Glucose: Normal and Lymphocytes: Increased. Findings are consistent with the diagnosis of:
a. Tubercular meningitis b. Viral meningitis
c. Cryptococcal meningitis d. Acute bacterial meningitis

Ans. b. Viral meningitis

254. Condition most commonly seen in African people:

a. Hypertrophic scar b. Keloid
c. Lupus vulgaris d. Marjolin ulcer

Ans. b. Keloid

255. Which of the following fracture is managed by tension band wiring?

a. Fracture patella
b. Fracture medial femoral condyle
c. Fracture lateral femoral condyle
d. Fracture intercondylar area femur

Ans. a. Fracture patella

256. Mechanism of action of local anesthetics:

a. Opening of sodium channels
b. Blockage of sodium voltage-gated channels
c. Opening of potassium channels
d. Blockage of potassium channels

Ans. b. Blockage of sodium voltage-gated channels

257. Necklace appearance in ovaries on ultrasound is suggestive of:

a. TB of ovary
b. Polycystic ovarian disease
c. Ovarian cyst
d. Adenomyosis

Ans. b. Polycystic ovarian disease

258. A patient presented to the Medical OPD with the complaints of miosis, loss of sweating and slight ptosis. Most likely diagnosis:

a. Acute congestive glaucoma
b. Acute anterior uveitis
c. Orbital cellulitis
d. Horner's syndrome

Ans. d. Horner's syndrome

259. Most widely used local anesthetic is:

a. Lignocaine b. Bupivacaine
c. Prilocaine d. Dibucaine

Ans. a. Lignocaine

260. Rice water stools are suggestive of:

a. Cholera b. Typhoid
c. Amoebic dysentery d. Pseudomembranous colitis

Ans. a. Cholera

261. Level of termination of spinal cord in infants/neonates:

a. L1 b. L2
c. L3 d. L4

Ans. c. L3

262. Mother is Rh negative and the fetus is Rh positive. What type of hypersensitivity reaction can occur in this (second) pregnancy, if Anti-D was not administered after first pregnancy:

a. Anaphylactic reaction
b. Cytotoxic reaction
c. Immune complex reaction
d. Delayed/cell mediated reaction

Ans. b. Cytotoxic reaction

263. A child presented to the Pediatric OPD in a restless and agitated state. He had stridor at rest and marked tachypnoea. There was chest retraction as well. Such a case of pneumonia would be classified as:

a. Mild pneumonia b. Moderate pneumonia
c. Severe pneumonia d. No pneumonia

Ans. c. Severe pneumonia

264. Air under diaphragm suggest:

a. Liver abscess b. Gut perforation
c. Pyloric stenosis d. Intestinal obstruction

Ans. b. Gut perforation

265. Most commonly involved nerve in leprosy:

a. Median nerve b. Ulnar nerve
c. Radial nerve d. Axillary nerve

Ans. b. Ulnar nerve

266. Swelling over scalp which is present at birth, may extend over suture lines and disappears spontaneously within 24 hours after birth:

a. Caput succedaneum
b. Cephalhematoma
c. Rupture of middle meningeal artery
d. Rupture of subdural veins

Ans. a. Caput succedaneum

267. Spaghetti and meatball appearance is related to which of the following organism?

a. Candida albicans b. Malassezia furfur
c. Pneumocystis jirovecii d. Cryptococcus neoformans

Ans. b. Malassezia furfur

268. Drug of choice for bacterial vaginosis:

a. Azithromycin b. Erythromycin
c. Metronidazole d. Ciprofloxacin

Ans. c. Metronidazole

269. Multiple perforation of tympanic membrane is characteristically seen in:

a. Acute otitis media
b. Chronic suppurative otitis media
c. Tubercular otitis media
d. Serous otitis media

Ans. c. Tubercular otitis media

270. Minimum number of antenatal visits must be:

a. 1 b. 2
c. 3 d. 4

Ans. d. 4

271. What would be the odour in acute arsenic poisoning?

a. Foul smell b. Garlic smell
c. Almond smell d. Odourless

Ans. b. Garlic smell

272. What is the most common cause of blindness in children in our country?

a. Vitamin A deficiency b. Cataract
c. Glaucoma d. Blunt injury to the eye

Ans. a. Vitamin A deficiency

273. Management of a male presenting to ENT department with bilateral abductor palsy:

a. Speech therapy
b. Tracheostomy
c. Lateralization of vocal cord
d. Wait and watch

Ans. b. Tracheostomy

274. Which of the following is NOT a complication of gestational diabetes?

a. Neonatal hyperglycaemia
b. Macrosomia
c. Sacral agenesis
d. Single umbilical artery

Ans. a. Neonatal hyperglycaemia

275. A male newborn was brought to the Pediatric surgery OPD with the complaint of abdominal distension and no passage of fecal matter since last 48 hours. What is the next best step in such a case?

a. Barium enema
b. Reassurance to the parents
c. Give high fibre diet
d. Submucosal suction biopsy

Ans. a. Barium enema

276. Snowstorm appearance on USG suggest the diagnosis of:

a. Ectopic pregnancy b. Polycystic ovarian disease
c. Intrauterine fetal death d. Hydatidiform mole

Ans. d. Hydatidiform mole

277. If the sex ratio is more than 1,000, it implies:

a. Females are more than males
b. Males are more than females
c. Males and females are equal
d. Cannot comment as data is insufficient

Ans. a. Females are more than males

278. What could be the reason for abdominal cramps in a breastfeeding mother?

a. Prolactin b. Oxytocin
c. Estrogen d. Progesterone

Ans. b. Oxytocin

279. Which of the following is NOT true for colostrum:

a. High chloride b. High protein
c. High IgA d. High Vitamin B

Ans. d. High Vitamin B

280. What would be the effect of low temperature on Oxygen Hemoglobin Dissociation curve?

a. Shift to left
b. Shift to right
c. Firstly, there is shift to right and then to left
d. Firstly, there is shift to left and then right

Ans. a. Shift to left

281. Which of the following is the most cost-effective way of screening carcinoma cervix?

a. Papanicolaou smear
b. Whole abdomen ultrasonography
c. Blood tests
d. Colposcopy examination

Ans. a. Papanicolaou smear

282. Dashboard injury is also known as:

a. Anterior dislocation of the hip joint
b. Posterior dislocation of the hip joint
c. Fracture neck of femur
d. Fracture acetabulum

Ans. b. Posterior dislocation of the hip joint

283. Effect of vitamin A over formation of urinary stones:

a. Prevents formation of urinary stones
b. Promotes formation of urinary stones
c. No effect on formation of urinary stones
d. Initial decrease, later increase in the formation of urinary stones

Ans. a. Prevents formation of urinary stones

284. All of the following anti-diabetic drug require dose-reduction in renal failure patients *except*:

a. Vildagliptin b. Sitagliptin
c. Sexagliptin d. Linagliptin

Ans. d. Linagliptin

285. A young male, who used to take non-vegetarian diet mostly, presently with redness and pain in right great toe. He had similar episodes in the past as well. His serum uric acid came out to be 10 mg/dL. Based on symptoms and uric acid levels, clinical diagnosis of gout was made. Along with analgesic, treating doctor prescribed one drug, which intends to decrease formation of uric acid in the body. Which of the following enzyme is likely to be inhibited by this anti-gout drug?

a. HMG CoA reductase
b. Xanthine oxidase
c. Dihydrofolate reductase
d. Enolase

Ans. b. Xanthine oxidase

286. A 25-years-old G1P1 woman came to the Gynecology OPD with the complaint of amenorrhoea of 6 months duration, since her full term normal vaginal delivery. What could be the probable cause of this amenorrhoea?

a. Hyperprolactinemia
b. Sheehan syndrome
c. Malnutrition
d. Polycystic ovarian disease

Ans. a. Hyperprolactinemia

287. A 35-years-old male with the complaints of itching, jaundice, mood disorder and tremors. Eye examination shows a golden-brown ring in Descemet's membrane. Most likely diagnosis:
a. Primary hemochromatosis
b. Parkinson disease
c. Obstructive jaundice
d. Wilson disease

Ans. d. Wilson disease

288. Enzyme deficiency in galactosemia:
a. Phosphofructokinase
b. Hexokinase
c. Galactose-1-phosphate uridyl transferase
d. HMG CoA reductase

Ans. c. Galactose-1-phosphate uridyl transferase

289. A patient who was on long-term steroid therapy presented to the Orthopedics OPD with the complains of pain in both the hip joints. Most likely condition:
a. Fracture neck of femur
b. Avascular necrosis of the head of femur
c. Posterior dislocation of the hip joint
d. Anterior dislocation of the hip joint

Ans. b. Avascular necrosis of the head of femur

290. A patient is having diabetes mellitus for more than 20 years. Fundus examination revealed microaneurysms. This is suggestive of:
a. CRAO b. CRVO
c. Proliferative diabetic retinopathy
d. Non-proliferative diabetic retinopathy

Ans. d. Non-proliferative diabetic retinopathy

291. Rouleaux formation of RBCs is seen in:
a. Multiple myeloma b. Thalassemia
c. Sickle cell anemia d. Iron deficiency anemia

Ans. a. Multiple myeloma

292. All of the following nerves can be injured in cases of fracture of humerus (any part) *except*:
a. Radial nerve b. Ulnar nerve
c. Median nerve d. Musculocutaneous nerve

Ans. d. Musculocutaneous nerve

293. Malar rash is found in:
a. Erythema infectiosum b. Photodermatitis
c. Bee sting d. SLE

Ans. d. SLE

294. Tense blisters on flexor surfaces and anti-BPAG1 and anti-BPAG2 antibodies suggest the diagnosis of:
a. Bullous pemphigoid b. Pemphigus vulgaris
c. Scalds d. Lupus vulgaris

Ans. a. Bullous pemphigoid

295. A three-years-old male boy does not make friends. He prefers to stay alone and likes to play with toys. His parents complains that he does not make any eye contact too. Most likely diagnosis:
a. Autism
b. Attention-deficit-hyperactivity disorder
c. Conduct disorder
d. Deaf and dumb child

Ans. a. Autism

296. True statement regarding action of dopamine at low doses:
a. Decreases renal blood flow
b. Increases renal blood flow
c. Renal blood flow remains unaffected with any alteration in dose
d. Initial decrease, then increase in renal blood flow

Ans. b. Increases renal blood flow

297. A child having diarrhoeal episodes, is irritable and thirsty. Such a case of diarrhoea is best managed by:
a. Wait and watch policy
b. Oral fluids
c. Intravenous fluid administration
d. Intra-osseous fluid administration

Ans. b. Oral fluids

298. A 60-years-old male presented to the Medicine OPD with the complaints of discomfort in the left upper quadrant of the abdomen. There is also associated history of fatigue and weight loss. Per abdomen examination revealed an enlarged spleen. Laboratory tests showed a hemoglobin of 8.5 gm%, total leucocyte count of 4.6 lakhs/cmm and platelet count of 5.1 lakhs/cmm. Differential leucocyte count revealed 6% basophils. Peripheral blood smear showed promyelocytes, metamyelocytes and blast forms. Findings are consistent with the diagnosis of:
a. Chronic myelogenous leukemia
b. Chronic lymphocytic leukemia
c. Hodgkin's lymphoma
d. Non-Hodgkin's lymphoma

Ans. a. Chronic myelogenous leukemia

299. Most probable site of lesion in a patient presenting with brain lesion and homonymous hemianopia with macular sparing:
a. Retina b. Optic nerve
c. Optic chiasm d. Occipital cortex

Ans. d. Occipital cortex

300. A 35-years-old smoker, alcoholic and hypertensive lady presented to Obstetrics OPD in 37th week of gestation. She complains of abdominal pain and bleeding per vaginum. On examination her blood pressure was 160/110 mm Hg. Per-abdomen examination revealed a tender abdomen and fetal parts can be felt superficially. Fetal heart sounds were not audible on auscultation. Most probable diagnosis could be:
a. Accidental hemorrhage
b. Placenta previa
c. Intrauterine fetal death
d. Intrauterine growth retardation

Ans. a. Accidental hemorrhage

301. **Kwashiorkor occurs because of:**
a. Less energy intake
b. Less protein intake
c. Excess energy intake
d. Excess protein intake

Ans. b. Less protein intake

302. **A post-covid diabetic patient, with uncontrolled blood sugar, presented to the casualty with the complaint of breathlessness. Most likely diagnosis:**
a. Mucormycosis
b. Kaposi sarcoma
c. Oral thrush
d. Diphtheria

Ans. a. Mucormycosis

303. **Which of the following condition presents with menstrual disturbances, infertility and recurrent abortions?**
a. Uterine fibroids
b. Carcinoma fallopian tube
c. Carcinoma ovary
d. Carcinoma cervix

Ans. a. Uterine fibroids

304. **A 12-years-old girl from Nigeria presented to the Pediatrics OPD with the complaints of night sweat, fever and loss of weight since last few months. There was an intra-abdominal mass and peripheral lymphadenopathy as well. Doctor advised for biopsy of the lymph node which showed sheets of lymphocytes with interspersed macrophages. Most probable diagnosis and associated translocation:**
a. Burkitt's lymphoma; t(9, 22)
b. Burkitt's lymphoma; t(8, 14)
c. CML; t(8, 14)
d. CML; t(9, 22)

Ans. b. Burkitt's lymphoma; t(8, 14)

305. **Fracture of which of the bone, does not require any specific treatment?**
a. Ulna
b. Humerus
c. Scapula
d. Radius

Ans. c. Scapula

306. **A child having diarrhoeal episodes is lethargic and floppy. He is drinking poorly and on pinching skin, skin goes back very slowly. Such a case of diarrhea is defined as:**
a. No dehydration
b. Some dehydration
c. Severe dehydration
d. None of the above

Ans. a. No dehydration

307. **A known case of diabetes presented with painless visual loss. Fundus examination shows blood and thunder fundus. Most likely diagnosis:**
a. Central retinal vein occlusion
b. Central retinal artery occlusion
c. Proliferative diabetic retinopathy
d. Non-proliferative diabetic retinopathy

Ans. a. Central retinal vein occlusion

308. **Which of the following anti-asthmatic drug does NOT cause bronchodilation?**
a. Hydrocortisone
b. Salbutamol
c. Deriphylline
d. Ipratropium bromide

Ans. a. Hydrocortisone

309. **An elderly patient complains of lower back pain. X-ray lumbar spine showed sclerotic lesions. What could be the most probable diagnosis?**
a. Osteoporosis
b. Osteomalacia
c. Carcinoma prostate
d. Carcinoma urinary bladder

Ans. c. Carcinoma prostate

310. **What could be the more likely malignancy in an elderly person who is an employee of a dye industry and now had developed urinary problems?**
a. Renal cell carcinoma
b. Hypernephroma
c. Squamous cell carcinoma of urinary bladder
d. Transitional cell carcinoma of urinary bladder

Ans. d. Transitional cell carcinoma of urinary bladder

311. **A female was on warfarin in the past 2 months, but she became pregnant during the course of treatment. As a doctor, what advice you would give regarding warfarin therapy now?**
a. Stop warfarin
b. Increase dose of warfarin
c. Lower dose of warfarin
d. Replace warfarin with heparin

Ans. d. Replace warfarin with heparin

312. **A female patient presented to the Medicine OPD with the complaints of restlessness, inability to concentrate on work and fatigue. On general examination, there was pallor. Neurological examination was normal. There was no neurological deficit. Laboratory tests shows a low hemoglobin, raised MCV, normal methyl malonic acid levels and raised homocysteine levels. Treatment of such a patient must include:**
a. Folic acid
b. Vitamin B_{12}
c. Thiamine
d. Niacin

Ans. a. Folic acid

313. **For measuring intra-ocular pressure, the gold standard method is:**
a. Schiotz tonometer
b. Goldmann applanation tonometer
c. Keratometer
d. Slit lamp

Ans. b. Goldmann applanation tonometer

314. **Multiple infection (more than one parasite invades RBC) is seen in:**
a. Plasmodium vivax
b. Plasmodium falciparum
c. Plasmodium malariae
d. Plasmodium ovale

Ans. b. Plasmodium falciparum

315. **A 33-years-old sexually active female came to the Gynecology OPD for routine screening for carcinoma cervix. Pap smear was done which showed dysplastic changes on histopathological examination. Organism responsible for such a presentation:**

a. Human immunodeficiency virus
b. Human papilloma virus
c. Hepatitis B virus
d. Ebstein Barr virus

Ans. b. Human papilloma virus

316. Which of the following is NOT associated with atrial septal defect?

a. Down syndrome
b. Pierre–Robin syndrome
c. Ehler–Danlos syndrome
d. Turner syndrome

Ans. d. Turner syndrome

317. An elderly diabetic male had Covid infection. Later on, he presented to ENT OPD with complaints of nasal obstruction. On endoscopic examination, black, friable mass was seen. Findings suggest the diagnosis of:

a. Mucormycosis
b. Malignant otitis externa
c. Atrophic rhinitis
d. Rhinoscleroma

Ans. a. Mucormycosis

318. What is the treatment of empyema?

a. Wait and watch
b. Chest drainage only
c. Antibiotics only
d. Chest drainage with antibiotics

Ans. d. Chest drainage with antibiotics

319. An old man, who is an employee of a dye industry presented to the Surgery OPD with the complaint of hematuria. There is no pain during micturition. This is accompanied by frequency and urgency lately during micturition. Imaging study revealed a bladder mass. Surgeon made a provisional diagnosis of urinary bladder carcinoma. Most likely type of bladder carcinoma in such a case:

a. Transitional cell carcinoma
b. Squamous cell carcinoma
c. Adenocarcinoma
d. Anaplastic carcinoma

Ans. a. Transitional cell carcinoma

320. A 65-years-old diabetic male with uncontrolled sugar levels presented to ENT OPD with the complaints of severe dyspnea, fever and generalized malaise. On examination, tachypnea was noted. He was ordered for nasopharyngeal swab RT-PCR, which was positive for SARS-CoV2 virus. 2 weeks later, he developed swelling in both the periorbital area and proptosis of right eye. Which micro-organism could be responsible for such a presentation?

a. Pseudomonas aeruginosa
b. Mucor
c. Candida albicans
d. Aspergillus

Ans. b. Mucor

321. A female patient presented to the ENT OPD with the complaints of fever, dysphagia and sore throat. X-ray of the neck region showed 'thumb sign'. Which of the micro-organism is responsible for such a clinical presentation?

a. Hemophilus influenzae
b. Neisseria gonorrhoeae
c. Pseudomonas aeruginosa
d. Staphylococcus aureus

Ans. a. Hemophilus influenzae

322. A 25-years-old male sustained injury to the left eye because of fist. What finding can be seen in such a case?

a. Fracture of superior orbital wall
b. Fracture of medial orbital wall
c. Fracture of inferior orbital wall
d. Fracture of lateral orbital wall

Ans. c. Fracture of inferior orbital wall

323. Which of the following is NOT a feature of HELLP syndrome?

a. Hemolysis
b. Elevated liver enzymes
c. Low platelets count
d. Pancytopenia

Ans. d. Pancytopenia

324. A person who had recently travelled to China, presented to Flu clinic with the complaints of fever, body-ache and cough. During the course of treatment, he developed dyspnea as well. Treating doctor advised for a test and made a clinical diagnosis of Covid infection. Which of the following test was most probably ordered?

a. Complete blood count
b. Chest X-ray
c. Liver function test
d. RT-PCR

Ans. d. RT-PCR

325. Cysts of which of the following can be detected by acid fast stain?

a. Cryptosporidium
b. Cryptococcus neoformans
c. Campylobacter jejuni
d. Clostridium botulinum

Ans. a. Cryptosporidium

326. A 25-years-old female with G3P0A2L0 came to the antenatal clinic for her second trimester follow-up. She was worried because she had two abortions in the past. Obstetrician found that the length of cervix is 18 mm. Based on this, the probable cause of previous abortions could be:

a. Short cervical length
b. Anti-sperm antibodies formation
c. Cervical incompetence
d. Anti-phospholipid antibody syndrome

Ans. a. Short cervical length

327. An eccentric, epiphyseal tumour, which can extend up to metaphysis:

a. Osteoblastoma
b. Osteosarcoma
c. Giant cell tumour
d. Osteoid osteoma

Ans. c. Giant cell tumour

328. Thyroid carcinoma with best prognosis:

a. Anaplastic carcinoma thyroid
b. Medullary carcinoma thyroid
c. Follicular carcinoma of thyroid
d. Papillary carcinoma thyroid

Ans. d. Papillary carcinoma thyroid

329. **Acute osteomyelitis is most commonly caused by:**
a. Staphylococcus aureus
b. Streptococcus pneumoniae
c. Pseudomonas aeruginosa
d. Corynebacterium diphtheriae

Ans. a. Staphylococcus aureus

330. **Which of the following is associated with mutation in ATP7B gene?**
a. Hepatocellular carcinoma
b. Arsenic poisoning
c. Parkinson's disease
d. Wilson's disease

Ans. d. Wilson's disease

331. **What could be the most probable diagnosis of a young female presenting with fatigue and limb weakness in the evening hours, which tend to improve on administration of edrophonium?**
a. Myasthenia gravis
b. Eaton–Lambert syndrome
c. Malingering
d. Botulism

Ans. a. Myasthenia gravis

332. **A 28-years-old lady presented to the Medicine OPD with the complaint of joint pains and rash over face. She did not have any history of fever. Serology revealed a raised ESR. She had small, warty vegetations on both sides of the heart valves. Findings are suggestive of:**
a. Libmann–Sac endocarditis
b. Rheumatic carditis
c. Non-bacterial thrombotic endocarditis
d. Subacute endocarditis

Ans. a. Libmann–Sac endocarditis

333. **Which of the following condition does NOT cause a grey-white membrane over the tonsils?**
a. Ludwig's angina
b. Diphtheria
c. Infectious mononucleosis
d. Malignancy of tonsil

Ans. a. Ludwig's angina

334. **Ascoli thermo-precipitation test is related to:**
a. Yersinia pestis
b. Staphylococcus aureus
c. Shigella
d. Bacillus anthracis

Ans. d. Bacillus anthracis

335. **Most visually handicapping type of cataract:**
a. Posterior polar cataract
b. Posterior subcapsular cataract
c. Anterior polar cataract
d. Anterior subcapsular cataract

Ans. b. Posterior subcapsular cataract

336. **Which condition can be managed by marsupialization?**
a. Bartholin gland cyst
b. Bartholin gland carcinoma
c. Bartholin gland adenoma
d. Skene's duct cyst

Ans. a. Bartholin gland cyst

337. **A substance was stained with Congo red stain and when visualized under normal light under microscope, shows red-pink colour. The substance is:**
a. Collagen
b. Cellulose
c. Amyloid
d. Starch

Ans. c. Amyloid

338. **A 30-years-old lady attended Medicine OPD with the complaints of difficulty in walking and tingling-burning sensation in her lower limbs. General examination showed pallor. Neurological examination revealed bilateral loss of proprioception and vibration senses in her lower limbs. Peripheral blood smear was done, the image of which is shown below. Findings suggest the diagnosis of:**
a. Thiamine deficiency
b. Niacin deficiency
c. Folate deficiency
d. Vitamin B_{12} deficiency

Ans. d. Vitamin B_{12} deficiency

339. **A young lady presented to the Endocrinology OPD with the complains of lethargy, increased sleep, weight gain and cold intolerance. Most likely diagnosis:**
a. Hyperparathyroidism
b. Hypoparathyroidism
c. Hyperthyroidism
d. Hypothyroidism

Ans. d. Hypothyroidism

340. **A male child was having recurrent episodes of tonsillitis. ENT surgeon advised tonsillectomy. After surgery, the patient started complaining of pain in his left ear. Nerve responsible for this referred otalgia is:**
a. Chorda tympani nerve
b. Auriculotemporal nerve
c. Glossopharyngeal nerve
d. Facial nerve

Ans. c. Glossopharyngeal nerve

341. **Which of the following structure is affected in an old male presenting with hearing loss?**
a. Apex of hair cells
b. Base of hair cells
c. Semi-circular canals
d. Utricle

Ans. b. Base of hair cells

342. **Which of the following is the most common congenital anomaly of larynx?**
a. Laryngomalacia
b. Laryngocele
c. Laryngeal web
d. Laryngeal agenesis

Ans. a. Laryngomalacia

343. **Recurrent pterygium is commonly managed by:**
a. Conjunctival autograft
b. Chemotherapy with Mitomycin-C
c. Excision only
d. Wait and watch

Ans. a. Conjunctival autograft

344. **Which of the following is evaluated by Berberios test?**
a. Semen
b. Sputum
c. Blood
d. Cerebrospinal fluid

Ans. a. Semen

345. A 65-years-old male patient had painless hematuria and pain in lumbar area. What can be the most probable diagnosis:

a. Multiple myeloma
b. Prolapsed intervertebral disc
c. Tuberculosis of spine
d. Renal cell carcinoma

Ans. d. Renal cell carcinoma

346. Effect of prolonged vomiting:

a. Respiratory acidosis
b. Respiratory alkalosis
c. Metabolic acidosis
d. Metabolic alkalosis

Ans. d. Metabolic alkalosis

347. A male patient developed high-grade fever, headache, vomiting and nuchal rigidity of sudden onset. Lumbar puncture was done and CSF sample showed the growth of lanceolate-shaped diplococci. Identify the organism:

a. Pseudomonas aeruginosa
b. Neisseria meningitidis
c. Staphylococcus aureus
d. Streptococcus pneumoniae

Ans. d. Streptococcus pneumoniae

348. A 22-years-old primigravida presented to the Obstetrics department with labor pain. On examination, fetus was found to be in occipito-posterior position. Obstetrician tried to manually reposition the fetus to occipito-anterior position but the attempt failed and the fetus continued to lied in occipito-posterior position. Such a clinical presentation is usually associated with which type of female pelvis?

a. Gynecoid
b. Platypelloid
c. Android
d. Anthropoid

Ans. d. Anthropoid

349. Which of the following inflammatory mediator has a major role in a patient presenting with swelling of the face and breathlessness after a bee-sting?

a. Histamine
b. Serotonin
c. Substance P
d. Bradykinin

Ans. a. Histamine

350. Most common bone to fracture in body:

a. Clavicle
b. Humerus
c. Radius
d. Calcaneum

Ans. a. Clavicle

351. Which of the following artery is ligated in a 32-years-old lady with post-partum hemorrhage?

a. Uterine artery
b. Ovarian artery
c. Internal iliac artery
d. External iliac artery

Ans. a. Uterine artery

352. A 29-years-old female, mother of 4 children, attended Medicine OPD with the complaint of tiredness. On examination, there was pallor. Hemoglobin level came out to be 6.5 gm%. Most likely diagnosis:

a. Arsenic poisoning
b. Iron deficiency anemia
c. Chronic liver disease
d. Chronic kidney disease

Ans. b. Iron deficiency anemia

353. Main lead of pacemaker is attached to which chamber of the heart?

a. Right atrium
b. Right ventricle
c. Left atrium
d. Left ventricle

Ans. b. Right ventricle

354. Fluid requirement is NOT increased in:

a. Severe vomiting
b. Bacterial endocarditis
c. Pulmonary hypertension
d. Constrictive pericarditis

Ans. d. Constrictive pericarditis

355. Best ways to manage carcinoma cervix stage IIIB:

a. Neoadjuvant chemotherapy followed by surgery/radiotherapy
b. Chemotherapy
c. Radiotherapy
d. Surgery

Ans. a. Neoadjuvant chemotherapy followed by surgery/radiotherapy

356. Stored hay is associated with which of the following pneumoconiosis?

a. Bagassosis
b. Byssinosis
c. Farmer's lung
d. Anthracosis

Ans. c. Farmer's lung

357. Lucid interval is seen in:

a. Subdural hemorrhage
b. Subarachnoid hemorrhage
c. Extradural hemorrhage
d. Parenchymal hemorrhage

Ans. c. Extradural hemorrhage

358. An 18-months-old female patient presented to ENT OPD with severe sensorineural hearing loss. She was advised hearing aids but there was no improvement. What is the next best step in managing such a case?

a. Continue with hearing aids
b. Cochlear implant
c. Stapedectomy
d. Myringotomy

Ans. b. Cochlear implant

359. Which of the following is the common set of finding in case of strangulation and low-level hanging?

a. Hand touching the floor
b. Blood stasis at dependent area of the body
c. Facial pallor
d. Transverse ligature mark

Ans. d. Transverse ligature mark

360. What could be the best treatment of a 11-years-old female child presenting to Ophthalmology OPD with unilateral amblyopia?

a. Wait and watch
b. Occlusion therapy
c. Surgery
d. Radiotherapy

Ans. b. Occlusion therapy

361. A young lady developed unilateral sudden visual loss which was painful. The pain worsened on moving the eyes. Perimetry showed central scotoma in the affected eye. A relative afferent pupillary defect was also present. Clinical diagnosis of such a case:

a. Papilledema
b. Optic neuritis
c. Retinal detachment
d. Acute congestive glaucoma

Ans. b. Optic neuritis

362. LEAST chances of recipient failure in transplant is seen in:

a. Allograft
b. Isograft
c. Xenograft
d. Heterotopic graft

Ans. b. Isograft

363. What could be the most likely diagnosis of a case in which ptosis improves on eating and drinking?

a. Horner syndrome
b. Mechanical ptosis
c. Marcus Gunn Jaw winking syndrome
d. Malingering

Ans. c. Marcus Gunn Jaw winking syndrome

364. Which vitamin deficiency is seen in short bowel syndrome?

a. Vitamin B_{12}
b. Vitamin B_6
c. Vitamin B_3
d. Vitamin B_1

Ans. a. Vitamin B_{12}

365. A young female sustained injury to the left eye with leaf a few days ago. Now she presented to the Ophthalmology OPD with complaints of pain in the eye and photophobia. Most possible diagnosis:

a. Acanthamoeba keratitis
b. Viral keratitis
c. Bacterial keratitis
d. Fungal keratitis

Ans. d. Fungal keratitis

366. Killian's dehiscence lies between:

a. Thyropharyngeus and cricopharyngeus muscles
b. Cricopharyngeus and esophagus laterally
c. Cricopharyngeus muscle and esophagus inferiorly
d. Two thyropharyngeus muscles

Ans. a. Thyropharyngeus and cricopharyngeus muscles

367. Which of the following type of shock will usually have warm peripheral extremities?

a. Hypovolemic shock
b. Anaphylactic shock
c. Neurogenic shock
d. Cardiogenic shock

Ans. c. Neurogenic shock

368. Drainage of cervical abscess is an example of:

a. Clean contaminated wound
b. Dirty infected wound
c. Clean uncontaminated wound
d. Unclean contaminated wound

Ans. b. Dirty infected wound

369. A person has a visual acuity of 3/60 in one eye and visual acuity of 1/60 in another eye. What kind of blindness is this?

a. Total blindness
b. Social blindness
c. Partial blindness
d. Legal blindness

Ans. b. Social blindness

370. Radiolucent renal stones are composed of:

a. Xanthine
b. Cysteine
c. Calcium phosphate
d. Calcium oxalate

Ans. a. Xanthine

371. High flying prostate is a sign of:

a. Bulbar urethral injury
b. Intraperitoneal bladder rupture
c. Membranous urethral injury
d. Extra-peritoneal bladder rupture

Ans. c. Membranous urethral injury

372. A 4-months-old female child presented with excessive watering from her right eye. On pressing the medial canthus of the right eye, there is an increase in discharge. What is the most appropriate treatment of such a case?

a. Dacryocystorhinostomy
b. Massaging of lacrimal sac
c. Probing
d. Syringing

Ans. b. Massaging of lacrimal sac

373. Which of the following is the most common cancer of 'Head and Neck' region in India?

a. Oral cavity
b. Nasopharynx
c. Oropharynx
d. Laryngopharynx

Ans. a. Oral cavity

374. Which of the following condition is managed by V-Y procedure?

a. Ankyloblepharon
b. Ptosis
c. Entropion
d. Ectropion

Ans. d. Ectropion

375. Transplanted kidney is relocated to which region in the recipient's body?

a. Retroperitoneal region
b. Epigastrium
c. Lumbar region
d. Pelvis

Ans. a. Retroperitoneal region

376. Subdural hematoma is due to rupture of:

a. Middle meningeal artery
b. Retromandibular vein
c. Communicating veins to superior sagittal sinus
d. Saccular Berry aneurysm

Ans. c. Communicating veins to superior sagittal sinus

377. A 55-years-old male, a known case of diabetes mellitus with poorly controlled sugar level developed right facial nerve palsy. He was also having severe pain in right ear. On examination, granulation tissue was found at the external auditory canal. Findings suggest the diagnosis of:
a. Acute suppurative otitis media
b. Chronic suppurative otitis media
c. Simple otitis externa
d. Malignant otitis externa

Ans. d. Malignant otitis externa

378. A 10-years-old female presented with complaints of hearing loss. Otoscopic examination showed a bulging tympanic membrane. Tympanometry showed a 'B' graph. Most likely diagnosis:
a. Acute otitis media
b. Serous otitis media
c. Chronic otitis media
d. Disruption of ossicular chain

Ans. b. Serous otitis media

379. Investigation of choice for dysphagia is:
a. Endoscopy b. Barium swallow
c. Manometry d. CT scan

Ans. a. Endoscopy

380. All of the following are removed in Whipple's procedure *except*:
a. Pylorus
b. Common bile duct
c. Proximal jejunum
d. Neck of pancreas

Ans. d. Neck of pancreas

381. Management of a patient with complete placenta previa at 38 weeks of gestation without any vaginal bleeding is:
a. Expectant treatment
b. McAfee and Johnson regimen
c. Elective caesarean section
d. Emergency caesarean section

Ans. c. Elective caesarean section

382. All are of value in modified Bishop score *except*:
a. Dilatation b. Cervical length
c. Effacement d. Consistency

Ans. c. Effacement

383. Funnelling in cervicogram is seen in:
a. Cervical cancer b. Normal cervix
c. During labor d. Cervical incompetence

Ans. d. Cervical incompetence

384. In a demographic cycle, low stationary phase is:
a. Phase 1 b. Phase 2
c. Phase 3 d. Phase 4

Ans. d. Phase 4

385. Out of the following features of ischemia, which presentations has the worst outcome?
a. Pulselessness b. Paralysis
c. Pallor d. Paresthesia

Ans. a. Pulselessness

386. Pregnancy occurred with IUCD in situ, the strings are however not visible. All of the following can be done *except*:
a. Leave in situ
b. Remove IUCD under USG guidance
c. Remove using IUCD hook
d. Remove IUCD using hysteroscope

Ans. c. Remove using IUCD hook

387. What do you mean by demographic bonus?
a. Increased fertility rate
b. Increased income
c. Increased density of the population
d. Reduction in population because of use of contraceptive measures

Ans. d. Reduction in population because of use of contraceptive measures

388. A 32-years-old female patient presented to Gynecology OPD with the complaints of amenorrhoea. She had a history of some procedure done for abortion 3 months back. FSH and LH levels were found to be normal. Most likely diagnosis of such a case:
a. Endometrial TB b. Premature ovarian failure
c. Asherman's syndrome d. Sheehan's syndrome

Ans. c. Asherman's syndrome

389. A 70-years-old male presented with complaints of imbalance while standing. On examination, it was found that there was loss of proprioception and vibration sense as well. What should be given to such a patient?
a. Thiamine b. Niacin
c. Folic acid d. Vitamin B_{12}

Ans. d. Vitamin B_{12}

390. Ortho-tolidine test measures:
a. Free chlorine
b. Combined chlorine
c. Free chlorine and combined chlorine
d. Chlorine demand

Ans. c. Free chlorine and combined chlorine

391. A 50-years-old lady has carcinoma cervix stage III (FIGO). What is the best possible management of such a case?
a. Chemotherapy
b. Radiotherapy
c. Concurrent chemoradiation
d. Surgery

Ans. c. Concurrent chemoradiation

392. In which of the following types of shock, there is an elevated central venous pressure (CVP)?
a. Cardiogenic shock b. Hypovolemic shock
c. Septic shock d. Neurogenic shock

Ans. a. Cardiogenic shock

393. **A young female presented to the medical OPD with the complaints of dyspnea on exertion and fatigue. Peripheral blood smear showed macrocytic RBCs. Serum methyl-cobalamin level were found to be within normal limits. What should be given to this patient?**
   a. Pyridoxine b. Folic acid
   c. Methyl-cobalamin d. Iron

Ans. b. Folic acid

394. **A female with 46XX karyotype has absent vagina and uterus. Ovary is present and secondary sexual characters are also normal. LH and FSH levels were found to be within normal limits. Most likely diagnosis:**
   a. PCOD
   b. Turner's syndrome
   c. MRKH syndrome
   d. Androgen insensitivity syndrome

Ans. c. MRKH syndrome

395. **A patient had developed arrhythmia. There is a history of long-term intake of digitalis. What is the best possible management of such a case?**
   a. Lignocaine b. Adenosine
   c. Verapamil d. Amiodarone

Ans. a. Lignocaine

396. **Which of the following is NOT increased in PCOD?**
   a. Estrogen
   b. Luteinizing hormone
   c. Sex hormone binding globulin
   d. Fasting insulin

Ans. c. Sex hormone binding globulin

397. **A known case of thyroiditis has low thyroxine and high thyroid stimulating hormone levels. He also has raised levels of anti-thyroperoxidase antibody. Findings are consistent with the diagnosis of:**
   a. Reidel's thyroiditis b. Hashimoto's thyroiditis
   c. Subacute thyroiditis d. Secondary hypothyroidism

Ans. b. Hashimoto's thyroiditis

398. **A 55-years-old lady presented with a mass of 5 × 6 cm in the right breast. On examination, a single hard axillary lymph node was found. What could be the best management of this case of breast carcinoma?**
   a. Simple mastectomy
   b. Interval mastectomy
   c. Radical mastectomy
   d. Neoadjuvant chemotherapy→Modified radical mastectomy→ Radiotherapy

Ans. d. Neoadjuvant chemotherapy→Modified radical mastectomy→ Radiotherapy

399. **Uterine height is greater than the gestational age of the patient in all the following cases *except*:**
   a. IUGR b. Fibroid uterus
   c. Wrong dates d. Polyhydramnios

Ans. a. IUGR

400. **Amniotic fluid is maximum at what gestational age?**
   a. 40 weeks b. 36 weeks
   c. 32 weeks d. 28 weeks

Ans. b. 36 weeks

401. **Set of arteries arising from second part of axillary artery:**
   a. Anterior circumflex humoral artery, Posterior circumflex humoral artery
   b. Lateral thoracic artery, Superior thoracic artery
   c. Subscapular artery, Thoracoacromial artery
   d. Lateral thoracic artery, Thoracoacromial artery

Ans. d. Lateral thoracic artery, Thoracoacromial artery

402. **Vocal cords are abducted by which of the following muscle?**
   a. Cricothyroid
   b. Posterior cricoarytenoid
   c. Lateral cricoarytenoid
   d. Thyroarytenoid

Ans. b. Posterior cricoarytenoid

403. **Which of the following is NOT a site of urinary extravasation in case of injury to bulbar urethra?**
   a. Superficial perineal pouch
   b. Deep perineal pouch
   c. Scrotum
   d. Thigh

Ans. b. Deep perineal pouch

404. **High volume of distribution of a drug depends upon:**
   a. Rate of elimination
   b. Half-life
   c. Lipid solubility
   d. High plasma protein binding

Ans. c. Lipid solubility

405. **Which of the following is NOT a site of avascular necrosis?**
   a. Humerus b. Femur
   c. Talus d. Scaphoid

Ans. a. Humerus

406. **Drug of choice for akathisia:**
   a. Central anticholinergic b. Dantrolene sodium
   c. Propranolol d. Levodopa

Ans. c. Propranolol

407. **What is the correct sequence of structures pierced by the needle, while giving epidural anesthesia?**
   a. Skin → Subcutaneous tissue → Supraspinous ligament → Interspinous ligament → Ligamentum flavum
   b. Skin → Subcutaneous tissue → Interspinous ligament → Supraspinous ligament → Ligamentum flavum
   c. Skin → Subcutaneous tissue → Supraspinous ligament → Ligamentum flavum→ Interspinous ligament
   d. Skin → Subcutaneous tissue → Ligamentum flavum → Interspinous ligament → Supraspinous ligament

Ans. a. Skin → Subcutaneous tissue → Supraspinous ligament → Interspinous ligament → Ligamentum flavum

408. Rokitansky protuberance is found in:
a. Leiomyoma b. Seminoma
c. Dermoid cyst d. Choriocarcinoma

Ans. c. Dermoid cyst

409. Which of the following can lead to adenocarcinoma of the urinary bladder?
a. Aniline dye
b. Cigarette smoking
c. Persistent urachal remnant
d. 2-naphthyl-amine toxicity

Ans. c. Persistent urachal remnant

410. Most common mediastinal tumour:
a. Thymoma b. Neuroblastoma
c. Lymphoma d. Rhabdomyoma

Ans. b. Neuroblastoma

411. Type of collagen found in bone is:
a. Type 5 b. Type 4
c. Type 2 d. Type 1

Ans. d. Type 1

412. What is the correct sequence of brain structures moving from outside to inside:
a. Insula → Caudate nucleus → Internal capsule → Lentiform nucleus → Thalamus
b. Insula → Internal capsule → Lentiform nucleus → Caudate nucleus → Thalamus
c. Insula → Lentiform nucleus → Caudate nucleus → Internal capsule → Thalamus
d. Insula → Lentiform nucleus → Internal capsule → Caudate nucleus → Thalamus

Ans. d. Insula → Lentiform nucleus → Internal capsule → Caudate nucleus → Thalamus

413. Anterior and middle layer of thoracolumbar fascia encloses which muscle?
a. Erector spinae b. Latissimus dorsi
c. Quadratus lumborum d. Serratus anterior

Ans. c. Quadratus lumborum

414. Lower limit of retropharyngeal space is:
a. C7 vertebra
b. 4th esophageal constriction
c. Bifurcation of trachea
d. Bifurcation of main bronchus

Ans. c. Bifurcation of trachea

415. All of the following are parts of bony labyrinth *except*:
a. Vestibule b. Cochlea
c. Utricle d. Semi-circular canals

Ans. c. Utricle

416. Which of the following vitamin helps in iron absorption?
a. Vitamin A b. Vitamin B
c. Vitamin C d. Vitamin D

Ans. c. Vitamin C

417. A person feel limb weakness and tiredness especially in the evening after working all day. This muscle weakness improved after Edrophonium test. Most likely diagnosis:
a. Eaton–Lambert syndrome
b. Guillain–Barre syndrome
c. Tetanus
d. Myasthenia gravis

Ans. d. Myasthenia gravis

418. All of the following cartilages are calcified *except*:
a. Epiglottis b. Thyroid
c. Arytenoid d. Cricoid

Ans. a. Epiglottis

419. Secondary oocyte contains:
a. 23X b. 46XY
c. 46XX d. 23Y

Ans. a. 23X

420. Site of decussation of corticospinal tract:
a. Lower medulla b. Upper medulla
c. Pons d. Midbrain

Ans. a. Lower medulla

421. The principle 'distractive forces are converted into compressive forces' can be used in managing the fracture of:
a. Head of radius b. Capitellum
c. Olecranon process d. Trochlea

Ans. c. Olecranon process

422. A 4-years-old child is admitted with fever, non-purulent conjunctivitis, rashes, cervical lymphadenopathy, hepatomegaly and desquamation of fingers and toes. Echocardiography shows coronary artery aneurysm. Findings are consistent with the diagnosis of:
a. German measles b. Kawasaki disease
c. Measles d. Rubella

Ans. b. Kawasaki disease

423. What stage is carcinoma cervix involving body of uterus?
a. Stage I b. Stage II
c. Stage III d. Stage IV

Ans. a. Stage I

424. Example of unpaired cartilage in larynx:
a. Cricoid b. Arytenoid
c. Corniculate d. Cuneiform

Ans. a. Cricoid

425. A male working in a cardboard manufacturing industry is at risk of developing:
a. Bagassosis b. Anthracosis
c. Asbestosis d. Byssinosis

Ans. a. Bagassosis

426. Amongst the following option, substance which acts as an iron chelator:
a. EDTA b. Penicillamine
c. Deferoxamine d. BAL

Ans. c. Deferoxamine

427. **What is the cause of death in Judicial hanging, which is a method of execution of criminals?**
a. Asphyxia
b. Fracture of upper cervical vertebrae
c. Myocardial infarction
d. Vagal inhibition

Ans. b. Fracture of upper cervical vertebrae

428. **Which of the following poison can cause cherry red colour post-mortem staining?**
a. Carbon monoxide
b. Carbon dioxide
c. Hydrogen sulphide
d. Cyanide

Ans. a. Carbon monoxide

429. **Which of the following enzyme is deficient in a case of Lesch-Nyhan syndrome?**
a. HMG CoA reductase
b. HGPRTase
c. Glucocerebrosidase
d. Sphingomyelinase

Ans. b. HGPRTase

430. **First sign of vulval cancer:**
a. Ulcerated lesion
b. Mass in the groin
c. White discharge per vaginum
d. Pruritis

Ans. d. Pruritis

431. **ATP 7A protein deficiency is found in:**
a. Minimata's disease
b. Wilson's disease
c. Hemochromatosis
d. Menke's kinky hair syndrome

Ans. d. Menke's kinky hair syndrome

432. **A patient of Maple syrup urine disease would excrete which of the following amino acid in urine?**
a. Leucine
b. Arginine
c. Phenylalanine
d. Glutamate

Ans. a. Leucine

433. **A farmer consumed some unknown poison. On examination, he was having dilated pupils and dry mouth. Which of the following is the most likely agent?**
a. Cannabis
b. Heroine
c. Cocaine
d. Dhatura

Ans. d. Dhatura

434. **A young male has consumed unknown poison. He was attended by emergency medicine physician, who noticed pin point pupils, sweating and increased saliva and tear secretion. Physician also noticed a garlic-like smell coming from the body. Which of the following drug can be used to treat such a patient?**
a. Flumazenil
b. N-acetyl-cysteine
c. Atropine
d. Deferoxamine

Ans. c. Atropine

435. **In a given case of Chronic Myelogenous Leukaemia, which of the following is the most sensitive test for monitoring treatment response?**
a. Complete blood count
b. Reverse transcriptase polymerase chain reaction (RT-PCR)
c. Fluorescence in-situ hybridization
d. Karyotyping

Ans. b. Reverse transcriptase polymerase chain reaction (RT-PCR)

436. **A young male who was riding his bike singly had a road traffic accident. He became unconscious and was taken by the local residents to a nearby hospital. Examining doctor found that this case needs an emergency operative procedure. But since the patient was not accompanied by any of his family members or friends, what the doctor should do, considering the need of emergency surgery?**
a. He must wait for family members to come before doing any surgical intervention as he had to take consent
b. Need to get consent from local police station first
c. Need to take consent of the hospital owner
d. He can do the surgery, if he feels that it is urgent, without waiting for consent

Ans. d. He can do the surgery, if he feels that it is urgent, without waiting for consent

437. **A 5-years-old male child was delivered normally at full term without any congenital anomalies. Now he is only 71% of the normal body weight for his age. On examination, he had a large and distended abdomen. He is also having dependent edema on both the lower extremities. Skin examination showed desquamation with multiple irregular areas of depigmentation and hyperpigmentation. Such a presentation indicates:**
a. Kwashiorkor
b. Marasmus
c. Rickets
d. Vitamin A deficiency

Ans. a. Kwashiorkor

438. **What is the upper age limit for prisoning in the Juvenile home (as per Indian constitution)?**
a. 14 years
b. 16 years
c. 18 years
d. 20 years

Ans. c. 18 years

439. **A 5-years-old child had frequent attacks of convulsions with unconsciousness. He had poor intake of food, loss of weight, difficulty in learning and fatigue. Urine examination showed formation of purple ring and a positive Rothera's test. Blood chemistry showed a plasma level of leucine in excess of 1000 micromoles/Litre. Such a clinical presentation is because of deficiency of:**
a. Branched chain alpha ketoacid dehydrogenase complex
b. Pyruvate dehydrogenase complex
c. Succinyl CoA thiokinase
d. Phosphofructokinase

Ans. a. Branched chain alpha ketoacid dehydrogenase complex

440. A patient had swelling in testes. What is the investigation of choice?

a. USG
b. FNAC
c. CECT scan
d. MRI

Ans. a. USG

441. A young male suffered from Covid-19 infection in 2020. Now, since last 4 months, he feels that still Covid-19 infection is continuing and he might die soon. Whenever he thinks so, he had palpitations and a fear of impending doom, lasting only for few minutes. Likely diagnosis:

a. Alzheimer's disorder
b. Bipolar disorder
c. Post-traumatic stress disorder
d. Panic disorder

Ans. d. Panic disorder

442. A 48-years-old male was a chronic alcohol drinker. He has stopped taking alcohol 3 days back. He is more likely to present with:

a. Delirium tremens
b. Hallucinosis
c. Fits
d. Unconsciousness

Ans. a. Delirium tremens

443. A young lady complains of hearing voices which usually are comments about her looks. She feels as if people are also inserting their thoughts in her mind. Most likely diagnosis:

a. Delusion
b. Mania
c. Depression
d. Schizophrenia

Ans. d. Schizophrenia

444. A farmer presented with acute intoxication of some unknown substance of abuse. He presented with arrhythmia, hypoglycemia, tremors and hyperthermia. Most likely substance is:

a. Alcohol
b. Cocaine
c. LSD
d. Amphetamine

Ans. b. Cocaine

445. A 40-years-old, widow female, staying alone, started believing that her relatives are planning to kill her, just to take her property. This is known as:

a. Persecutory delusion
b. Post-traumatic stress disorder
c. Depression
d. Mania

Ans. a. Persecutory delusion

Quick Review Points

Quick Review Points

ANATOMY

No.	Question	Answer
1.	Cholecystocaval line separates	*Right and left lobe of liver*
2.	Last fontanelle to fuse in a child	*Anterior fontanelle*
3.	Neurovascular bundle lies in which compartment of leg	*Superficial posterior*
4.	Capacitation of sperm means	*Improvement in motility for fertilization*
5.	Spring ligament is also known as	*Plantar calcaneonavicular ligament*
6 .	Right coronary artery is a branch of	*Right aortic sinus*
7.	Tensor of vocal cord	*Cricothyroid*
8.	Epithelial lining of vagina	*Squamous epithelium*
9.	Cutaneous nerve supply of medial side of leg is through	*Saphenous nerve, femoral nerve*
10.	Primary auditory area is present in which lobe	*Superior temporal gyrus*
11.	Dangerous area of face is drained by which vein	*Angular facial vein*
12.	Inferior rectal artery is a branch of	*Internal pudendal artery*
13.	Gastroduodenal artery is a branch of	*Hepatic artery*
14.	Most commonly injured ligament of knee in injury	*Medial collateral ligament*
15.	Peroneal tubercle is present on which bone	*Calcaneum*
16.	What is the level of pulmonary valve	*3rd costal cartilage*
17.	Which tendon is affected in lateral epicondylitis	*Extensor carpi radialis brevis*
18.	Action of anconeus	*Extension of elbow joint*
19.	Mastoid process is which type of epiphyses	*Traction*
20.	Only pharyngeal muscle which is innervated by glossopharyngeal nerve	*Stylopharyngeus*
21.	Lacrimation is lost in injury to which nerve	*Greater petrosal nerve*
22.	Inferior parathyroid gland develops from which pharyngeal pouch	*3rd*
23.	Carotid artery is palpated by	*Cricoid cartilage*
24.	Sensory supply of parotid gland	*Auriculotemporal nerve*
25.	Descending fibers in genu of internal capsule is	*Cortico-nuclear tract*
26.	Double aortic arch arises from	*Right 4th aortic arch*
27.	Muscle derived from third pharyngeal arch	*Stylopharyngeus*
28.	Differentiation of the genital ridge into testes occurs at	*6–10 weeks*
29.	Sweat glands are which type of glands	*Simple coiled tubular*
30.	Corpora amylacea is histological finding of	*Prostate*
31.	Ansa nephroni is lined by	*Cuboidal and squamous*
32.	Proprioception is carried by	*Fasciculus cuneatus and fasciculus gracilis*
33.	Upper 3/4th of vagina develops from	*Mullerian duct*
34.	Tensor tympani is derived from which pharyngeal arch	*1st*

PHYSIOLOGY

No.	Question	Answer
1.	Which hormone is responsible for breast cramp during breastfeeding	***Oxytocin***
2.	Ovulation occurs after .... hours of LH surge	***36***
3.	Serum calcium level in body is regulated by	***PTH, calcitonin and vitamin D***
4.	Injury to which neurological structure results in increased sexual activity, increased appetite, increased anger and absence of fear in experimental animals	***Amygdala***
5.	Which reflex is associated with both neurological and cardiovascular system	***Bezold–Jarisch reflex***
6.	Which substance is reabsorbed almost 100% in PCT	***Glucose and amino acids***
7.	Free hemoglobin molecule is not able to pass through glomerulus is because of	***Negative charge of Bowman's capsule and large molecule bounded with protein cannot pass***
8.	Effect of low dose of dopamine on renal blood vessels	***Vasodilator***
9.	In gestational life, source of surfactant	***Type II pneumocytes***
10.	Hormone secreted by parafollicular cells of thyroid	***Calcitonin***
11.	Increased pH shifts the oxygen-dissociation curve to which side	***Left***
12.	A child presented to the Pediatrics OPD with the complaints of vomiting and diarrhoea. He was given ORS. Mechanism of absorption of glucose	***Secondary active transport***
13.	Estimation of total body fat can be done by measuring	***Total body water***
14.	Nitric oxide produces its action via	***cGMP***
15.	Endothelin acts through	***IP_3-DAG system***
16.	Factor which stimulates aldosterone secretion	***Angiotensin II***
17.	Isovolumetric ventricular contraction produces which wave in jugular venous pulse	***C wave***
18.	Counter current multiplier system occurs in which part of kidney	***Loop of Henle***
19.	Glucose absorption in intestine occurs by	***Secondary active transport***
20.	Inability to identify faces is known as	***Prosopagnosia***
21.	Alpha waves on EEG are seen during	***Relaxed state and eyes closed***
22.	Which ions helps in absorption of glucose in intestine	***Sodium***
23.	Spermatozoa gets its nutrition from	***Fructose***
24.	Mullerian inhibiting substance is secreted by	***Sertoli cells***
25.	Motor aphasia is due to damage to Brodmann area	***44***
26.	Functional residual capacity is the amount of air remaining in lungs at the end of	***Normal expiration***
27.	Which segment of the nephron is also known as diluting segment	***Ascending limb of loop of Henle***
28.	Major thyroxine binding protein in serum is	***Globulin***
29.	Climbing fiber inputs in the cerebellum stimulate	***Purkinje fibers***
30.	Half-life of T_4 is	***6 days***
31.	Effect of hypovolemia on ADH	***Secretion of ADH is increased***
32.	Location of GLUT-5	***Intestine***
33.	Event occurring before start of isovolumetric contraction of ventricle	***Closure of AV valve***
34.	Contralateral loss of pain and temperature is seen in injury to which tract	***Lateral spinothalamic tract***

BIOCHEMISTRY

No.	Question	Answer
1.	A patient with intellectual disability was found to have raised serum uric acid levels. He also showed self-mutilating behaviour. Such a presentation is seen in deficiency of which enzyme	***Hypoxanthine guanine, Phosphoribosyl transferase***
2.	Amino acid excreted in urine in Maple syrup urine disease	***Leucine***
3.	Enzyme deficiency seen in Lesch-Nyhan syndrome	***HGPRTase***
4.	A 6-years-old child presented with history of frequent attacks of convulsions followed by unconsciousness. Child's food intake is poor and he is having loss of weight, fatigue and poor learning ability. Urine was found to have a burnt sugar odour. Plasma leucine concentration was more than 1100 micromoles/L. Such a presentation is seen in deficiency of which enzyme	***Branched chain alpha keto acid dehydrogenase complex***
5.	In which of the following disorder, ATP 7A is deficient	***Menke's kinky hair syndrome***
6.	A patient has macrocytic anemia and raised homocysteine levels but normal methyl malonyl CoA levels. He is having deficiency of which vitamin	B_9
7.	Bony change seen in a patient with fluorosis	***Osteosclerosis***
8.	Which metal is present in the enzyme glutathione peroxidase	***Selenium***
9.	A patient presented with fatigue and weakness. Serum iron level and hemoglobin was low. He also observed that a wound in his left leg took a long time to heal. Such a presentation is observed in deficiency of which vitamin	***Vitamin C***
10.	A patient presented with pain in right first metatarsophalangeal joint. His serum uric acid level was high. The drug which would be prescribed to such a patient would inhibit which enzyme	***Xanthine oxidase***
11.	Most sensitive test for monitoring treatment response in CML	***RT-PCR***
12.	Fat is stored in tissues as	***Triglycerides***
13.	Mechanism associated with Xeroderma pigmentosa	***Nucleotide excision repair***
14.	Enzyme deficient in Von-Gierke's disease	***Glucose-6-phosphatase***
15.	Deficiency of which vitamin results in development of neurological symptoms in an alcoholic patient	B_1
16.	Which metabolic cycle does NOT occur in muscle	***Ketosis***
17.	Sunlight helps in conversion of 7-dehydrocholesterol to	***Vitamin*** D_3 ***(Cholecalciferol)***
18.	Short chain fatty acids are absorbed in which part of gastrointestinal tract	***Large intestine***
19.	Decrease in body temperature shifts the oxygen-dissociation curve to	***Left***
20.	A person has a history of alcoholism for 25 years. He had stopped taking alcohol 48 hours back. Now he had presented with global confusion, disorientation, agitation, hallucinations, hypertension, excessive sweating and autonomic hyperactivity. Such a presentation is suggestive of the diagnosis of	***Delirium tremens***
21.	A 3-months-old male child presented with ambiguous genitalia. Blood pressure was within normal range. Dihydrotestosterone level was low. Such a presentation is associated with deficiency of which enzyme	***17-alpha-hydroxylase***
22.	Fat sugar baby is associated with	***Kwashiorkor***
23.	Glycemic index of sweet corn	***Low***
24.	Deficiency of which micronutrient is observed post-ileal resection	***Vitamin*** B_{12}
25.	A strict vegetarian presented with features of anemia. Peripheral blood smear showed hypersegmented neutrophils. Most likely diagnosis	***Megaloblastic anemia***
26.	A male presented with dermatitis, diarrhoea and dementia. Such a presentation is seen in	***Pellagra***
27.	Menke's disease is caused by deficiency of	***Copper***
28.	Cholesterol is synthesized from	***Acetyl CoA***
29.	Changes in insulin and glucagon in fed state	***Increased insulin and decreased glucagon***
30.	A patient underwent cholecystectomy. What metabolic change can be seen	***Steatorrhoea***
31.	Activity of which enzyme is low in deficiency of riboflavin	***Glutathione reductase***
32.	Creatinine, nitric oxide and urea are synthesized from which amino acid	***Arginine***
33.	Collagen defect in Menke's disease is due to defect in which enzyme	***Lysyl oxidase***
34.	Excessive ammonia is dangerous as it depletes one intermediate of Kreb's cycle. That intermediate is	***Alpha-ketoglutarate***

PATHOLOGY

No.	Question	Answer
1.	Someone working in cardboard factory is at risk of developing which pneumoconiosis	***Bagassosis***
2.	Causative agent of oral hairy leukoplakia	***Epstein–Barr virus***
3.	ATP 7A protein is deficient in	***Menke's kinky hair syndrome***
4.	An 18-years-old male has a progressively enlarging abdominal swelling with peripheral lymphadenopathy. He has night sweats, fever, weight loss of over 6 kilograms over the last few months. Genetic analysis shows t(8;14) translocation. Most likely diagnosis	***Burkitt's lymphoma***
5.	A 69-years-old male had lower back pain. Serum electrophoresis was done which showed raised level of IgG-kappa monoclonal proteins. He is anemic as well. Calcium and creatinine levels were also raised. Skull X-ray showed multiple punched out lytic lesions. Findings are suggestive of	***Multiple myeloma***
6.	Amyloid when stained with Congo red stain and visualized under polarizing microscope shows	***Apple green birefringence***
7.	Auer rods are hallmark of	***Acute myeloblastic leukemia***
8.	A young lady presented with neurological deficit and pallor. Peripheral blood smear showed hypersegmented neutrophils. Most likely diagnosis	***Vitamin B_{12} deficiency (Megaloblastic anemia)***
9.	A young male had a history of bee-sting. Now he had developed swelling over face and breathlessness. Which inflammatory mediator might have caused such a presentation	***Histamine***
10.	Takayasu arteritis type II, involve which arteries commonly	***Aortic arch and descending aorta***
11.	Malignancy commonly associated with asbestosis is	***Adenocarcinoma***
12.	A 30-years-old lady presented with thyroid swelling for the past 1 year. Histological examination showed Orphan Annie eye nuclei. Most likely diagnosis	***Papillary carcinoma of thyroid***
13.	Small or medium sized, sterile vegetations found on both sides of the heart valve seen in a known case of SLE is most likely	***Libman–Sacks endocarditis***
14.	A patient with past history of Covid-19 infection presented with headache and a black discharge from nose. Most likely diagnosis	***Mucormycosis***
15.	A tall stature male patient presented with enlargement of breast and absence of secondary sexual characters. His genetic analysis showed a Barr body. Most likely diagnosis	***Klinefelter's syndrome***
16.	An 18-years-old child presented with pain in abdomen on the left side. His father also had same problem, who later developed some gastrointestinal malignancy. Colonoscopy showed many polyps. Most likely diagnosis	***Familial adenomatous polyps***
17.	Supravital staining is used for	***Reticulocytes***
18.	A 30-years-old male presented with a painless testicular mass but normal AFP levels. Most likely diagnosis	***Seminoma***
19.	A 65-years-old male, working in dye industry for more than 35 years, presented with hematuria, increased frequency and urgency. Most likely diagnosis	***Transitional cell carcinoma***
20.	A 40-years-old male presented with swelling around the knee joint. X-ray showed soap bubble appearance and the biopsy of the bony lesion showed multiple giant cells. Most likely diagnosis	***Osteoclastoma/Giant cell tumour***
21.	Most likely diagnosis in a female with raised T3, raised T4 and low TSH	***Grave's disease***
22.	A young female had history of weight gain and constipation. There was lymphocytic infiltration in thyroid gland and anti-TPO antibodies were seen. Most likely diagnosis	***Hashimoto thyroiditis***
23.	A lady had breast carcinoma. Biopsy showed Indian file pattern. Most likely diagnosis	***Invasive lobular carcinoma***
24.	Aflatoxin is associated with development of which tumour	***Hepatocellular carcinoma***
25.	A 2-years-old child presented with recurrent episodes of diarrhoea and abdominal distension. He also had failure to thrive. Upper GI endoscopic biopsy showed villous atrophy and elongated crypts. Most likely diagnosis	***Celiac sprue***

No.	Question	Answer
26.	A female patient presented to the Medicine OPD with the clinical features of anemia. There is a past history of gastrectomy few months back. Tongue showed macroglossia. Such a presentation could be because of deficiency of	***Vitamin B_{12}***
27.	A patient is having an abdominal tumour, which on biopsy showed tissue having origin from all the three germ layers. Most likely tumour	***Teratoma***
28.	A young male was operated. After few days of surgery, there was a raised scar which was limited to suture line. This is known as	***Hypertrophic scar***
29.	Prognosis of Luminal A type of breast carcinoma	***Best prognosis***
30.	Calcitonin is secreted by which cells of thyroid gland	***Parafollicular/C cells***
31.	Mother is Rh +ve and the fetus is Rh –ve. There is Rh mismatch reaction. Coomb's test was positive. Mechanism of this type of hypersensitivity reaction in fetus	***Cytotoxic/Antigen-antibody mediated/Type II hypersensitivity reaction***
32.	A 10-years-old male child presented to the OPD with the features of anemia. There is past history of multiple blood transfusions. Peripheral blood smear showed features of microcytic and hypochromic anemia. RBC indices were Hemoglobin: 9 gm%, MCV: 70 fL, MCHC: 27 g/dL and MCH: 24 pg. Such a case is best diagnosed by	***Hemoglobin electrophoresis (Thalassemia)***
33.	A young female presented to the OPD with malar rash. She was also positive for anti-Sm antibody. Most likely diagnosis	***SLE***
34.	A 50-years-old male presented with fever, weight loss and fatigue. On examination, pallor was noted. Blood parameters showed hemoglobin: 9 g/dL, raised total lymphocyte count, myeloid cells: Less than 9% and Basophils: 4%. Such a case is usually associated with which translocation	***t(9;22) {CML}***

PHARMACOLOGY

No.	Question	Answer
1.	Anti-diabetic drug which does not require dose reduction in renal failure patient	*Linagliptin*
2.	Which anti-asthmatic drug does NOT act by causing bronchodilatation	*Hydrocortisone*
3.	An example of iron chelator	*Desferrioxamine*
4.	In a dose-response curve, if the graph of a drug is on the left-most side, it indicates it is more	*Potent*
5.	Drug of choice for mountain sickness	*Acetazolamide*
6.	Which anti-depressant drug act by inhibiting the re-uptake of both non-adrenaline and serotonin	*Venlafaxine*
7.	Fluoroquinolone contraindicated in liver disease	*Pefloxacin*
8.	Action of low levels of dopamine on renal blood flow	*Increases renal blood flow*
9.	Anti-hypertensive drug contraindicated in a patient with high serum uric acid level	*Hydrochlorothiazide*
10.	Drug used in managing anaphylactic shock	*Adrenaline*
11.	One of the longest acting phospho-di-esterase drugs	*Tadalafil*
12.	Allopurinol is used for chronic gout. Which enzyme is inhibited by allopurinol	*Xanthine oxidase*
13.	Drug of choice for invasive aspergillosis	*Voriconazole*
14.	Mechanism of action of 6-Mercaptopurine	*Inhibits DNA replication*
15.	Use of Granisetron	*Chemotherapy-induced vomiting*
16.	Drug of choice for digitalis-induced ventricular tachycardia	*Lidocaine*
17.	Mechanism of action of oseltamivir	*Neuraminidase inhibitor*
18.	Antidepressant which is selective serotonin and norepinephrine reuptake inhibitor (SSNRI)	*Duloxetine*
19.	One of the absolute contraindications to the use of oral contraceptive pills/OCPs	*Deep venous thrombosis/DVT*
20.	Antimalarial drug used for radical cure of malaria	*Primaquine*
21.	Amphotericin-B acts on	*Fungal cell membrane*
22.	Mechanism of action of muscle relaxant tizanidine	*Alpha-2 adrenergic agonist*
23.	Which anti-tubercular drug can cause peripheral neuropathy due to deficiency of pyridoxine	*INH*
24.	Colchicine acts in acute gout by inhibiting	*Leucocytic migration*
25.	Use of anti-cholinergic drug pirenzepine	*Gastric ulcer*
26.	Which drug acts primarily by reducing pre-load	*Nitroglycerine*
27.	Topical antibiotic of choice for MRSA infection	*Mupirocin*
28.	One of the contraindications of Levodopa	*Angle closure glaucoma*
29.	Mechanism of action of cyclosporine	*IL-2 transcription inhibition*
30.	One of the serious and characteristic adverse effect of Metformin	*Lactic acidosis*
31.	Antitubercular drug with prominent visual side effects	*Ethambutol*
32.	QT prolongation is caused by	*Quinidine*
33.	pKa of a drug refers to	*pH at which 50% of the drug is ionized*
34.	Cephalosporin having anti-pseudomonal activity	*Cefepime*

MICROBIOLOGY

No.	Question	Answer
1.	Gp120 is present in which virus	***HIV***
2.	A male had sudden onset of high-grade fever. He also had vomiting and headache. On clinical examination, nuchal rigidity was noticed. CSF examination was done and microscopy revealed the presence of Gram-negative bacteria. Most likely bacteria responsible for this presentation	***Neisseria meningitidis***
3.	In which sexually transmitted disease, safety pin appearance is seen under microscope	***Donovanosis (caused by Klebsiella granulomatosis)***
4.	Schizont stage is not seen in	***Plasmodium falciparum***
5.	A 35-years-old prostitute attended a pap smear camp for screening of carcinoma cervix. Her histopathology report was suggestive of dysplastic changes. Which organism is responsible for these changes	***Human papilloma virus***
6.	Causative agent of Donovanosis	***Klebsiella granulomatosis***
7.	A known patient of HIV-AIDS developed severe diarrhoea. Most likely agent responsible for this presentation	***Cryptosporidium***
8.	Vector for Zika virus	***Aedes aegypti***
9.	Sterilization of plasma is done by	***Hydrogen peroxide***
10.	Dose of Diphtheria toxin in a suspected case if diphtheria	***10,000 – 1,00,000 IU***
11.	Ziemann's stippling in infected RBCs is a feature of which species of plasmodium	***P. malariae***
12.	Acute prostatitis is commonly caused by	***Neisseria gonorrhoeae***
13.	Transfer of genetic material in transduction involves	***Bacteriophage***
14.	Sabin-Feldman dye test is used for	***Toxoplasmosis***
15.	Longest pre-erythrocytic schizogony is seen in which species of plasmodium	***P. malariae***
16.	Microbe likely to be acquired by traumatic inoculation	***Sporothrix schenkii***
17.	Immunity to a particular infectious organism after recovery from that infection is a type of	***Active adaptive immunity***
18.	Acute hemorrhagic conjunctivitis is caused by which enterovirus	***Enterovirus 70***
19.	Rubella virus belongs to which family	***Rheovirus***
20.	Which gram-negative bacillus can grow in acidic medium	***H. pylori***
21.	Superantigen is produced by	***Streptococcus pyogenes***
22.	EBV causing oral hairy leukoplakia is included in which stage of AIDS	***Stage 3***
23.	Serological test used for diagnosing leptospirosis is	***Microscopic agglutination test (MAT)***
24.	Urea breath test is used for diagnosis of	***Helicobacter pylori***
25.	Shingles is caused by	***Varicella zoster virus (VZV)***
26.	Most common complement component deficiency is	C_2
27.	Structure which helps in bacterial adhesion	***Fimbriae***
28.	Neurocysticercosis is caused by which parasite	***Cysticercosis cellulosae***
29.	Flask-shaped ulcer in intestine is caused by	***Entamoeba histolytica***
30.	Cryoglobulinemia is seen in infection with which hepatitis virus	***HCV***
31.	Treatment of choice for carriers of typhoid fever	***Ciprofloxacin***
32.	Myasthenia gravis is which type hypersensitivity reaction	***Type II***
33.	Special stain commonly used for cryptococcus	***Mucicarmine stain***
34.	Culture media used for diagnosis of EHEC O157:H7 is	***Sorbitol MacConkey media***

FORENSIC MEDICINE

No.	Question	Answer
1.	Which organism produces catecholamine storm, as seen with scorpion sting also	*Spider*
2.	A cricketer got hit by the ball over his head and he fainted. After some time, he gained consciousness but then after some time, again fainted. Such a phenomenon is suggestive of	*Extradural hemorrhage*
3.	Gender estimation in a 12-years-old child is best done by	*Pelvis (hip)*
4.	A gunshot case is brought to the forensic department for autopsy. It shows an entry wound with inverted margins, surrounded by tattooing, without burning and singeing of hairs. What is the range of firearm weapon	*Near*
5.	Which IPC is related to medical negligence	*IPC 304-A*
6.	A newly wed female committed suicide and she left a suicide note mentioning that she was tortured for dowry. Who will carry out inquest in such a case	*Magistrate*
7.	A female faked pregnancy and later on presented with a real child to blackmail her boyfriend. Such a child is known as	*Suppositious child*
8.	In case a minor is raped, what happens to hymen	*It remains intact (and deep)*
9.	Stains over clothes showed yellow coloured needle-shaped crystals. What is the nature of stain examined	*Semen*
10.	In sodomy, passive agent is labelled as catamite, when he/she is	*A young child*
11.	Difference between strangulation and hanging	*There is more extensive local damage in strangulation than hanging*
12.	The onus of proof in civil negligence case, against a doctor, lies with	*Patient*
13.	Cherry red spot inside the track of bullet is seen in which range of gunshot injury	*Contact shot*
14.	After postmortem examination of stomach, it is ......ligated	*Doubly*
15.	A man continues to make phone call to females, achieves sexual gratification by talking obscenity and sharing obscene pictures. This is known as	*Scatalogia*
16.	Hemodialysis is particularly useful in poisoning with overdose of	*Phenobarbitone*
17.	Use of Locard's exchange principle of	*Identification of rape accused*
18.	Principle of confidentiality (professional secrecy) is **NOT** applicable in	*Criminal case*
19.	On voluntary admission, the maximum number of days, a person can be admitted, as per Mental Health Care Act is	*30 days*
20.	Well-marked iliopectineal line in pelvis suggest that the pelvis is of	*Male*

PREVENTIVE AND SOCIAL MEDICINE

No.	Question	Answer
1.	Which centre is considered as the first referral centre	***Community Health Centre***
2.	Which type of surveillance is done for malaria	***Active surveillance***
3.	Definition of social blindness	***Vision of 3/60***
4.	Yellow bag biomedical waste should be disposed by	***Incineration***
5.	Most common cause of blindness among children in India	***Vitamin A deficiency***
6.	Under Ayushman package, insurance amount given to a family is	***5 lakhs/year***
7.	Which organization provides fund for TB program	***World Health Organization***
8.	Which vaccine does **NOT** follow open vial policy	***BCG***
9.	A pregnant female got infected with rubella virus at 22 weeks of pregnancy. The management of such a case	***Reassurance***
10.	Average number of children that are born to a woman during her reproductive life span is known as	***Total fertility rate (TFR)***
11.	Inter-sectoral coordination is one of the principles of	***Primary Health Care***
12.	Sullivan Index measures	***Disability rate***
13.	Most sensitive indicator of health status of a community is	***Infant mortality rate***
14.	Children welfare program is funded by	***UNICEF***
15.	Total iron requirement during the whole period of pregnancy	***1000 mg***
16.	Most important single determinant of infant mortality is	***Birth weight***
17.	Denominator in calculation of case fatality rate	***Total number of cases due to the disease concerned***
18.	Farmer's lung is caused due to the inhalation of	***Grain dust with actinomycetes***
19.	An important measure of communicability of a disease is	***Secondary attack rate***
20.	Risk of a disease is measured by	***Incidence rate***
21.	While testing a BP lowering drug, BP was measured before and after the use of the drug. Which test is best suited for this type of study	***Paired t-test***
22.	Health assistant (female) functions at the level of	***PHC***
23.	Best method of teaching villagers about how to make ORS solution	***Demonstration***
24.	Due to a measles outbreak in a community, a medical officer decided to immunize a child aged 7 months with measles vaccine. When should the next measles vaccine be given	***At the age of 9 months***
25.	Severe disease results as a result of antibody response in secondary or re-infection with some virus. Which virus is this	***Dengue virus***
26.	To control Mansonoides mosquitoes, the most effective method is	***Removal of water plants***
27.	Which vitamin can prevent hemorrhagic disease of newborn	***Vitamin K***
28.	Which fertility indicator gives the approximate magnitude of completed family size	***Total fertility rate***
29.	First step in carrying out an Adverse Events Following Immunization (AEFI)	***Confirm information in report***
30.	Most important sign in deciding severe pneumonia in a child	***Chest indrawing***
31.	What is likely diagnosis of a child who had swelling over parotid region and in scrotal area	***Mumps***
32.	How would you pictorially demonstrate a balance diet to illiterate relatives of a patient	***Pie chart***
33.	As per Factory Act, maximum working hours in a factory, per week is	***48 hours***
34.	As per MTP Act 2021, now MTP is permitted up to	***24 weeks of pregnancy***
35.	What will be the colour of the solution after adding Orthotolidine, which indicates presence of free chlorine	***Yellow***
36.	A person was exclusively fed on maize. Now he presents with diarrhoea, dermatitis and some mental issue. Most likely diagnosis	***Pellagra***
37.	A patient is showing resistance to Isoniazid, Rifampicin, Ofloxacin and Kanamycin. Such a resistance is known as	***Extensive drug resistance (XDR)***

No.	Question	Answer
38.	What study design is best to study the incidence of ear problem in members of a Band party	*Cohort*
39.	Caisson's disease is usually seen in which workers	*Construction workers under sea level*
40.	A person presented with bleeding from gums. Which vitamin deficiency is most likely	*Vitamin C*
41.	Sodium content of loaf of bread	*1.13 g/100 gram*
42.	What is the colour code of the STD kit used for treating a female presenting to STD clinical with lower abdominal pain and discharge per vaginum	*Yellow (Kit-6)*
43.	What dose of folic acid should be given to pregnant women, who had a past history of a baby with neural tube defect	*4 mg*
44.	Condition which can be screened during neonatal screening by biochemical tests	*Congenital hypothyroidism*
45.	What is the oral dose of vitamin A for a 12-months-old child weighing less than 8 kilogram and showing signs of malnutrition and vitamin A deficiency	*1 Lakh IU*
46.	A married couple has 1 child in the family. Such a pair belong to which phase of family cycle	*Formation*
47.	Minimum number of antenatal visits as per WHO	*4*
48.	Who have the responsibility of data collection for active malaria surveillance at PHC level	*Medical Officer-PHC*
49.	Number of maternal deaths (due to pregnancy-related causes) divided by 1,00,000 live births is known as	*Maternal mortality ratio*
50.	Manual Vacuum Aspiration (MVA) is introduced in primary health centres as it helps in reducing	*Maternal mortality*
51.	Agreement (yes/ no) between two observers is statistically measured by	*Kappa coefficient*
52.	What was the duration of quarantine for ship sailors during Plague outbreak in 14th century	*40 days*
53.	How much land area is needed per year to construct trench method sanitary landfill pit with a depth of 2 meters for a village of 10,000 population	*1 acre*
54.	How many post-natal visits should be made by the ANM to the house of a low-birth-weight baby	*6*
55.	Which type of screening method is least useful	*Mass screening*
56.	Indicator for evaluation of impact of family planning	*Family size*
57.	Test applied to compare mean hemoglobin level of two groups of antenatal mothers	*Unpaired t-test*
58.	Chemoprophylactic agent of choice for health care personnel and close contacts of suspected/confirmed case of pandemic influenza A (H1N1)	*Oseltamivir*
59.	Glycemic index of sweet corn	*53*
60.	A female of 30 years, educated till 9th class, of divorced status having good communication skills is eligible to work as ...... in her village	*ASHA (Accredited Social Health Activist)*
61.	Burden of disease in a community is best described by	*DALY*
62.	Recommended site for immunization with hepatitis B vaccine in young children, for ensuring reliable absorption	*Deltoid region*
63.	Government of India provides kit for home-based pregnancy test. The name of the kit is	*NISCHAY*
64.	Vaccine Associated Paralytic Poliomyelitis/VAPP is mostly observed due to which isolate type strain of polio virus	*Type-3*
65.	Association between hardness of drinking water and death rate from cardiovascular disease	*Inverse*
66.	Number of antenatal mothers included in focal group discussion by a medical officer of PHC	*6–12*
67.	Oil containing high mono-unsaturated fatty acid and moderate linoleic acid	*Groundnut oil*
68.	Deficiency of which trace element in diet results in low birthweight, preterm delivery, spontaneous absorption or even congenital malformation like anencephaly	*Zinc*
69.	A contraindication for BCG vaccination in a new born	*HIV infection—symptomatic*
70.	Which coloured bag is used to dispose cotton swab contaminated with patient's blood	*Yellow*

EAR, NOSE AND THROAT

No.	Question	Answer
1.	An old diabetic patient with poor sugar control had nasal congestion and fever. He also had headache on right side. Later on, he developed numbness and pain on face. Blackish discharge was noticed from the nasal cavity. Findings are suggestive of	***Mucormycosis***
2.	A 65-years-old diabetic woman had foul smelling discharge from the ear, which is greenish black in colour. She is also having fever and itching in the external auditory canal. Most likely diagnosis	***Malignant otitis externa***
3.	Most common cause of acute epiglottitis	***Hemophilus influenzae type B***
4.	A 15-years-old boy had sore throat accompanied by fever, difficulty in swallowing and muffled voice. Lateral X-ray of the neck region showed thumb sign. Most likely diagnosis	***Epiglottitis***
5.	Most common cause of inspiratory stridor in children	***Laryngomalacia***
6.	Brown sign is seen in	***Glomus tumour***
7.	Most common malignant tumour of parotid gland	***Mucoepidermoid cancer***
8.	Edema over mastoid process is seen in	***Lateral sinus thrombophlebitis***
9.	Picket fence fever is a feature of	***Lateral sinus thrombophlebitis***
10.	Tripod fracture is seen in which bone	***Zygoma***
11.	Another term for Schwartz operation	***Simple mastoidectomy***
12.	Type of voice in antrochoanal polyp	***Hyponasal voice***
13.	Facial nerve lies with which other nerve in internal auditory meatus	***Vestibulocochlear nerve***
14.	Passavant's ridge is formed by	***Palatopharyngeus and superior constrictor***
15.	Recruitment is seen in which type of hearing loss	***Cochlear sensorineural hearing loss***
16.	A 25-years-old male after adenoidectomy developed hypernasality, difficulty in chewing and swallowing. Most likely reason	***Velopharyngeal insufficiency***
17.	Treatment of choice for nasal synechiae	***Surgical removal of adhesions***
18.	Clinical sign seen in thrombosis of mastoid emissary veins	***Griesinger's sign***
19.	Radiologically, which paranasal air sinus appears last	***Frontal sinus***
20.	A 53-years-old male complain of pain around his cheek and neck. On examination, there is pus pouring out from Stenson's duct. Most likely involved gland is	***Parotid gland***
21.	Pott's puffy tumour is	***Osteomyelitis/subperiosteal abscess of frontal bone***
22.	In cold caloric stimulation test, cold water induces movement of the eyeball in which direction	***Towards the opposite side***
23.	Embryological basis of pre-auricular sinus	***Develops due to faulty fusion between hillocks of first and second pharyngeal arches***
24.	Location of organ of Corti	***Membranous labyrinth***
25.	Another name of oral thrush	***Candidiasis***
26.	Most common cause of trigeminal neuralgia	***Vascular compression***
27.	Mini tracheostomy is performed through which structure	***Cricothyroid membrane***
28.	Turban epiglottitis is a clinical finding of	***Tubercular laryngitis***
29.	Positive head impulse test is suggestive of	***Injury to peripheral vestibular nerve***
30.	Inspiratory stridor is usually found in disease, which are ...... the level of vocal cord	***Above (supraglottic)***

OPHTHALMOLOGY

No.	Question	Answer
1.	Cobblestone papilla is a feature of	***Vernal keratoconjunctivitis***
2.	Best management for a diabetic patient presenting with visual loss and hemorrhage, exudates and new vessels formation of fundus examination	***Pan retinal photocoagulation***
3.	A 3-months-old female was brought to the Ophthalmology OPD with the complaints of excessive watering from right eye. Initial treatment of such a case	***Lacrimal sac massaging***
4.	Management of Pterygium	***Conjunctival limbal graft***
5.	A 45-years-old farmer presented to the Ophthalmology OPD with complains of redness and discharge from eye. Ophthalmological examination revealed dry and rough ulcers with unsterile hypopyon and satellite nodules. Most common organism implicated in such a clinical condition	***Aspergillus fumigatus***
6.	One of the best ways of treating amblyopia	***Occlusion of the normal eye***
7.	Posterior cerebral artery lesion may lead to which type of visual field defect	***Homonymous hemianopia with macular sparing***
8.	A 6-years-old child has ptosis in left eye, which corrects on eating food. Most likely diagnosis	***Marcus Gunn Jaw winking syndrome***
9.	Vossius ring is seen in	***Blunt injury***
10.	Type of refractive error seen in keratoconus	***Irregular astigmatism***
11.	Muscae volitantes is seen in	***Remains of primitive hyaloid vasculature***
12.	Uveitis as a result of lens tissue-induced inflammation following cataract surgery is known as	***Phacoanaphylactic uveitis***
13.	Most common age-related change in vitreous	***Posterior vitreous detachment***
14.	Rigid gas permeable lens is made up of	***Copolymer of PMMA, silicon containing monomer and cellulose acetyl butyrate***
15.	Antiglaucoma drug that needs to be avoided in hypertensives is	***Apraclonidine***
16.	Which instrument uses the principle of total internal reflection	***Ophthalmoscope***
17.	Keratic precipitates are most commonly seen in	***Uveitis***
18.	Unilateral frontal blisters with upper lid edema and conjunctivitis are seen in	***Herpes zoster ophthalmicus***
19.	Correct power of a pair of glasses is checked by	***Lensometer***
20.	Zonules suspending the lens are attached to	***Ciliary body***
21.	Purtscher's retinopathy is associated with	***Head trauma***
22.	Diplopia in left gaze is a manifestation of paralysis of	***Sixth cranial nerve of left side***
23.	In case of myopia, LASIK will provide correction up to	***12D***
24.	Most common site of anterior staphyloma	***Corneal ulcer***
25.	Most powerful refractory surface of eye	***Cornea***
26.	Muscarinic agonist used in the treatment of angle closure glaucoma	***Pilocarpine***
27.	A child had unilateral proptosis and restricted movements of the eye on the same side. Ophthalmologist noticed chemosis as well. Most likely diagnosis	***Orbital cellulitis***
28.	Haab's striae is a feature of	***Buphthalmos***
29.	Collection of emulsified silicon oil in anterior chamber is known as	***Reverse hypopyon***
30.	Silk retina is a feature of	***Hypermetropia***

MEDICINE

No.	Question	Answer
1.	HFE gene mutation is associated with which condition	***Hemochromatosis***
2.	A 12-years-child presented with facial puffiness and cola-coloured urine. The child was hypertensive. Microscopic examination of urine showed proteinuria and hematuria. Most likely diagnosis	***Post-streptococcal glomerulonephritis (PSGN)***
3.	A masonry worker presented with the complaints of chest tightness and difficulty in breathing. He is also a patient of tuberculosis. Most likely condition	***Silicosis***
4.	Early inflammatory cells in acute inflammation are	***Neutrophils***
5.	A young male was having testicular tumour which was OCT-4 positive. What type of tumour is this	***Seminoma***
6.	A young male had a history of bee-sting. Now he had developed swelling and redness over face and breathlessness. Which type of antibody might have caused such a presentation	***IgE***
7.	An old female, a known case of urinary bladder carcinoma was planned for radiotherapy. Which pelvic structures would be affected most by radiation	***Ovary***
8.	Function of selectin	***Adhesion of leucocyte to the endothelium***
9.	Tetralogy of Fallot is most commonly associated with which aneuploidy	***Down syndrome***
10.	Ileal resection will affect absorption of	***Vitamin B_{12}***
11.	An elderly male presented to the OPD with fatigue, weight loss, pallor and fever. Laboratory report shows hemoglobin: 8.5 gm%, TLC: 17,000/cmm, Basophils: 4%, Myeloid blasts: Less than 10 and a platelet count of 1,60,000/cmm. Most likely diagnosis	***CML***
12.	An elderly male presented to the OPD with fatigue, weight loss, pallor and fever. Laboratory report shows hemoglobin: 7.5 gm%, TLC: 2,900/cmm and a platelet count of 90,000/cmm. There was no associated hepatosplenomegaly. Most likely diagnosis	***Aplastic anemia***
13.	A child has presented with pain in abdomen, joint pains and rash on lower limbs. He is also having hematuria. Platelet count was normal. Most likely diagnosis	***Henoch–Schonlein purpura***
14.	A patient having jaundice, pruritis, tremors and mood changes, is found to have Kayser–Fleischer rings in the eyes. Most likely diagnosis	***Wilson disease***
15.	Single lead pacemaker connects to which chamber of the heart	***Right ventricle***
16.	Which is the most sensitive test for monitoring treatment response in CML	***Reverse transcriptase PCR test***
17.	A 35-years-old female presented with fatigue and weakness in limbs. Symptoms were more pronounced in the evening time. When she was given Edrophonium, she felt better and her symptoms improved. Findings are consistent with the diagnosis of	***Myasthenia gravis***
18.	A 65-years-old diabetic patient was admitted to the hospital with the complaints of fever and breathlessness. Few days later, he developed periorbital puffiness and pain. It was also noticed that there is some black colour growth in the nasal cavities and around the orbital cavity. Most likely diagnosis	***Mucormycosis***
19.	Type of tremor seen in Wilson disease	***Wing beat tremor***
20.	Best management of empyema thoracis	***Chest drainage and antibiotic coverage***
21.	A person had a history of visit to China. Now he had fever, cough and body ache for 7 days. Recently he developed dyspnea and his SpO_2 is found to be less than 90. Which test should be done to make a diagnosis	***RT-PCR***
22.	A young lady presented to Medicine OPD with complaints of weakness and easy fatiguability. Pallor was present. Her nails were spoon-shaped. She had a hemoglobin value of 6.5 gm/dL. Most likely diagnosis	***Iron deficiency anemia***
23.	A 12-years-old boy from Nigeria presented with progressive intra-abdominal mass and enlargement of peripheral lymph nodes. He also had fever and sweating at night. He also had lost around 7 kg weight in last 7 months. Biopsy of the lymph node was done and it showed starry sky appearance. Findings are suggestive of	***Burkitt's lymphoma***
24.	A young female presented to the Medicine OPD with the complaints of fatigue, restlessness and inability to concentrate in work. She also had pallor but there was no neurological deficit. Blood tests revealed a decreased hemoglobin, increased homocysteine and increased MCV levels. Methyl malonic acid level is normal. What should be given to such a patient	***Folic acid***

No.	Question	Answer
25.	A lady with fever and rashes was found to have small, warty vegetations on either side of the heart valves. There is no history of fever. ESR was raised. Most likely diagnosis	*Libman–Sacks endocarditis*
26.	Antidote for acute iron poisoning	*Desferroxamine*
27.	Edrophonium test is done for	*Myasthenia gravis*
28.	A young male presented to the Endocrinology clinic with the complaints of gain in weight and lethargy. He also had intolerance to cold. Most likely diagnosis	*Hypothyroidism*
29.	A 30-years-old lady presented to Medicine OPD with complaints of tingling and burning sensation in both the lower limbs. She also felt as if she is having difficulty in walking. She was also having pallor. Neurological examination demonstrated that she had loss of vibration sense and proprioception in both the lower limbs. Findings are suggestive of deficiency of which vitamin	*Vitamin B_{12}*
30.	Treatment of Falciparum malaria	*Artemether + Primaquine + Lumifantrine*
31.	A patient in ICU had developed shortness of breath, which is not responding to oxygen therapy. Most likely diagnosis	*Atelectasis*
32.	Drug used in managing digoxin-induced ventricular arrhythmia	*Lidocaine*
33.	Management of constrictive pericarditis	*Pericardial stripping*
34.	A patient had many episodes of vomiting. This might lead to	*Metabolic alkalosis*
35.	A 60-years-old male presented to the Medicine OPD with the complains of weight loss and fatigue. He is also having discomfort in the left upper quadrant of the abdomen for the past 9 months. Per-abdomen examination revealed an enlarged spleen. Blood tests showed a hemoglobin of 8.9 gm%, TLC of 4.6 lakhs/mm^3 with DLC showing 7% basophils and a platelet count of 5.1 lakhs/mm^3. Peripheral blood smear showed blast forms, metamyelocytes and promyelocytes. Most likely diagnosis:	*Chronic myelogenous leukemia*
36.	Locked-in state is characterized by	*Paralysis of all voluntary muscles except ocular muscles*
37.	Complication of diabetes which can not be prevented by strict control of blood sugar	*Macular edema*
38.	Most reliable investigation in amyloid disease is	*Abdominal fat pad biopsy*
39.	Shelf-life of blood in blood bank in CPDA buffer is	*35 days*
40.	An obese patient presented in casualty with random blood sugar of 400 mg%, urine sugar +++ and ketone bodies 1+. Drug useful in managing such a case	*Insulin*
41.	Which antibody correlates with disease activity in SLE	*Anti-dsDNA*
42.	Contractile dysfunction is the dominant feature of which type of cardiomyopathy	*Dilated cardiomyopathy*
43.	A patient presents with recurrent episodes of sharp pain over his right cheek that is precipitated on chewing, between attacks, patient is otherwise normal. Most likely diagnosis	*Trigeminal neuralgia*
44.	Pressure difference of 5 mm Hg between the two upper limbs is seen in which congenital heart disease	*Supravalvular aortic stenosis*
45.	A male presents with headache, profuse sweating and palpitations with a BP of 180/120 mm Hg. Drug of choice in such a case	*Phenoxybenzamine (for pheochromocytoma)*
46.	Most suitable drug for a 45-years-old diabetic patient with BP of 150/94 mm Hg	*Lisinopril*
47.	Which factor can differentiate primary polycythemia from secondary polycythemia	*Arterial oxygen tension <90% on room air*
48.	An adult patient presents with normal to enlarged kidneys with massive proteinuria. Most likely diagnosis	*Amyloidosis*
49.	Treatment of choice in a patient with massive pulmonary embolism in shock is	*Thrombolytic therapy*
50.	Number of café au lait spots as one of the diagnostic criteria for adult neurofibromatosis	*>6*
51.	Which ECG lead is most sensitive in determining intra-operative myocardial ischemia	*Lead V_5*
52.	The term 'ragged red fibers' is applied to describe the skeletal muscle fibers in	*Mitochondrial myopathy*
53.	Oral anti-diabetic drug of choice in a diabetic patient with renal failure	*Glipizide*
54.	Dose of streptokinase to be used in MI	*1.5 million units*

No.	Question	Answer
55.	First drug to be started in Sheehan's syndrome	***Corticosteroids***
56.	Initial treatment recommended for newly diagnosed patient with CML	***Imatinib mesylate therapy***
57.	Initial treatment of tumour lysis syndrome	***Allopurinol + Hydration + Potassium binder + Alkalinization***
58.	Steroids are prescribed in rheumatic fever if there is development of	***Carditis***
59.	Dementia in a patient of chronic renal failure with chronic haemodialysis is due to	***Aluminum toxicity***
60.	Osmotic demyelination syndrome develops due to rapid correction of hyponatremia at a level exceeding	***0.5 mEq/hour***
61.	Both PT and aPTT are prolonged in deficiency of clotting factor	***II***
62.	Presence of erythematous flat-topped papules over knuckle (Gottron's sign) is a characteristic finding of	***Dermatomyositis***
63.	Test predicting the return of renal function in a patient with tumour lysis syndrome	***Serum uric acid***
64.	Most common antecedent infection associated with Guillain–Barre syndrome	***Campylobacter jejuni***
65.	Most common presentation of sick euthyroid state	***Low T3 and normal T4***
66.	Recurrent spontaneous hemarthrosis is commonly seen in patients with hemophilia when factor VIII levels are below	***5%***
67.	Most common initial presenting feature of multiple sclerosis	***Optic neuritis***
68.	An 18-years-old male presented with acute onset of history of blurring of vision. Patient also had quadriparesis and areflexia. Both the pupils are non-reactive. Most likely diagnosis	***Botulism***
69.	A patient with hypertension presents with hypokalemia. Aldosterone level and renin level both were elevated. Most likely diagnosis	***Renal artery stenosis***
70.	Initial anti-hypertensive agent of choice in a patient with stable ischemic heart disease	***Beta-blockers***

SURGERY

No.	Question	Answers
1.	Multicentric and bilateral type of breast carcinoma	***Lobular***
2.	A 32-years-old female had a slow-growing thyroid swelling for the last 1 year. Surgeon performed FNAC of the swelling. Histopathology report of the swelling showed Orphan Annie eyed nuclei. Most probable variety of thyroid carcinoma	***Papillary carcinoma of thyroid***
3.	Most common location of carcinoma breast	***Upper outer quadrant***
4.	Respiratory distress, scaphoid abdomen and mediastinal shift suggest the diagnosis of:	***Congenital diaphragmatic hernia***
5.	Peau'd Orange suggest which stage of carcinoma breast	***Stage 4B***
6.	A 60-years-old male had painless hematuria and pain in lumbar region. Most likely diagnosis	***Renal cell carcinoma***
7.	Non-small cell carcinoma of lung 3 cm lesion is best managed by	***Surgery alone***
8.	6 weeks, post-burn, now patient is posted for surgery. Increased potassium intraoperatively may be due to	***Succinylcholine***
9.	Open biopsy is done for salivary gland tumours unless they are arising from	***Parotid gland***
10.	What could be the most probable diagnosis of an elderly male patient presenting to the Surgery OPD with low back pain and sclerotic lesions in lumbar vertebrae	***Carcinoma prostate***
11.	A young male had a road traffic accident (RTA), and had raised intracranial tension but without cerebral hemorrhage. Which drug is useful in managing such a case	***Mannitol***
12.	A 78-years-old male known case of prostate cancer is having multiple painful vertebral metastasis. Ideal management of such a case	***Androgen ablation with orchidectomy***
13.	A 19-years-old girl sustained blunt abdominal trauma. She is diagnosed of having splenic rupture. Her pulse is 110/minute and BP is normal. She is having a respiratory rate of 22/minute. She is anxious also. Her approximate blood loss is	***750–1500 mL***
14.	A case of polytrauma with blunt abdominal injury presents to the casualty. The first investigation to evaluate his abdomen is	***USG***
15.	A young female presented to the surgery OPD with the complaint of painless enlargement of the thyroid for the past 7 months. She is also having tiredness, hair loss, cold intolerance and fatigue since last 7 months. She also informed that she had gained more than 10 kg weight in the past 7 months. Blood test showed a low T3 and T4 value and raised TSH. TPO antibodies were also demonstrated. Most likely diagnosis:	***Hashimoto's disease***
16.	Positive Homan's sign is seen in	***Deep venous thrombosis***
17.	A known alcoholic presents to the emergency department with hematemesis. On examination, he has ascites and splenomegaly and gynecomastia. Most likely diagnosis	***Portal hypertension due to alcoholic cirrhosis***
18.	An employee of dye industry presented to the Surgery OPD with symptoms of painless hematuria along with frequency and urgency. Cystoscopy revealed a urinary bladder mass. What could be the most likely pathology	***Transitional cell carcinoma of urinary bladder***
19.	A 27-years-old lady having a 3-months-old child presented to the Surgery OPD with complaints of breast pain. She was also having fever with chills. On examination, swelling and redness was noticed. Most likely diagnosis	***Breast abscess or mastitis***
20.	A 34-years-old male presented to the Surgery OPD with the complaints of a painless testicular tumour. Blood tests revealed a normal beta-HCG and increased LDH levels and was managed by orchidectomy. Most likely diagnosis	***Seminoma testis***
21.	A 22-years-old female with blunt injury to her head and face presents with subconjunctival hemorrhage. Posterior media was not visible. Likely cause	***Zygomatic and orbital blow out fracture***
22.	Most common immune-suppressant regime used in renal transplant for maintenance	***Calcineurin inhibitors + Purine antagonists + Glucocorticoids***
23.	BI-RADS score is designed to	***Maintain uniformity in the reporting of imaging findings of various breast diseases***
24.	A 57-years-old male suffering from acute pancreatitis develops sudden onset of breathlessness with a CVP <18 mm Hg. The chest X-ray shows bilateral infiltrates. The possible diagnosis is	***ARDS***

No.	Question	Answers
25.	A 70-years-old male, chronic smoker is having carcinoma in situ of urinary bladder. TUR is done. Now there is recurrence with the tumour extending into the muscle. Treatment of such a case	*Radical cystectomy*
26.	A 24-years-old female, with suspected appendicitis is taken up for surgery. However, during surgery, the appendix appears to be normal. Instead, the ileum is inflamed, enlarged with multiple adhesions. Surrounding flat is also involved. Most likely diagnosis	*Ileocecal TB*
27.	A 40-years-old woman undergoing laparoscopic cholecystectomy is found to have a mass suspicious of carcinoma gallbladder. It appears to have permeated through the entire thickness but there is no involvement of overlying serosa. Next surgical step would be	*Extended cholecystectomy*
28.	Transplantation of an organ at site other than its original site is known as	*Heterotopic graft*
29.	In a post-menopausal woman with ER positive breast carcinoma, most appropriate drug would be	*Aromatase inhibitor*
30.	A 40-years-old male with chest trauma presents with breathlessness, decreased respiratory sounds on the right side, hyper-resonance on percussion and distended neck veins. Most likely diagnosis	*Tension pneumothorax*
31.	A 40-years-old male presented with a penetrating trauma to chest. He is dyspneic with distended neck veins with hypotension and mediastinum is shifted to opposite side. There is a sucking wound over the chest. Most appropriate management would be	*Insertion of a large bore needle in the 2nd intercostal space in the mid-clavicular line*
32.	A 45-years-female underwent modified radical mastectomy with axillary clearance for carcinoma breast. After surgery, she could not lift her arm above head. Which nerve is likely to be injured	*Long thoracic nerve of Bell*
33.	A 45-years-old male is diagnosed with carcinoma penis. The surgeon must look out for which lymph nodes	*Inguinal*
34.	A 70-years-old male chronic smoker is diagnosed of having cancer of urinary bladder. It is confined to the trigone of bladder and is extending up to the submucosa. Management of such a case	*Complete transurethral resection with intravesical chemotherapy*
35.	A 45-years-old male presenting with penile cancer extending up to the glans penis is treated with	*Partial penectomy with 2 cm margin*
36.	A 29-years-male complains of pain in the flank that radiates from the loin to the groin region. The first investigation to be done is	*Plain CT scan*
37.	A young male presents with a testicular mass on the right side. AFP is elevated while the HCG is normal. Most appropriate next step is	*USG*
38.	Prostate cancer that is limited to the capsule and not involving the urethra is staged as	*T2*
39.	A 60-years-old alcoholic who sustained blunt trauma to his head due to assault appears confused. He opens his eyes and speaks incomprehensible words on when the sternum is pressed. He withdraws his hand when approached. His Glasgow Coma Score is	*8*
40.	In case of polytrauma with multiple injuries to the chest, neck and abdomen, highest priority is given to	*Stabilization of the cervical spine*
41.	A 54-years-old woman is diagnosed as having carcinoma of the renal pelvis of size less than 4 cm without any metastasis. Best treatment option is	*Partial nephrectomy*
42.	A patient presents with difficulty in swallowing liquids but not solids. Best investigation to make a diagnosis	*Manometry (for achalasia cardia)*
43.	A 78-years-old male presents with jaundice associated with increased itching and a palpable gallbladder. Most likely diagnosis	*Peri-ampullary carcinoma*
44.	Most tissue reaction is seen with which type of suture	*Silk*
45.	What is the most common malignant tumour of parotid gland	*Mucoepidermoid carcinoma*
46.	Best investigation to visualize posterior urethra is	*Cystoscopy*
47.	Most common infantile tumour is	*Teratoma*
48.	Mode of healing of a incisional wound	*Primary healing*
49.	Most common type of bladder rupture is	*Extra-peritoneal*
50.	Battle's sign is	*Ecchymosis over the mastoid*

No.	Question	Answers
51.	Paraneoplastic syndrome manifestation of small carcinoma of lung	***Secretion of ACTH***
52.	Significance of hepatorenal pouch of Morrison	***It is the most dependent space in the abdomen and fluid from ascites first accumulates here***
53.	Treatment of choice for carcinoma head of pancreas	***Whipple's surgery***
54.	Most common complication of siding hernia	***Esophagitis due to continuous reflux***
55.	During renal transplantation, the renal vein is connected to	***External iliac vein***
56.	Best investigation for prostate cancer	***PSA velocity***
57.	Nerve of Latarjet is spared in which type of vagotomy	***Highly selective vagotomy***
58.	Full form of ATLS	***Advanced trauma life support***
59.	Needle for thoracocentesis is inserted most commonly at	***5th intercostal space in the midaxillary line***
60.	A 4-years-old child presents with shock and circulatory collapse. It is not possible to get intravenous access. What should be done	***Intraosseous cannulation***
61.	What is addressed first in a case of polytrauma	***Airway***
62.	What is flail chest	***Fracture of three or more ribs at 2 or more places***
63.	Venous embolism during craniotomy occurs most commonly in which position	***Sitting***
64.	Most common pituitary adenoma is	***Prolactinoma***
65.	The term universal tumour refers to	***Lipoma***
66.	Recurrent infection of urinary bladder leads to which type of malignancy	***Squamous cell carcinoma***
67.	Management of Barrett's esophagus	***Endoscopy and biopsy at regular intervals***
68.	What is Cock's peculiar tumour	***Ulceration of sebaceous cyst on the scalp***
69.	Most common CNS tumour in adults	***Metastasis***
70.	Cyst coming from an unerupted tooth	***Dentigerous cyst***

OBSTETRICS

No.	Question	Answer
1.	Components of HELLP syndrome	***Hemolysis, elevated liver enzymes and low platelets (thrombocytopenia)***
2.	A 28-years-old lady with $G_3P_0A_2L_0$ is having 19 weeks pregnancy. She presented to the antenatal centre for her second trimester check-up. Obstetrician performed per vagina examination and found that the length of cervix is only 18 mm. What could be the most probable reason for her previous 2 abortions	***Short length of cervix***
3.	A 32-years-old chronic smoker lady with 37 weeks pregnancy presented to the labor room with abdominal pain and bleeding per vaginum. On examination, her blood pressure was 154/102 mm Hg. Per abdominal examination revealed a tender-abdomen and fetal parts were felt superficially. Fetal heart sounds were not heard. Findings are consistent with the diagnosis of	***Accidental hemorrhage/Abruptio placentae***
4.	Most common cause of late post-partum hemorrhage in clinical practice	***Uterine atony***
5.	21-years-old primigravida was detected to have low amniotic fluid on routine USG. What could be the commonest cause for this low amniotic fluid	***Fetal renal dysfunction***
6.	24-years-old G_1P_1 lady presented with the complaints of crampy abdominal pain and hypomenorrhoea. She had a previous history of Dilatation and Curettage. Moreover after her first child, she had 2 pregnancies but they aborted. Most likely diagnosis	***Asherman syndrome***
7	20-years-old, primigravida is in labor and the fetus is in occipito-posterior position. All attempts to change the position of the head failed. Such type of failure of manipulation is encountered most commonly in which type of female pelvis	***Anthropoid***
8.	A young female patient was on warfarin therapy but during the course of the treatment, she became pregnant. What advice should be given to this lady now about her warfarin therapy	***Stop warfarin and start heparin***
9.	Which drug, if given to pregnant lady, can cause Ebstein's anomaly in fetus	***Lithium***
10.	A young woman is married last year. Now she presented to the Obstetrics department with the complaints of amenorrhoea since last 2 months. What investigation should be offered early	***Urinary pregnancy test***
11.	19-years-old primigravida, residing in a far village went into labor. Delivery was conducted by Trained Birth Dai in the village. But after delivery of the baby, the lady has severe bleeding and she went into shock after which she died. Most probable cause of her death	***Uterine inversion***
12.	Presence of two fetus in a womb of different age is known as	***Superfetation***
13.	What could be the effect on mother, if injection Oxytocin is given as a bolus rather than infusion during labor	***Hypotension***
14.	Which vaccine should NOT be given to a pregnant lady	***Measles (live vaccine)***
15.	Engaging diameter in brow presentation	***Mento-vertical***
16.	In cervical incompetence, diameter of internal os of cervix is	***1 cm***
17.	Maximum duration of ectopic pregnancy is seen in	***Ampulla***
18.	Lovset's manoeuvre is done for	***Extended arm***
19.	Crowning means	***Biparietal diameter at the vulval outlet***
20.	Quickening in multipara is felt at what period of gestation	***16 weeks***
21.	Most common presentation in twin pregnancy	***Both vertex***
22.	Plane of cleavage during placental separation runs through	***Deep spongy layer of decidua basalis***
23.	Following delivery, tear involves perineum and external anal sphincter with intact mucosa. Degree of tear is	***Third degree***
24.	There is overlapping of skull sutures which can be reduced with gentle pressure. What is the grade of moulding	***Grade 2***
25.	Vasa previa is associated with which type of placental anomaly	***Velamentous placenta***
26.	Engaging diameter of well-flexed head in vertex presentation is	***Suboccipitobregmatic***
27.	Mother with chicken pox, delivers after 2 weeks if acquisition. What intervention is necessary for the new born	***Varicella zoster immunoglobulin***
28.	Confirmation of cervical pregnancy is done by	***Histology (showing presence of villi inside the cervical stroma)***
29.	Maximum chances of amniotic fluid embolism are seen at	***Labor***
30.	In pregnant females, surgery for heart disease like mitral stenosis is to be performed at	***14–16 weeks***

GYNECOLOGY

No.	Question	Answer
1.	Bartholin cyst is best managed by	*Marsupialization*
2.	Most of the fibromas are initially	*Intramural/Interstitial*
3.	Best management for carcinoma cervix stage 3B	*Neoadjuvant chemotherapy followed by radiation or surgery*
4.	25-years-old G_1P_1 presented to the Gynecology department with 6 months amenorrhoea. She had a child of 6 months also. Most likely reason for this amenorrhoea	*Hyperprolactinemia*
5.	A 32-years-old lady is not interested in keeping the IUCD anymore. She decided to go for IUCD removal. But it was found to be missing on USG. Which investigation can help in removal of IUCD	*Hysteroscopy*
6.	Most cost-effective method of screening for carcinoma of cervix is	*Pap smear*
7.	A 23-years-old lady attended Gynecology OPD with complaints of amenorrhoea for last 8 months. Ratio of LH:FSH was found to be elevated. Most likely diagnosis	*Polycystic ovarian syndrome*
8.	Endometrial repair after menstrual bleeding is under the influence of which hormone	*Estrogen*
9.	Which fibroid is commonly associated with inversion of uterus	*Submucosal fundal fibroid with sarcomatous change*
10.	Ideal treatment of imperforate hymen	*Cruciate incision*
11.	Method employed to differentiate between acute pelvic inflammatory disease and ectopic gestation	*Laparoscopic examination*
12.	Emergency contraception should be started with in how many hours of unprotected intercourse	*72 hours*
13.	Young woman presents with low back pain, fever and leucocytosis. She was having last menstrual period (LMP) 2 weeks back. Likely diagnosis	*Mittelschmerz*
14.	Woman presents with 6 weeks amenorrhoea and bleeding per vaginum. What is the screening test for this case	*Urine pregnancy test*
15.	Source of anti-mullerian hormone	*Sertoli cells, Granulosa cells*
16.	Primary amenorrhoea refers to failure of menstruation beyond the age of	*16 years*
17.	Most common tumour associated with delayed puberty	*Craniopharyngioma*
18.	Mifepristone is used as abortifacient till	*9 weeks*
19.	Staging of cervical cancer is mainly by	*Clinical staging*
20.	Which hormone is increased in premature ovarian failure	*Serum FSH*
21.	Primary amenorrhoea, absent uterus and normal pubic hairs. Likely diagnosis	*Mullerian agenesis*
22	40 years female with abnormal cervical cytology. Pap smear is suggesting CIN III. Next step in management	*Colposcopy and biopsy*
23	Condition presenting with greenish discharge per vaginum	*Trichomoniasis*
24	Lowermost amount of estrogen in OCP	*20 micrograms*
25	LeFort repair is done for	*Uterovaginal descent*
26	Krukenberg tumour is	*Metastatic ovarian tumour*
27	Ectopic endometrial glands within the myometrium	*Adenomyosis*
28	Management of Theca lutein cyst	*Spontaneous regression once the underlying cause is treated*
29	Both uterus and vagina come outside through the introitus	*Procidentia*
30	Which theory explains umbilical endometriosis	*Coelomic metaplasia*

DERMATOLOGY

No.	Question	Answer
1.	Which condition can cause both cicatricial as well as non-cicatricial alopecia	***SLE***
2.	IgA deposition in dermo-epidermal junction of skin is seen in	***Linear IgA disease***
3.	Antigen defect in pemphigus vulgaris	***Desmoglein-3***
4.	Pseudo-Koebner's phenomenon is seen in	***Plane warts***
5.	Most likely diagnosis of a child presenting with white umbilicated lesions over face	***Molluscum contagiosum***
6.	Flaccid bullae with mucosal involvement and intra-epidermal acantholysis are characteristic of	***Pemphigus vulgaris***
7.	Sexually transmitted disease with pseudo-bubo formation	***Granuloma inguinale***
8.	Drug of choice for genital warts	***Podophyllin***
9.	Most important cytokine for type II lepra reaction	***TNF-alpha***
10.	Onychomycosis is most commonly caused by	***Trichophyton rubrum***

ANESTHESIA

No.	Question	Answer
1.	While giving epidural anesthesia, order of structures pierced are	***Skin, subcutaneous tissue, supraspinous ligament, interspinous ligament, ligamentum flavum***
2.	Structure NOT pierced during spinal anesthesia	***Intervertebral disc space***
3.	A patient suffering from COVID-19 infection requires oxygen therapy. Doctor ordered the ward boy to bring oxygen cylinder. How the ward boy would identify the oxygen cylinder	***Black body, white shoulder***
4.	Main indication of endotracheal tube	***Secure definitive airway***
5.	A patient was given halothane for general anesthesia. But later on, he developed hyperthermia and rigidity. This presentation occurred due to which ion	***Calcium***
6.	What is the next step in managing a child with difficult intubation with 4 failed attempts at intubation	***Use laryngeal mask airway***
7.	Standard method to differentiate between endotracheal and esophageal intubation	***End-tidal carbon dioxide***
8.	Most appropriate circuit for ventilating a spontaneously breathing infant during anesthesia is	***Jackson–Rees modification of Ayre's T piece***
9.	Characteristic EEG pattern seen in surgical tolerance stage of anesthesia	***Delta***
10.	Most sensitive method of non-invasive monitoring of cardiovascular ischemia in peri-operative period is	***Transesophageal echocardiography (TEE)***

RADIOLOGY

No.	Question	Answer
1.	Lenticular hyperdensity on skull CT scan suggest	***Extradural hemorrhage***
2.	Best X-ray view to visualize maxillary sinus	***Water's view***
3.	Isotope of iodine used in treating thyroid disorders	***Iodine-131***
4.	Most sensitive investigation for minimum gas in abdomen	***CT scan***
5.	Chest X-ray showing opacity in the lung with irregular calcification suggest	***Hamartoma***
6.	The first investigation of choice in a patient with suspected subarachnoid hemorrhage should be	***Non-contrast computed tomography***
7.	Christmas tree appearance of bladder on intravenous pyelography is suggestive of	***Neurogenic bladder***
8.	Best imaging study for earliest diagnosis of cerebral infarct	***Diffusion weighted MRI***
9.	Investigation of choice for solitary pulmonary nodule	***CT scan***
10.	Radium emits	***Alpha, beta and gamma rays***

PSYCHIATRY

No.	Question	Answer
1.	A chronic drug addict of some unknown substance presented to the OPD with rashes and ulceration of the skin. Patient had severe itching. He was agitated. On examination, there was tachycardia, hypertension and mydriasis. Which substance is responsible for such a presentation	***Cocaine***
2.	Markedly inappropriate sensitivity, self-importance and suspiciousness are clinical features of	***Paranoid***
3.	Elderly patient awakens scared at night and he mistake rope for a snake. This is	***Illusion***
4.	A neurodevelopmental disorder characterized by impaired social interaction, verbal and non-verbal communication and restricted and repetitive behaviour is best description for	***Autism***
5.	Man taking haloperidol for 5 days presents with grimacing, torticollis and abnormal posture. Most likely diagnosis	***Acute muscular dystonia***
6.	Patient on anti-psychotic for 3 weeks presents with high-grade fever, raised CPK and myoglobinuria. Most likely diagnosis	***Neuroleptic malignant syndrome***
7.	A 10-years-old child presents with impaired social interaction, communication and stereotyped behaviour. He has normal IQ and language skills. Most likely diagnosis	***Asperger's syndrome***
8.	A man with intermittent hiccups feels that he is about to die because he is suffering from gastric carcinoma. All his X-rays and other investigations proved to be contrary. Most likely diagnosis	***Hypochondriasis***
9.	Patient presents with depressed mood, loss of sleep, loss of hope, feeling of worthlessness and diminished concentration for last 1 month. Drug of choice for such patient	***SSRI (for depression)***
10.	Balance between REM and NREM sleep is maintained by	***Suprachiasmatic nuclei***

ORTHOPEDICS

No.	Question	Answer
1.	A male who used to consume lot of non-vegetarians developed redness and painful swelling in great toe. His serum uric acid level came out to be 9.4 mg/dL. Most likely diagnosis	***Gout***
2.	A 7-years-old child was brought to the Orthopedics OPD with the complaint of difficulty in walking and progressive muscle weakness. His elder sister is also having the same problem. On examination, the calf muscles were hypertrophied but with less power. Thigh muscles were atrophied. Most likely diagnosis	***Duchenne muscular dystrophy***
3.	A 29-years-old male had swelling in the left knee joint. X-ray of the left knee showed lytic lesion, causing erosion of the bony cortex leading to soap bubble appearance. Most likely diagnosis	***Giant cell tumour***
4.	A 4-years-old child presented with a history of fall on outstretched hand. Radiograph showed a broken anterior cortex with an intact posterior cortex of the radius with an exaggeration bowing of the radius. Such a fracture is known as	***Greenstick fracture***
5.	Fracture neck of femur in a 80-years-old male, sustained 1 week back is best managed by	***Hemi-arthroplasty***
6.	While performing a total hip replacement, the surgeon found destruction of the articular cartilage and multiple wedge-shaped subchondral depressions. This is known as	***Osteonecrosis***
7.	A child presented with a limp. The surgeon suspected him to have a fixed, flexion deformity of the hip joint. Which test should the surgeon perform to confirm his finding	***Thomas test***
8.	Which type of fracture neck of the femur is associated with maximal compromise in the blood supply to the head of femur	***Subcapital fracture***
9.	Most common cause of carpal tunnel syndrome	***Idiopathic***
10.	Investigation of choice to detect a prolapsed intervertebral disc	***MRI***

PEDIATRICS

No.	Question	Answer
1.	Cause of kwashiorkor	***Less protein intake***
2.	Bull neck appearance suggest	***Diphtheria***
3.	A 6-years-old child had history of frequent attacks of convulsions and unconsciousness. Child also had poor food intake, loss of weight, poor learning abilities and fatigue. Urine examination showed a positive Rothera's test and there is formation of a purple ring. Blood tests showed elevated levels of plasma leucine (>1000 micromol/L). Findings are suggestive of the diagnosis of	***Maple syrup urine disease (deficiency of branched chain alpha ketoacid dehydrogenase complex)***
4.	A 5-years-old child has now only 70% of the normal body weight. He was born full term and without any congenital anomalies. Clinical examination revealed, dependent edema on lower extremities, large distended abdomen and desquamating skin showing irregular areas of hyperpigmentation and depigmentation. Findings are suggestive of	***Kwashiorkor***
5.	Palmar grasp reflex is present by	***1 month***
6.	Holt-Oram syndrome is associated with which congenital heart disease	***ASD***
7.	Pulmonary hypoplasia with uropathy. Likely diagnosis	***Potter syndrome***
8.	Child with proteinuria, generalised edema, hypoproteinemia and hyper-lipidemia. Most likely diagnosis	***Minimal change nephrotic syndrome***
9.	A child is suffering from dry skin and is mentally retarded. Likely diagnosis	***Hypothyroidism***
10.	Which vaccine is contraindicated in a baby with history of convulsions	***DPT***
11.	A 3-years-old child presented to the Pediatrics OPD with diarrhoeal episodes. He is now lethargic and floppy. He is not drinking fluids properly and skin goes back very slowly when pinched. What type of dehydration is this	***Severe dehydration***
12.	An 18-months-old child has cellulitis of leg. SpO_2 is 88%. There is no past history of hospitalization or any illness. Most likely organism	***Streptococcus pyogenes***
13.	A 2-weeks-old baby is having scrotal pigmentation along with hyponatremia, hypoglycemia and hyperkalemia. Which enzyme is deficient	***21-alpha hydroxylase***
14.	Drug used for closure of patent ductus arteriosus	***Indomethacin***
15.	A child presented to the Pediatrics OPD with diarrhoea episodes. Now he is feeling thirsty. On examination he seems to be irritated. Such a patient is best managed by	***Oral fluids***
16.	Mid-arm circumference in severe acute malnutrition	***<11.5 cm***
17.	Type of cerebral palsy in which upper limb is less affected than the lower limb	***Spastic diplegia***
18.	A child of 6 weeks is having hemoglobin of 10 gram%. He is pale on examination. Most likely diagnosis	***Physiological anemia***
19.	A 4-months-old infant with cough, respiratory rate >60/minutes and without any chest retraction. Management as per IMNCI protocol	***Oral antibiotic, explain danger sign and follow-up***
20.	Protein requirement for 2-years-old child	***20 gram/day***
21.	Apnea of prematurity	***>20 seconds***
22.	Commonest cause of female pseudo-hermaphroditism	***Congenital adrenal hyperplasia***
23.	A 15-months-old child feeding on cow milk with water developed severe wasting and bipedal edema with poor appetite. Likely diagnosis	***Kwashiorkor***
24.	In congenital adrenal hyperplasia, most common deficiency enzyme is	***21-alpha hydroxylase***
25.	A 2-weeks-old neonate with history of stridor in prone position. Management	***Wait and watch (laryngomalacia)***
26.	A 4-years-old child with severe wasting and voracious appetite without pedal edema is having	***Marasmus***
27.	A 6-years-old drowsy child came in emergency with history of vomiting, loose motion for 3 days. On examination, he had sunken eyes, hypothermia and skin on pinching takes time to revert. Likely diagnosis	***Severe dehydration***
28.	4-days-old newborn baby having icterus involving the sole. Bilirubin level would be	***15 mg/dL***
29.	10-days-old baby develops swelling in left posterior cervical area which is bluish in appearance, increases in size on crying and is brilliantly transilluminant. Likely diagnosis	***Cystic hygroma***
30.	A 10-years-old boy presents with gross hematuria, loin pain and diarrhoea. Urine examination is normal. Serum C_3 levels are also normal. Likely diagnosis	***Berger's disease***